Extracorporeal Membrane Oxygenation

Extracorporeal Membrane Oxygenation

Editor: Sandra Williams

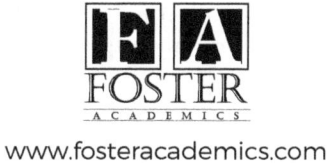

www.fosteracademics.com

www.fosteracademics.com

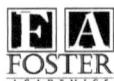

Cataloging-in-Publication Data

Extracorporeal membrane oxygenation / edited by Sandra Williams.
    p. cm.
Includes bibliographical references and index.
ISBN 978-1-63242-919-3
1. Extracorporeal membrane oxygenation. 2. Respiratory therapy. 3. Blood--Circulation, Artificial.
4. Membrane oxygenators. 5. Emergency medicine. 6. Critical care medicine. I. Williams, Sandra.
RJ312 .E98 2020
615.836--dc23

Foster Academics,
118-35 Queens Blvd., Suite 400,
Forest Hills, NY 11375, USA

ISBN 978-1-63242-919-3 (Hardback)

Contents

Preface

This book aims to highlight the current researches and provides a platform to further the scope of innovations in this area. This book is a product of the combined efforts of many researchers and scientists, after going through thorough studies and analysis from different parts of the world. The objective of this book is to provide the readers with the latest information of the field.

Extracorporeal membrane oxygenation (ECMO) is the clinical technique by which cardiac and respiratory support is provided to patients whose heart and lungs are deemed incapable of maintaining an adequate gas exchange or perfusion, for the sustenance of life. This technology is mostly used in children but also in adults with respiratory and cardiac failure. There are several forms of ECMO. Veno-venous ECMO and veno-arterial ECMO are the common forms. In ECMO, blood is removed from a person's body, the carbon dioxide is removed artificially and the red blood cells are oxygenated. It is performed either after a cardiopulmonary bypass or in the later stages in the treatment of lung or heart failure. This book aims to shed light on some of the unexplored aspects of extracorporeal membrane oxygenation and the recent researches in this domain. The various studies that are constantly contributing towards advancing technologies and evolution of this field are examined in detail. It aims to equip students and experts with the advanced topics and upcoming concepts in this area.

I would like to express my sincere thanks to the authors for their dedicated efforts in the completion of this book. I acknowledge the efforts of the publisher for providing constant support. Lastly, I would like to thank my family for their support in all academic endeavors.

Editor

Venoarterial Extracorporeal Membrane Oxygenation in Refractory Cardiogenic Shock and Cardiac Arrest

Marie-Eve Brunner , Carlo Banfi and Raphaël Giraud

Abstract

The aim of this chapter is to discuss the indication and the role of a venoarterial extracorporeal membrane oxygenation (VA-ECMO) in the refractory cardiogenic shock and cardiac arrest.

Cardiogenic shock occurs in 5–10% of patients following acute myocardial infarction, and mortality remains high at 50–80% when using only medical treatment, while cardiac arrest has a poor prognosis, and despite conventional cardiopulmonary resuscitation maneuvers, only a few patients can fully return to a normal lifestyle.

VA-ECMO is a rapidly deployable temporary system for supporting the circulatory and respiratory systems. It allows time for reversible cardiac failure to recover and can prevent end-organ damage from hypoperfusion. Emergency VA-ECMO has been described for the treatment of refractory cardiogenic shock following acute myocardial infarction, electrical storm, myocarditis, and pulmonary embolism as well as in refractory cardiac arrest. VA-ECMO is used as bridge to decision to sustain life until a full clinical evaluation can be completed, as bridge to recovery until intrinsic cardiac function recovers, as bridge to candidacy to make an ineligible patient eligible for transplantation/LVAD, and sometimes as direct bridge to transplantation.

However, morbidity on VA-ECMO is rather high and has an impact on the outcome. Bleeding, lower limb ischemia, infections, and irreversible central nervous system damage still remain as serious complications.

After a few days of mechanical assistance, patients implanted with VA-ECMO for cardiogenic shock or cardiac arrest can sometimes be successfully weaned from the device, when they have partially or fully recovered from the condition that indicated ECMO use. Weaning parameters are discussed.

Finally, prognosis and survival of patients on VA-ECMO are discussed as well as the ethical aspects.

Keywords: venoarterial extracorporeal membrane oxygenation, VA-ECMO, refractory cardiogenic shock, refractory cardiac arrest, ECLS - Extracorporeal Life Support

1. Introduction

Venoarterial extracorporeal membrane oxygenation (VA-ECMO) is a temporary technique for supporting the cardiac and the pulmonary system in patients suffering from refractory cardiogenic shock [1]. It allows time for reversible forms of cardiac failure to recover and can prevent end-organ damage from under perfusion.

Cardiogenic shock (CS) is defined as critical end-organ hypoperfusion due to low cardiac output and myocardial contractile dysfunction without hypovolemia [2]. CS has a broad spectrum from mild hypoperfusion to refractory CS. Experts' recommendations for the management of adult patients with cardiogenic shock from the French-Language Society of Intensive Care (Société de Réanimation de Langue Française), with the participation of the French Society of Anesthesia and Intensive Care, the French Cardiology Society, the French Emergency Medicine Society, and the French Society of Thoracic and Cardiovascular Surgery recommend the use of peripheral VA-ECMO if temporary circulatory support is needed with a strong agreement [3]. Five percent of patients with acute myocardial infarction (AMI) develop a CS, with high mortality rates [4]. Despite optimal maximal therapy such as inotropes, Vasoconstrictors, intra-aortic balloon pump (IAPB), revascularization techniques, and mechanical circulatory support, CS remains the most frequent source of hospital death ranging between 60 and 70% compared to patients with AMI without advanced CS which is about 10% [5]. Cardiac arrest (CA) is the main cause of sudden death and occurs in almost 22% of patients with AMI [6]. CA has obviously a poor prognosis, and only a small percentage of the patients can return to a normal lifestyle. The principal causes for very poor outcome and prognosis in CA are an absence of return of spontaneous circulation (ROSC), long CPR, hypoxic encephalopathy, and out-of-hospital CA. In both refractory CS and CA following AMI, which are very critical circumstances, VA-ECMO has been proposed and utilized during the last decades to obtain rapid resuscitation, stabilization, and subsequent triage to bridge treatment. ECMO has remarkably progressed over the recent years; it became an invaluable tool in the care of adults with severe CS refractory to conventional management [7, 8].

The aim of this chapter is to describe VA-ECMO techniques, the more recent indications, and results in the use of the VA-ECMO in patients with refractory CS and CA.

2. ECMO techniques in CS and CA

VA-ECMO drains blood from the vascular system, which circulates outside the body by a mechanical pump, and is then re-infused into the circulation. In the circuit, hemoglobin becomes fully saturated with O_2, and CO_2 is removed. Oxygenation is determined by flow rate, and CO_2 elimination can be controlled by adjusting the rate of countercurrent gas flow through the oxygenator.

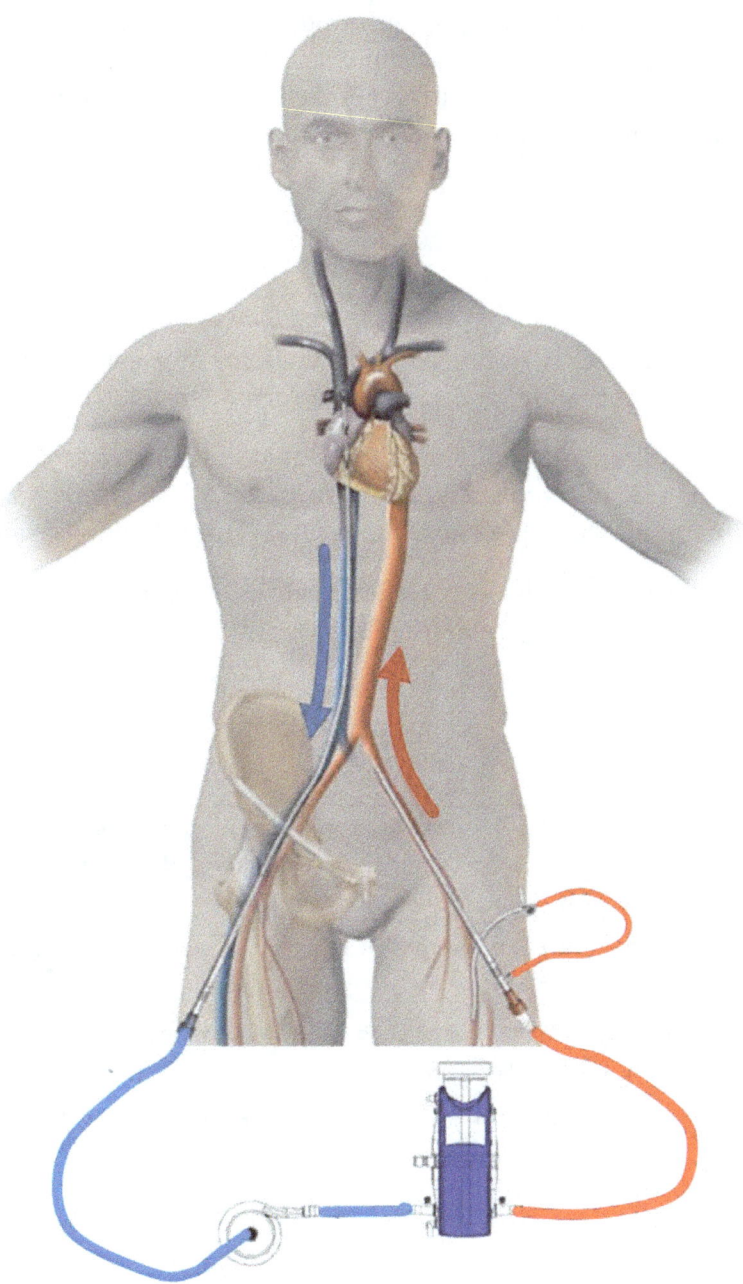

Figure 1. Percutaneous femoro-femoral VA-ECMO cannulation.

In CS and CA, where the cardiac circulation needs to be supported, a venoarterial configuration is required. This system includes a membrane oxygenator and a centrifugal pump to supply up to 5 L/min of support. VA-ECMO can be performed either peripherally or centrally. In peripheral VA-ECMO, a venous cannula is inserted via the femoral vein to the right atrium for drainage and an arterial cannula is inserted via the femoral artery into the ascending aorta for perfusion [9] (**Figure 1**).

Peripheral VA-ECMO cannulation can be performed both surgically by semi-Seldinger cut down and percutaneously. Intensive care physicians, interventional cardiologists, and obviously cardiac surgeons can perform the percutaneous technique whereas only cardio-thoracic surgeons can perform central VA-ECMO [10].

3. Indications

There are a number of emergency indications. CS can occur in previously healthy patients or patients with chronic cardiac failure and with acute decompensation.

Refractory CS can take place after a myocardial infarction [11], any cardiomyopathy [12], a fulminant myocarditis [13, 14], intoxication with cardiotoxic drugs, electrical storm [15, 16], valvular insufficiency, massive pulmonary embolism [17], or CA with certain conditions.

Post cardiotomy CS (PCCS) can also occur after a cardiac surgery (heart transplantation for example) when it is not possible to wean from bypass [18].

Four types of situations can be described and are resumed in **Table 1**: bridge to decision, bridge to recovery, bridge to candidacy , and bridge to transplantation.

Bridge to decision (BTD)	Use of VA-ECMO in patients with drug-refractory acute circulatory collapse and at immediate risk of death to sustain life until a full clinical evaluation can be completed and additional therapeutic options can be evaluated.
Bridge to recovery (BTR)	Use of VA-ECMO to keep patient alive until intrinsic cardiac function recovers sufficiently to remove VA-ECMO.
Bridge to candidacy (BTC)	Use of VA-ECMO to improve end-organ function in order to make an ineligible patient eligible for transplantation/LVAD.
Bridge to transplantation (BTT)	Use of VA-ECMO to keep a patient at high risk of death before transplantation alive until a donor organ becomes available.

Table 1. VA-ECMO: Types of situations.

Before VA-ECMO implantation, we should have several considerations. First of all, the likelihood of organ recovery has to be weighted. Initiation of VA-ECMO is appropriate only if the organ failure is thought to be reversible. When recovery is not expected, others options as transplantation or long term assist device as bridge to transplant versus destination therapy may be considered. The place of VA-ECMO in CS is shown in **Figure 2**.

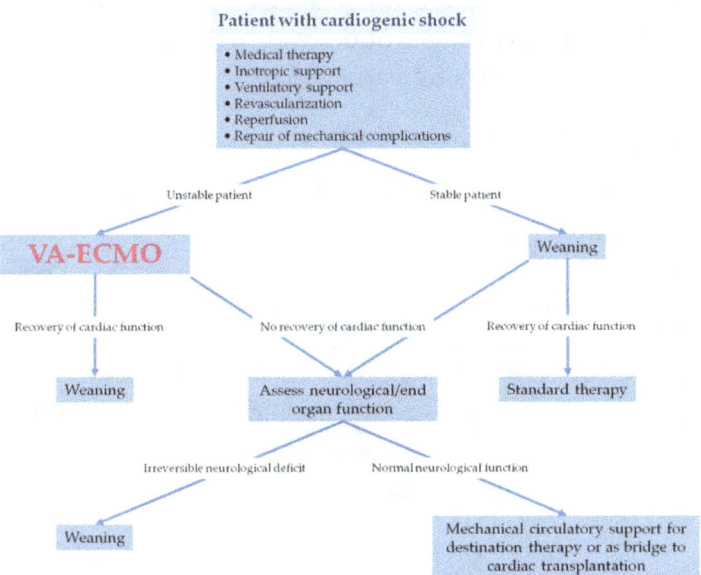

Figure 2. Place of VA-ECMO in CS.

Cardiogenic shock / Severe cardiac failure due to almost any cause	Myocardialinfarction
	Cardiacarrhythmicstorm refractory to other measures
	Fulminant myocarditis
	Massive pulmonary embolisms
	Drug overdose/toxicity with profound cardiac depression
	Septic cardiomyopathy
Post-cardiotomy	Inability to wean from cardiopulmonary bypass after cardiac surgery
Post heart transplant	Primary graft failure after heart or heart-lung transplantation
Refractory cardiac arrest (No ROSC despite 30 min of optimal CPR)	Indications:
	• Age < 65 years
	• First rhythm: "shockable" rhythm
	• No flow ≤ 5 min
	• Witnessed cardiac arrest
	• $EtCO_2$ per CPR > 10 mmHg
	• Time to ECMO < 60–90 min

Table 2. Main VA-ECMO indications for cardiogenic shock and cardiac arrest.

Advanced age, severe brain injury, long time cardiac arrest, disseminated malignancy are considered as contraindications to the institution of VA-ECMO. Finally, aortic insufficiency or aortic dissection are both major contraindications.

Indications for VA-ECMO are resumed in **Table 2**.

Clinical and biological signs as well as therapeutic measures leading to VA-ECMO implantations in cardiogenic shock are resumed in **Table 3**.

Clinical and biological signs	Therapeutic measures
SBP < 90 mmHg OR MAP < 60 mmHg	Fluid for optimal preload
	Vasoactive drugs (first choice: norepinephrine)
CI <2.2 l/min/m^2	Inotropes (first choice: dobutamine)
S(c)vO$_2$ < 50%	IABP
LVEF < 20%	
VTI < 10 cm	
SaO$_2$ < 92%	Mechanical ventilation + sedation
Urine output < 30 ml/h	
Malignant arrhythmia	IV Loading of amiodarone and/or lidocaïne
	External electric shock
If despite these measures lactate levels significantly still increase within 2 hours	
→ Consider VA-ECMO implantation	

SBP: Systolic blood pressure, MAP: Mean arterial blood pressure, CI: Cardiac index, S(c)vO2: Mixed/central venous saturation, LVEF: Left ventricular ejection fraction, VTI: Velocity time integral, SaO2: Arterial oxygen saturation, IABP: Intra aortic balloon pump.

Table 3. Clinical and biological signs of cardiogenic shock as well as therapeutic measures leading to VA-ECMO implantations.

A. Refractory CS post myocardial infarction

Refractory CS post myocardial infarction is the main cause of death in hospitalized patients with acute myocardial infarction. It occurs in 5–10% of patients [19]. The use of early PCI in those patients was associated with improved survival [11]. No randomized controlled trials compare VA-ECMO with other mechanical supports, but non-randomized studies show a survival benefit with the early use of VA-ECMO. One study tested the hypothesis that early ECMO offered additional benefits in improving 30-day survival in patients with acute myocardial infarction complicated by profound CS undergoing primary percutaneous coronary intervention. The VA-ECMO group had a significantly lower 30-day mortality (39.1% versus 72%, p=0.008). This study was limited by the fact that the two cohorts were enrolled in two different periods (Non-VA-ECMO Group: 1993–2002, versus VA-ECMO group: 2002–2009) and also because coronary stents were unavailable until 1998 [20]. To date, only case reports or case series showed a benefit in implanting VA-ECMO in refractory cardiogenic shock. It appears essential to implant VA-ECMO before multiorgan failure but no defined criteria are yet available to decide exactly when the device should be implanted. Randomized controlled trials are needed to determine if there is a true benefit in the use of VA-ECMO in CS post myocardial infarction to determine if early VA-ECMO in conjunction with optimal medical treatment would improve clinical outcomes at 30 days as compared with optimal medical treatment alone.

B. Electrical storm induced CS

In electrical storm induced CS, appropriate and timely VA-ECMO support helps to maintain and preserve vital organ perfusion. The period of stability offered by VA-ECMO support can allow optimization of anti-arrhythmic medication particularly the use of anti-arrhythmic agents most of whom have profound negative inotropic and hypotensive effects, and prevents left ventricular dilation [15]. It also prevents the low flow syndrome and multi-organ failure. VA-ECMO implantation should be considered early when conventional maneuvers fail to control the cardiac rhythm [21]. Early-onset VA-ECMO support may be lifesaving and should be considered in the management of hemodynamically unstable arrhythmias when conventional therapy fails to convert refractory ventricular tachycardia [16, 22]. While recommendations for VA-ECMO to handle refractory ventricular tachycardia remain to be set, success in using VA-ECMO in this case rely upon the correct selection of patients in the emergency department, and the prompt implantation before multiple organ failure occurs. Prompt institution of VA-ECMO support achieves the best outcome [21].

C. Fulminant myocarditis

Fulminant myocarditis is a non-ischemic, clinical manifestation of cardiac inflammation with rapid onset and severe hemodynamic compromise. Infective etiologic process is usually the most frequent finding. Inotropic therapy and intra-aortic balloon pump might not be sufficient to treat the pump failure. VA-ECMO support may be required to provide time to enhance heart recovery in this normally self-limiting disease. A recent 5-Year Multi-Institutional Experience showed a VA-ECMO weaning rate of 81% and discharge rate of 72% in the overall patient population [13]. Mirabel et al. shows that patients with fulminant myocarditis, who would have died without emergent initiation of circulatory support, had favorable short- and long-term outcomes with 68% hospital survivors and 46% partial or complete native heart function recovery [14]. In both studies, VA-ECMO implantations were performed when maximal medical therapy failed to improve hemodynamic status. In the study of Lorusso et al., pre-ECMO patient characteristics showed a systolic blood pressure at 61.8 ± 30.4 mmHg, pH at 7.2 ± 0.1 and lactate levels at 12.0 ± 4.6 mmol/L, corresponding to severe cardiogenic shock states [13].

D. Massive pulmonary embolism

A pulmonary embolism (PE) is a common illness that can cause death [23]. Massive acute PE (MAPE) results in CA in 41% of cases and is associated with a high mortality rate [24, 25]. Clinical practice guidelines recommend fibrinolytic therapy for patients with MAPE and CA, although few data are available to guide decisions about the agent, dose, rate, and frequency of administration [26, 27]. Fibrinolysis offers a rapid onset of action and ease of administration, and it is readily available in most hospital settings. The use of fibrinolysis during CPR in patients with presumed pulmonary embolism may improve survival [28, 29]. Fibrinolytic therapy is the first-line treatment in patients with high-risk pulmonary embolism presenting with CS in absence of contraindications. However, in several cases, there are absolute contraindications for this therapy. Catheter-based intervention is recommended for patients with circulatory collapse due to MAPE and is equivalent to surgical embolectomy [30]. Emergent VA-ECMO provides an opportunity for improving the prognosis of an otherwise near-fatal condition and should be considered in the algorithm for managing MAPE in an unstable patient [31]. The survival rate in patients with MAPE who receive VA-ECMO and anticoagulation or surgical embolectomy was 62% [31]. Thus, ECMO can provide lifesaving hemodynamic and respiratory support in critically ill patients with MAPE in patients hemodynamically unstable to support any other interventions or have not responded to medical therapies. Success in ECMO for MAPE is determined by the return of sufficient RV function [32]. ECMO may be considered in early management of patients with MAPE unresponsive or contraindicated to pharmacological treatment [33].

E. Pulmonary arterial hypertension

In addition, VA-ECMO is also a supportive option for patients with decompensated pulmonary arterial hypertension. In fact, pulmonary arterial hypertension is associated with high morbidity and mortality, particularly in patients with progressive RV failure. In this case, VA-ECMO can be used as a bridge to lung transplant or bridge to recovery when medical therapy is not sufficient to prevent cardiopulmonary failure in the acute setting [34].

F. Post-cardiotomy CS

Post-cardiotomy CS (PCCS) is very rare, but is a lethal complication in post cardiac surgery. PCCS occurs in 2–6% of patients undergoing surgical revascularization or valvular surgery [35, 36]. Approximately 0.5–1.5% of patients is refractory to maximal inotropic and intra-aortic balloon pump (IABP) support [37]. Post-cardiotomy CS occurs in perioperative cardiac surgery in patients with normal preoperative myocardial function as well as those with pre-existing impaired function [38]. Refractory PCCS leads rapidly to multi-organ dysfunction and is nearly always fatal without the use of advanced mechanical circulatory support [35]. VA-ECMO is used to salvage patients who develop refractory PCCS [39]. However, even if outcomes in patients requiring such support for PCCS continue to be poor [40], VA-ECMO may be used as temporary post-operative cardiovascular support.

G. Primary graft failure

Primary graft failure (PGF) after heart transplantation is a detrimental complication, and carries high morbidity and mortality. In a study involving 114 consecutive patients receiving orthotopic heart transplantation, 18 (15.7%) developed PGF requiring VA-ECMO support. Thirteen patients (72.2%) were able to be weaned from the support, and eight of them (44%)

were discharged [41]. Thus, as in PGF recovery is usually more frequent than in other cases of PCCS, due to the more probable reversibility of the damage, ECMO support could be used as bridge to graft recovery [42, 43].

H. Septic cardiomyopathy

Septic cardiomyopathy occurs with severe myocardial depression in septic shock. In a retrospective observational study, 14 patients with septic shock refractory to conventional treatment all had a severe myocardial dysfunction at VA-ECMO implantation. Mean LV ejection fraction (LVEF) was 16% and cardiac index was 1.3 L/min/m^2 in these patients. At ECMO implantation, mean pH was 7.16 and blood lactate was 9 mmol/L. Twelve patients were weaned off VA-ECMO. Ten patients survived after a follow-up of 13 months and recover a normal LVEF [44]. VA-ECMO may provide benefit to patients with a cardiac failure in the setting of a septic shock, but larger studies are needed.

I. Refractory cardiac arrest

Increasing number of papers has reported encouraging results on the use of VA-ECMO for refractory CA. Extracorporeal circulation ensures an adequate blood flow, time to perform diagnostic and therapeutic interventions even before a return of spontaneous circulation is achieved [43]. For patients with whom conventional advanced life support maneuvers are insufficient and/ or to make specific interventions possible (e.g., coronary angiography and percutaneous coronary intervention (PCI) or pulmonary embolectomy for MAPE), extracorporeal CPR (eCPR) has to be considered as a lifesaving therapy [45]. This practice is evolving and is used for both in-hospital (IHCA) and out-of-hospital (OHCA) CA despite few observational statistics. Observational studies suggest that eCPR for CA is correlated with enhanced survival [46] in case of reversible cause of CA, few comorbidity, witnessed CA, immediate high-quality CPR, and eCPR early implanted (e.g., within 1 h of CA) as well as when VA-ECMO is implanted by emergency physicians and intensivists [47–50]. eCPR involves significant resource and training. It has been correlated with enhanced survival after IHCA in selected patients [47, 51] when compared with manual or mechanical CPR. After OHCA, survival after eCPR is less favorable [52]. However, when deployed during and/or soon after resuscitation attempts, despite variations in practice and heterogeneity of outcomes, these interventions yield a good neurological survival in 12% of adults suffering a refractory OHCA [53]. In a retrospective observational study dividing CA patients in two groups (shockable rhythm and non-shockable rhythm), the authors found that non-shockable rhythms could be considered as a formal contraindication allowing a concentration of efforts on the shockable rhythms, where the chances of success are substantial. They conclude that VA-ECMO for refractory OHCA should be limited due to a very poor neurological outcome [54]. Indications for eCPR are detailed in **Table 2**. However, there is an urgent need for randomized studies of eCPR and large eCPR registries to identify the circumstances in which it works best, establish guidelines for its use and identify the benefits, costs and risks of eCPR.

4. Complications

Not surprisingly, VA-ECMO is associated with a lot of possible complications that can be lethal. This is why VA-ECMO must be done by well-trained teams in reference centers.

The most common complications listed with the use of VA-ECMO are: major or significant bleeding, re-thoracotomy for bleeding or tamponade, vascular complications as lower limb ischemia, lower limb ischemia requiring fasciotomy or compartment syndrome, lower extremity ischemia requiring amputation, neurologic complications like stroke, acute kidney injury requiring renal replacement therapy, and significant infection.

A. Bleeding

In a recent meta-analyze, 20 studies were analyzed including 1866 patients. Bleeding was the most frequent complications with an estimated rate of 41%. The most frequent source of hemorrhage is the femoral cannula insertion site [55]. In central ECMO, the rate of re-thora-cotomy for bleeding or tamponade was 42%. The average number of units of packed red blood cells transfused ranged from 12.7 to 29.0 units. Indeed, bleeding, thrombosis, and hemolysis remain the most common causes of morbidity and mortality for patients receiving ECMO therapy. These adverse effects have to be considered and should be monitored during ECMO therapy. Apart from surgical hemostasis problems, coagulation and inflammatory systems are immediately activated when blood comes in contact with the ECMO circuit, which necessitates systemic anticoagulation [56]. In a recent single center prospective randomized study on adult patients requiring ECMO therapy, hemostasis, anticoagulation, hemolysis, and inflammatory parameters were monitored. The results showed that median platelet count had dropped, prothrombin fragment 1.2, thrombin-antithrombin complex, and D-dimers increased, whereas fibrinogen values dropped [57]. However, antithrombotic therapy is necessary to maintain patency with the ECMO circuit and ultimately reduce the risk of clotting while decreasing the probability of hemorrhage. Currently, the most commonly used antithrombotic therapy is systemic anticoagulation with unfractionated heparin, which is associated with its well-known complications inclusive of bleeding (patient) and clotting (circuit). Systemic anticoagulation complications in ECMO support have not really reduced despite developments in technology and monitoring methods over the last few years.

Moreover, bleeding and thrombosis comprise majority of all side effects that can occur on ECMO, and the inability to mediate and control this effectively can lead to catastrophic complications and increases mortality. Heparin monitoring is very challenging on ECMO. There are actually no universal protocols concerning anticoagulation management; however, some centers propose to target 45–60 s for aPTT and 0.2–0.3 IU/ml for heparinemia (anti-Xa activity) [58]. Hemoglobin threshold for red cell transfusion should be 7–8 g/dl and only severe thrombocytopenia complicated by bleeding should be corrected. There is no single test that correctly monitors all of the factors influencing the anticoagulation, including the hepariniza-tion. As a result, over time and experience, a variety of tests are used. More recently, the Extracorporeal Life Support Organization (ELSO) proposed guidelines for management of the anticoagulation with ECMO. The main parameters monitored during ECMO are the activated coagulation time (ACT), the antifactor Xa assay (anti-Xa), and the activated partial thrombo-plastin time (aPTT). More recently, the thromboelastography (TEG) or the thromboelastometry (ROTEM) have been introduced to monitor ECMO patients. These tests add information about the phases of coagulation, platelet function, and fibrinolysis, which is very relevant in ECMO patients as they have coagulation abnormalities. While many centers have integrated those tests into their ECMO anticoagulation guidelines, more research is needed to understand the place of TEG and ROTEM monitoring in ECMO patients [59].

B. Vascular complications

Vascular issues are the second more frequent complication. The cumulative rate of lower extremity ischemia is around 17%. The cumulative rate of lower extremity fasciotomy or compartment syndrome is around 10%. The cumulative rate of lower extremity amputation occurs to 7 of 192 (5%) [60]. In another retrospective study, statistics of 100 patients with VA-ECMO inserted via percutaneous femoral approach for CS or refractory CA were examined. A 7-9 Fr percutaneous reperfusion catheter, distal to the arterial cannula, was positioned into the artery, if the leg showed sign of under-perfusion. Thirty patients with early ischemia benefited from a reperfusion cannula to improve perfusion of the limb and it succeeded in 26 of them. Seven patients suffered a compartment syndrome of the leg necessitating urgent fasciotomy. In two of those patients, the ischemia moved to irreversible ischemia necessitating amputation of the limb. The authors concluded that the majority of ischemic episodes were resolved with the insertion of a distal perfusion catheter. They did not observe any mortal vascular complication, nor was any of the observed complications related to increased mortality [61]. However, in another recent study, 84 peripheral VA-ECMO patients were separated into two groups depending on the presence of major vascular complications, defined as patients who required surgical intervention. The authors found that vascular complications negatively affect survival in patients receiving VA-ECMO support by means of femoral cannulation and that distal perfusion catheter can decrease the incidence of complications [62].

C. Hemolysis

Hemolysis during ECMO therapy remains of concern with a reported incidence between 5 and 18% [63–65]. Major contributors are technical-induced hemolysis that may consist of sub lethal damage to erythrocytes by shear stress, high ECMO blood flow particularly high flow velocity through small cannulas, cavitation particularly in case of hypovolemia, pressure changes within the oxygenator particularly in case of fibrin/thrombosis upon the membrane [66–72]. Free plasma hemoglobin (fHb) and lactate dehydrogenase can increase significantly during ECMO support [73, 74] because of red blood cell (RBC) destruction. fHb is cytotoxic causing cell necrosis [73, 75]. It also scavenges nitric oxide, leading to vasoconstriction, endothelial dysfunction, and platelet aggregation [76, 77]. Consequently, renal insufficiency or multiple organ failure can appear [78–80]. Then, prevention and rapid identification of hemolysis are crucial for ECMO patients.

D. Neurological complications

Neurological complications are rather common in patients on VA-ECMO [81]. These complications are generally related to thrombosis with cerebral infarction and intracranial hemorrhage [82]. Intracranial hemorrhage (ICH) in particular has been associated with higher rates of mortality [83]. A review on a large, multihospital database, the Nationwide Inpatient Sample of the Healthcare Cost and Utilization Project of the Agency for Healthcare Research and Quality reviewed patients between 2001–2011 receiving ECMO [84]. The authors showed that 10.9% suffered from neurological complications including seizure (4.1%), stroke (4.1%), and intracranial hemorrhage (3.6%). The outcome between seizure patients and patients without neurological complications did not differ. Patients with stroke or hemorrhage have a higher hospital length of stay, higher probability of discharge to a long-term facility, and patient who suffered of intracranial hemorrhage have a higher mortality rate. More research is still needed to prevent neurologic complications.

E. Infections

The ELSO registry found an overall prevalence of infection of 11.7%, ranging from 7.6% in neonates to 20.9% in adults, with little variation during the 11-year span of the registry data [85]. An increased rate of death was found in patients who acquired infection during VA-ECMO. Bloodstream infections were predominant in most studies that reported the site of infection, followed by surgical site infections, urinary tract infections, and respiratory tract infections [86]. A fungal infection developed in 12% of patients, with surgical site infections reported most commonly [87]. Currently, the ELSO Infectious Disease Task Force does not recommend routine antimicrobial prophylaxis during ECMO. This is confirmed by a recent review stating that there is no evidence to defend prophylactic antibiotics in most patients, even if infections during ECMO are serious complications. Infections should be prevented [86].

F. Refractory pulmonary edema

In case of peripheral VA-ECMO for refractory CS, patients with very low residual cardiac contractility and elevated afterload due to the ECMO can lead to an inadequate decompression of the left ventricle resulting in a refractory pulmonary edema, fatal pulmonary hemorrhage, and left ventricle (LV) clotting [88]. Various methods for left heart decompression are known, but there is no consensus about the appropriate method and timing of decompression. However, in this situation, the first therapeutic measures are the introduction of inotropic drugs associated with an intra-aortic balloon pump to help increase LV contractility allowing the opening of aortic valve, to decrease left ventricular afterload, and thus to unload the LV. Minimally invasive strategies such as percutaneous transseptal left atrial decompression [89] and subxiphoid surgical approaches to drain the left ventricle [90] have been described to reduce LV distension. The residual atrial defect may require correction once the patient has been weaned from mechanical support. Use of a percutaneously inserted VAD (Impella™; Abiomed, Aachen, Germany) to decompress the left ventricle has also been reported in this setting [91], alleviating the need for a high-risk septostomy or surgical venting. However, in some circumstances depending of the patient's state and local resources, central cannulation with left ventricular decompression may be indicated [92].

G. Harlequin syndrome

Harlequin syndrome is a hypoxemia of the upper body due to a competition of the VA-ECMO flow with the systolic function of the native heart. In a femoro-femoral VA-ECMO, when the heart function recovers, there is a competition between VA-ECMO flow and native cardiac flow in the aorta. In case of significant impairment of pulmonary gas exchange leading to an upper body hypoxemia, despite optimization of the ventilator settings, ECMO configuration has to be adapted. VA ECMO flows can be increased in an attempt to better perfuse the aortic root with retrograde arterialized blood. In addition, the arterial outflow cannulation site can be switched from the femoral artery to the axillary or carotid artery. As they are in closer proximity to the aortic arch, these cannulation sites may be more effective in washing the root with oxygenated blood. However, cannulation of these smaller vessels will require a smaller cannula, which will decrease the maximum achievable flows. A VA-V-ECMO circuit can also be created where a portion of arterialized blood from the arterial outflow cannula is diverted via the right internal jugular artery to the right heart. This enriches the blood traveling through the pulmonary circulation and to the left ventricle to provide better oxygen delivery to the coronary and cerebral circulations. Finally, if cardiac function has recovered sufficiently, VA-ECMO can be converted to VV-ECMO to provide only gas exchange support until the lungs fully recover its function [93].

5. Weaning

After a few days of mechanical assistance, patients implanted with VA-ECMO for CS or CA can sometimes be successfully weaned from the device, when they have partially or fully recovered from the condition that indicated ECMO use. Hemodynamic parameters such as invasive arterial pressure and heart rate, intravenous inotropes and vasoactive drugs, blood lactate and blood gas analyses should be monitored. A daily echocardiography should be performed and those criterions are evaluated: LVEF; aortic time–velocity integral (VTI); transmitral early peak (E) and late diastolic velocities; spectral tissue Doppler lateral mitral annulus peak systolic (TDSa); and early diastolic (Ea) annular velocities. LV filling pressures are estimated with the E/Ea ratio. First of all, the patient has to be considered as hemodynamically stable: baseline MAP > 60 mmHg with no or low-dose vasoactive agents and a pulsatile arterial waveform present for at least 24 h, and no compromising of the pulmonary blood oxygenation. Only in these conditions, an ECMO weaning trial can be attempted. ECMO flow is gradually reduced to 66% for 10–15 min, then to 33% and/or to a minimum of 1–1.5 L/min for another 10–15 min. If the patient begins to present hemodynamical instability (MAP dropped under 60 mmHg), the trial is stopped, and ECMO flow has to return to the initial flow. In a study upon 51 patients, the authors assessed a weaning strategy following support for refractory CS to recognize clinical, hemodynamic, and Doppler echocardiography parameters predictive for efficacious ECMO removal. Patients who were considered as hemodynamically stable underwent ECMO flow decrease trials to <1.5 L/min under clinical and Doppler echocardiography monitoring. Patients with partially or fully recovery from severe cardiac failure, weaning trial tolerance, LVEF >20–25% and VTI >10 cm under minimal ECMO support, had ECMO support removed. In this study, 38 patients endured the weaning trial and 20 were finally weaned of the ECMO support.

This study showed that echocardiographic parameters determine weaned and non-weaned patients more than all other factors examined. The authors concluded that patients who tolerate a full ECMO weaning trial and have aortic VTI ≥10 cm, LVEF >20–25%, and TDSa ≥6 cm/s at minimal ECMO flow can be weaned [94].

6. Predictors of survival and outcome

Survival after VA-ECMO for refractory CS depends on etiology and severity of the patient at the implantation of the VA-ECMO support.

Mirabel et al. described factors associated with unfavorable outcomes in myocarditis related CS as higher body mass index; severe comorbidity; ICU admission Simplified Acute Physiology Score II, Sepsis-Related Organ Failure Assessment, and Glasgow Coma Scale; VA-ECMO placed under cardiopulmonary resuscitation; elevated sodium, troponin Ic and blood lactate; and low hematocrit and arterial pH [14].

Health-related quality of life was also evaluated in those survivors and revealed persistent difficulties with work or other daily activities. Mental health and vitality were deemed satisfactory. Severe anxiety, depression, and PTSD symptoms were reported by 27–38% of the patients after a median follow-up of 18 months.

Despite the high number of refractory CS requiring VA-ECMO, predictive survival modeling has not been reported till 2015 with the SAVE Score: Predicting survival after VA-ECMO for refractory CS [95]. Using a large international cohort of 3846 patients treated with VA-ECMO for CS (Extracorporeal Life Support Organization: ELSO), prognostic factors were identified for hospital survival and created a well-calibrated and reasonably discriminatory in-hospital survival prediction score comprising 13 pre-VA-ECMO variables. Parameters are Acute CS diagnosis group (myocarditis, arrhythmias, post heart of lung transplantation, congenital heart disease or others diagnoses leading to refractory CS), age, weight, acute pre-VA-ECMO organ failure, chronic renal failure, and time of intubation before VA-ECMO implantation. All of them determine a 5-class survival risk with survival rate. A SAVE-score of zero is approximately equivalent to 50% survival with positive scores representing higher chances of survival [95].

While inappropriate VA-ECMO use raises resource utilization and hospital costs and is associated with unacceptably high mortality, early identification of mortality risk factors and detailed analyses of survivors' long-term outcomes are needed. A two-center retrospective study was designed to identify pre-ECMO factors associated with in-ICU death and then derive a practical mortality risk score that might help physicians to select appropriate acute myocardial infarction (AMI) patients for VA-ECMO.

A study concerning 138 ECMO supporting AMI patients analyzed long-term survivors' health-related quality of life (HRQOL) and frequencies of anxiety, depression, and post-traumatic stress disorder (PTSD). The survivors were evaluated for HRQOL, psychological and PTSD status 6 months after discharge of ICU. This study showed that nearly 50% of all patients were still alive. The authors developed the ENCOURAGE score on the basis of multivariable logistic regression analyses including seven pre-ECMO parameters: age >60, female sex, body mass index >25 kg/m2, Glasgow coma score < 6, creatinine >150 μmol/L, lactate (<2, 2–8, or >8 mmol/L), and prothrombin activity < 50%. Six months after ECMO, probabilities of survival were 80, 58, 25, 20, and 7% for ENCOURAGE score classes 0–12, 13–18, 19–22, 23–27, and ≥ 28, respectively. The ENCOURAGE score ROC AUC (0.84) was significantly better than those of the SAVE, SAPS II, and SOFA scores. Survivors' HRQOL evaluated after median follow-up of 32 months revealed satisfactory mental health but persistent physical and emotional related difficulties, with 34% anxiety, 20% depression, and 5% PTSD symptoms reported. The authors concluded that the ENCOURAGE score might be a useful tool to predict mortality of severe CS in AMI patients who received VA-ECMO. However, it now needs prospective validation on other populations than AMI patients [96].

Prognosis is quite different regarding refractory CA patients. Early VA-ECMO implantation has been shown to give a better outcome in patient with CA. Low flow longer than 90 minutes offers a very bad prognosis [47].

In 2008, a French group proposed recommendations to limit the VA-ECMO implantation in case of refractory CA [97]. Our local ECMO alarms criteria for refractory cardiac arrest are shown in **Table 4**. Patients are evaluated according to these criteria by a multidisciplinary team including emergency physicians, intensivists, anesthesiologists, cardiologists, and cardiac surgeons. A consensual decision to implant a VA-ECMO or not is taken.

ECMO alarm criteria	
Indications	**Contraindications**
No-flow ≤ 3 min	No-flow > 5 min
OR immediate CPR by professional **OR** signs of life per CPR **OR** hypothermia	
Age ≤ 65 years	Obvious sign of death
First rhythm ≠ asystole	Comorbidities +++ → Futility
EtCO$_2$ ≥ 10 mmHg (≥ 1.3 kPa) under CPR	Time from cardiac arrest to ECMO > 100 min
Projected arrival at the hospital ≤ 60 min	

Table 4. E-CPR Geneva University Hospitals: refractory cardiac arrest algorithm (CPR ≥ 30 min).

Finally, some papers are now published about the ethical dimension of ECMO support [98]. In fact, ECMO technology now allows prolonged support with decreased complications, and the need of early implantation, have led to a significant increase in the use of ECMO worldwide. This increasing use of a technology that is not a destination device in itself introduces many ethical dilemmas specific to this technology.

7. Conclusion

The use of VA-ECMO in patients with refractory cardiogenic shock and cardiac arrest is widely increasing and is now recognized as a standard technique because in these patients the mortality without the ECMO support would be dramatically higher. It seems essential to determine whether ECMO support should be initiated before organ dysfunction advances to preserve organ function. However, even if data in the literature show a progressive increase in the overall outcome, these devices are associated with serious complications such as bleeding, lower limb ischemia, infections, and CNS irreversible damage that remain problematic issues. Efforts to reduce or prevent them are necessary and strongly recommended to improve the outcome. Finally, as inappropriate VA-ECMO use raises resource utilization and hospital costs and is associated with unacceptably high mortality, early identification of mortality risk factors and detailed analyses of survivors' long-term outcomes are needed.

Author details

Marie-Eve Brunner[1*], Carlo Banfi[2] and Raphaël Giraud[3]

*Address all correspondence to: marie-eve.brunner@hcuge.ch

1 Geneva University Hospitals, Intensive Care, Department of Anesthesiology, Pharmacology and Intensive Care, Genève, Switzerland

2 University Hospitals, Division of Cardiovascular Surgery, Department of Surgery, Geneva, Switzerland

3 Geneva University Hospitals, Intensive Care, Department of Anesthesiology, Pharmacology and Intensive Care, Genève, Switzerland

References

[1] Makdisi G, Wang IW. Extra Corporeal Membrane Oxygenation (ECMO) review of a lifesaving technology. J Thorac Dis. 2015;7(7):E166-76.

[2] Authors/Task Force m, Windecker S, Kolh P, Alfonso F, Collet JP, Cremer J, et al. 2014 ESC/EACTS Guidelines on myocardial revascularization: The Task Force on Myocar-

dial Revascularization of the European Society of Cardiology (ESC) and the European Association for Cardio-Thoracic Surgery (EACTS)Developed with the special contribution of the European Association of Percutaneous Cardiovascular Interventions (EAPCI). Eur Heart J. 2014;35(37):2541-619.

[3] Levy B, Bastien O, Karim B, Cariou A, Chouihed T, Combes A, et al. Experts' recommendations for the management of adult patients with cardiogenic shock. Ann Intensive Care. 2015;5(1):52.

[4] Shah RU, de Lemos JA, Wang TY, Chen AY, Thomas L, Sutton NR, et al. Post-Hospital outcomes of patients with acute myocardial infarction with cardiogenic shock: findings from the NCDR. J Am Coll Cardiol. 2016;67(7):739-47.

[5] Goldberg RJ, Spencer FA, Gore JM, Lessard D, Yarzebski J. Thirty-year trends (1975 to 2005) in the magnitude of, management of, and hospital death rates associated with cardiogenic shock in patients with acute myocardial infarction: a population-based perspective. Circulation. 2009;119(9):1211-9.

[6] Brady WJ, Gurka KK, Mehring B, Peberdy MA, O'Connor RE, American Heart Association's Get with the Guidelines I. In-hospital cardiac arrest: impact of monitoring and witnessed event on patient survival and neurologic status at hospital discharge. Resuscitation. 2011;82(7):845-52.

[7] MacLaren G, Combes A, Bartlett RH. Contemporary extracorporeal membrane oxygenation for adult respiratory failure: life support in the new era. Intensive Care Med. 2012;38(2):210-20.

[8] Shekar K, Mullany DV, Thomson B, Ziegenfuss M, Platts DG, Fraser JF. Extracorporeal life support devices and strategies for management of acute cardiorespiratory failure in adult patients: a comprehensive review. Crit Care. 2014;18(3):219.

[9] Abrams D, Combes A, Brodie D. Extracorporeal membrane oxygenation in cardiopulmonary disease in adults. J Am Coll Cardiol. 2014;63(25 Pt A):2769-78.

[10] Conrad SA, Grier LR, Scott LK, Green R, Jordan M. Percutaneous cannulation for extracorporeal membrane oxygenation by intensivists: a retrospective single-institution case series. Crit Care Med. 2015;43(5):1010-5.

[11] Babaev A, Frederick PD, Pasta DJ, Every N, Sichrovsky T, Hochman JS, et al. Trends in management and outcomes of patients with acute myocardial infarction complicated by cardiogenic shock. JAMA. 2005;294(4):448-54.

[12] Bermudez CA, Rocha RV, Toyoda Y, Zaldonis D, Sappington PL, Mulukutla S, et al. Extracorporeal membrane oxygenation for advanced refractory shock in acute and chronic cardiomyopathy. Ann Thorac Surg. 2011;92(6):2125-31.

[13] Lorusso R, Centofanti P, Gelsomino S, Barili F, Di Mauro M, Orlando P, et al. Venoarterial extracorporeal membrane oxygenation for acute fulminant myocarditis in adult patients: a 5-year multi-institutional experience. Ann Thorac Surg. 2016;101(3):919-26.

[14] Mirabel M, Luyt CE, Leprince P, Trouillet JL, Leger P, Pavie A, et al. Outcomes, long-term quality of life, and psychologic assessment of fulminant myocarditis patients rescued by mechanical circulatory support. Crit Care Med. 2011;39(5):1029-35.

[15] Brunner ME, Siegenthaler N, Shah D, Licker MJ, Cikirikcioglu M, Brochard L, et al. Extracorporeal membrane oxygenation support as bridge to recovery in a patient with electrical storm related cardiogenic shock. Am J Emerg Med. 2013;31(2):467 e1-6.

[16] Pagel PS, Lilly RE, Nicolosi AC. Use of ECMO to temporize circulatory instability during severe Brugada electrical storm. Ann Thorac Surg. 2009;88(3):982-3.

[17] Pavlovic G, Banfi C, Tassaux D, Peter RE, Licker MJ, Bendjelid K, et al. Peri-operative massive pulmonary embolism management: is veno-arterial ECMO a therapeutic option? Acta Anaesthesiol Scand. 2014;58(10):1280-6.

[18] Bakhtiary F, Keller H, Dogan S, Dzemali O, Oezaslan F, Meininger D, et al. Venoarterial extracorporeal membrane oxygenation for treatment of cardiogenic shock: clinical experiences in 45 adult patients. J Thorac Cardiovasc Surg. 2008;135(2):382-8.

[19] Jeger RV, Radovanovic D, Hunziker PR, Pfisterer ME, Stauffer JC, Erne P, et al. Ten-year trends in the incidence and treatment of cardiogenic shock. Ann Intern Med. 2008;149(9):618-26.

[20] Sheu JJ, Tsai TH, Lee FY, Fang HY, Sun CK, Leu S, et al. Early extracorporeal membrane oxygenator-assisted primary percutaneous coronary intervention improved 30-day clinical outcomes in patients with ST-segment elevation myocardial infarction complicated with profound cardiogenic shock. Crit Care Med. 2010;38(9):1810-7.

[21] Tsai FC, Wang YC, Huang YK, Tseng CN, Wu MY, Chang YS, et al. Extracorporeal life support to terminate refractory ventricular tachycardia. Crit Care Med. 2007;35(7): 1673-6.

[22] Ricciardi MJ, Moscucci M, Knight BP, Zivin A, Bartlett RH, Bates ER. Emergency extracorporeal membrane oxygenation (ECMO)-supported percutaneous coronary interventions in the fibrillating heart. Catheter Cardiovasc Interv. 1999;48(4):402-5.

[23] Beckman MG, Hooper WC, Critchley SE, Ortel TL. Venous thromboembolism: a public health concern. Am J Prev Med. 2010;38(4 Suppl):S495-501.

[24] Bailen MR, Cuadra JA, Aguayo De Hoyos E. Thrombolysis during cardiopulmonary resuscitation in fulminant pulmonary embolism: a review. Crit Care Med. 2001;29(11): 2211-9.

[25] Kurkciyan I, Meron G, Sterz F, Janata K, Domanovits H, Holzer M, et al. Pulmonary embolism as a cause of cardiac arrest: presentation and outcome. Arch Intern Med. 2000;160(10):1529-35.

[26] Kearon C, Akl EA, Comerota AJ, Prandoni P, Bounameaux H, Goldhaber SZ, et al. Antithrombotic therapy for VTE disease: Antithrombotic Therapy and Prevention of

Thrombosis, 9th ed: American College of Chest Physicians Evidence-Based Clinical Practice Guidelines. Chest. 2012;141(2 Suppl):e419S-94S.

[27] Vanden Hoek TL, Morrison LJ, Shuster M, Donnino M, Sinz E, Lavonas EJ, et al. Part 12: cardiac arrest in special situations: 2010 American Heart Association Guidelines for Cardiopulmonary Resuscitation and Emergency Cardiovascular Care. Circulation. 2010;122(18 Suppl 3):S829-61.

[28] Bottiger BW, Bode C, Kern S, Gries A, Gust R, Glatzer R, et al. Efficacy and safety of thrombolytic therapy after initially unsuccessful cardiopulmonary resuscitation: a prospective clinical trial. Lancet. 2001;357(9268):1583-5.

[29] Fatovich DM, Dobb GJ, Clugston RA. A pilot randomised trial of thrombolysis in cardiac arrest (The TICA trial). Resuscitation. 2004;61(3):309-13.

[30] Jaff MR, McMurtry MS, Archer SL, Cushman M, Goldenberg N, Goldhaber SZ, et al. Management of massive and submassive pulmonary embolism, iliofemoral deep vein thrombosis, and chronic thromboembolic pulmonary hypertension: a scientific statement from the American Heart Association. Circulation. 2011;123(16):1788-830.

[31] Maggio P, Hemmila M, Haft J, Bartlett R. Extracorporeal life support for massive pulmonary embolism. J Trauma. 2007;62(3):570-6.

[32] Giraud R, Banfi C, Siegenthaler N, Bendjelid K. Massive pulmonary embolism leading to cardiac arrest: one pathology, two different ECMO modes to assist patients. J Clin Monit Comput. 2015.

[33] Lebreton G, Bouabdallaoui N, Gauduchon L, Mnif MA, Roques F. Successful use of ECMO as a bridge to surgical embolectomy in Life-Threatening Pulmonary Embolism. Am J Emerg Med. 2015;33(9):1332 e3-4.

[34] Abrams DC, Brodie D, Rosenzweig EB, Burkart KM, Agerstrand CL, Bacchetta MD. Upper-body extracorporeal membrane oxygenation as a strategy in decompensated pulmonary arterial hypertension. Pulm Circ. 2013;3(2):432-5.

[35] Mohite PN, Sabashnikov A, Patil NP, Saez DG, Zych B, Popov AF, et al. Short-term ventricular assist device in post-cardiotomy cardiogenic shock: factors influencing survival. J Artif Organs. 2014;17(3):228-35.

[36] Muehrcke DD, McCarthy PM, Stewart RW, Foster RC, Ogella DA, Borsh JA, et al. Extracorporeal membrane oxygenation for postcardiotomy cardiogenic shock. Ann Thorac Surg. 1996;61(2):684-91.

[37] Rastan AJ, Dege A, Mohr M, Doll N, Falk V, Walther T, et al. Early and late outcomes of 517 consecutive adult patients treated with extracorporeal membrane oxygenation for refractory postcardiotomy cardiogenic shock. J Thorac Cardiovasc Surg. 2010;139(2):302-11, 11 e1.

[38] Delgado DH, Rao V, Ross HJ, Verma S, Smedira NG. Mechanical circulatory assistance: state of art. Circulation. 2002;106(16):2046-50.

[39] Khorsandi M, Shaikhrezai K, Prasad S, Pessotto R, Walker W, Berg G, et al. Advanced mechanical circulatory support for post-cardiotomy cardiogenic shock: a 20-year outcome analysis in a non-transplant unit. J Cardiothorac Surg. 2016;11(1):29.

[40] Pokersnik JA, Buda T, Bashour CA, Gonzalez-Stawinski GV. Have changes in ECMO technology impacted outcomes in adult patients developing postcardiotomy cardiogenic shock? J Card Surg. 2012;27(2):246-52.

[41] Santise G, Panarello G, Ruperto C, Turrisi M, Pilato G, Giunta A, et al. Extracorporeal membrane oxygenation for graft failure after heart transplantation: a multidisciplinary approach to maximize weaning rate. Int J Artif Organs. 2014;37(9):706-14.

[42] Chung JC, Tsai PR, Chou NK, Chi NH, Wang SS, Ko WJ. Extracorporeal membrane oxygenation bridge to adult heart transplantation. Clin Transplant. 2010;24(3):375-80.

[43] Patroniti N, Sangalli F, Avalli L. Post-cardiac arrest extracorporeal life support. Best Pract Res Clin Anaesthesiol. 2015;29(4):497-508.

[44] Brechot N, Luyt CE, Schmidt M, Leprince P, Trouillet JL, Leger P, et al. Venoarterial extracorporeal membrane oxygenation support for refractory cardiovascular dysfunction during severe bacterial septic shock. Crit Care Med. 2013;41(7):1616-26.

[45] Wallmuller C, Sterz F, Testori C, Schober A, Stratil P, Horburger D, et al. Emergency cardio-pulmonary bypass in cardiac arrest: seventeen years of experience. Resuscitation. 2013;84(3):326-30.

[46] Xie A, Phan K, Tsai YC, Yan TD, Forrest P. Venoarterial extracorporeal membrane oxygenation for cardiogenic shock and cardiac arrest: a meta-analysis. J Cardiothorac Vasc Anesth. 2015;29(3):637-45.

[47] Chen YS, Lin JW, Yu HY, Ko WJ, Jerng JS, Chang WT, et al. Cardiopulmonary resuscitation with assisted extracorporeal life-support versus conventional cardiopulmonary resuscitation in adults with in-hospital cardiac arrest: an observational study and propensity analysis. Lancet. 2008;372(9638):554-61.

[48] Stub D, Bernard S, Pellegrino V, Smith K, Walker T, Sheldrake J, et al. Refractory cardiac arrest treated with mechanical CPR, hypothermia, ECMO and early reperfusion (the CHEER trial). Resuscitation. 2015;86:88-94.

[49] Maekawa K, Tanno K, Hase M, Mori K, Asai Y. Extracorporeal cardiopulmonary resuscitation for patients with out-of-hospital cardiac arrest of cardiac origin: a propensity-matched study and predictor analysis. Crit Care Med. 2013;41(5):1186-96.

[50] Sakamoto T, Morimura N, Nagao K, Asai Y, Yokota H, Nara S, et al. Extracorporeal cardiopulmonary resuscitation versus conventional cardiopulmonary resuscitation in

adults with out-of-hospital cardiac arrest: a prospective observational study. Resuscitation. 2014;85(6):762-8.

[51] Shin TG, Choi JH, Jo IJ, Sim MS, Song HG, Jeong YK, et al. Extracorporeal cardiopulmonary resuscitation in patients with inhospital cardiac arrest: a comparison with conventional cardiopulmonary resuscitation. Crit Care Med. 2011;39(1):1-7.

[52] Le Guen M, Nicolas-Robin A, Carreira S, Raux M, Leprince P, Riou B, et al. Extracorporeal life support following out-of-hospital refractory cardiac arrest. Crit Care. 2011;15(1):R29.

[53] Ortega-Deballon I, Hornby L, Shemie SD, Bhanji F, Guadagno E. Extracorporeal resuscitation for refractory out-of-hospital cardiac arrest in adults: a systematic review of international practices and outcomes. Resuscitation. 2016;101:12-20.

[54] Pozzi M, Koffel C, Armoiry X, Pavlakovic I, Neidecker J, Prieur C, et al. Extracorporeal life support for refractory out-of-hospital cardiac arrest: should we still fight for? A single-centre, 5-year experience. Int J Cardiol. 2016;204:70-6.

[55] Paden ML, Conrad SA, Rycus PT, Thiagarajan RR, Registry E. Extracorporeal Life Support Organization Registry Report 2012. ASAIO J. 2013;59(3):202-10.

[56] Esper SA, Levy JH, Waters JH, Welsby IJ. Extracorporeal membrane oxygenation in the adult: a review of anticoagulation monitoring and transfusion. Anesth Analg. 2014;118(4):731-43.

[57] Malfertheiner MV, Philipp A, Lubnow M, Zeman F, Enger TB, Bein T, et al. Hemostatic Changes During Extracorporeal Membrane Oxygenation: A Prospective Randomized Clinical Trial Comparing Three Different Extracorporeal Membrane Oxygenation Systems. Crit Care Med. 2015.

[58] Combes A, Bacchetta M, Brodie D, Muller T, Pellegrino V. Extracorporeal membrane oxygenation for respiratory failure in adults. Curr Opin Crit Care. 2012;18(1):99-104.

[59] Annich GM. Extracorporeal life support: the precarious balance of hemostasis. J Thromb Haemost. 2015;13 Suppl 1:S336-42.

[60] Cheng R, Hachamovitch R, Kittleson M, Patel J, Arabia F, Moriguchi J, et al. Complications of extracorporeal membrane oxygenation for treatment of cardiogenic shock and cardiac arrest: a meta-analysis of 1,866 adult patients. Ann Thorac Surg. 2014;97(2): 610-6.

[61] Avalli L, Sangalli F, Migliari M, Maggioni E, Gallieri S, Segramora V, et al. Early vascular complications after percutaneous cannulation for extracorporeal membrane oxygenation for cardiac assist. Minerva Anestesiol. 2016;82(1):36-43.

[62] Tanaka D, Hirose H, Cavarocchi N, Entwistle JW. The Impact of Vascular Complications on Survival of Patients on Venoarterial Extracorporeal Membrane Oxygenation. Ann Thorac Surg. 2016.

[63] Lubnow M, Philipp A, Foltan M, Bull Enger T, Lunz D, Bein T, et al. Technical com-plications during veno-venous extracorporeal membrane oxygenation and their relevance predicting a system-exchange--retrospective analysis of 265 cases. PLoS One. 2014;9(12):e112316.

[64] Murphy DA, Hockings LE, Andrews RK, Aubron C, Gardiner EE, Pellegrino VA, et al. Extracorporeal membrane oxygenation-hemostatic complications. Transfus Med Rev. 2015;29(2):90-101.

[65] Zangrillo A, Landoni G, Biondi-Zoccai G, Greco M, Greco T, Frati G, et al. A meta-analysis of complications and mortality of extracorporeal membrane oxygenation. Crit Care Resusc. 2013;15(3):172-8.

[66] Green TP, Kriesmer P, Steinhorn RH, Payne NR, Irmiter RJ, Meyer CL. Comparison of pressure-volume-flow relationships in centrifugal and roller pump extracorporeal membrane oxygenation systems for neonates. ASAIO Trans. 1991;37(4):572-6.

[67] Lehle K, Philipp A, Zeman F, Lunz D, Lubnow M, Wendel HP, et al. Technical-Induced Hemolysis in Patients with Respiratory Failure Supported with Veno-Venous ECMO - Prevalence and Risk Factors. PLoS One. 2015;10(11):e0143527.

[68] Leverett LB, Hellums JD, Alfrey CP, Lynch EC. Red blood cell damage by shear stress. Biophys J. 1972;12(3):257-73.

[69] Shimono T, Makinouchi K, Nose Y. Total erythrocyte destruction time: the new index for the hemolytic performance of rotary blood pumps. Artif Organs. 1995;19(7):571-5.

[70] Vercaemst L. Hemolysis in cardiac surgery patients undergoing cardiopulmonary bypass: a review in search of a treatment algorithm. J Extra Corpor Technol. 2008;40(4): 257-67.

[71] Wielogorski JW, Cross DE, Nwadike EV. The effects of subatmospheric pressure on the haemolysis of blood. J Biomech. 1975;8(5):321-5.

[72] Williams DC, Turi JL, Hornik CP, Bonadonna DK, Williford WL, Walczak RJ, et al. Circuit oxygenator contributes to extracorporeal membrane oxygenation-induced hemolysis. ASAIO J. 2015;61(2):190-5.

[73] Rother RP, Bell L, Hillmen P, Gladwin MT. The clinical sequelae of intravascular hemolysis and extracellular plasma hemoglobin: a novel mechanism of human disease. JAMA. 2005;293(13):1653-62.

[74] Skogby M, Mellgren K, Adrian K, Friberg LG, Chevalier JY, Mellgren G. Induced cell trauma during in vitro perfusion: a comparison between two different perfusion systems. Artif Organs. 1998;22(12):1045-51.

[75] Cappellini MD. Coagulation in the pathophysiology of hemolytic anemias. Hematol-ogy Am Soc Hematol Educ Program. 2007:74-8.

[76] Jeney V, Balla J, Yachie A, Varga Z, Vercellotti GM, Eaton JW, et al. Pro-oxidant and cytotoxic effects of circulating heme. Blood. 2002;100(3):879-87.

[77] Schaer DJ, Buehler PW, Alayash AI, Belcher JD, Vercellotti GM. Hemolysis and free hemoglobin revisited: exploring hemoglobin and hemin scavengers as a novel class of therapeutic proteins. Blood. 2013;121(8):1276-84.

[78] Betrus C, Remenapp R, Charpie J, Kudelka T, Brophy P, Smoyer WE, et al. Enhanced hemolysis in pediatric patients requiring extracorporeal membrane oxygenation and continuous renal replacement therapy. Ann Thorac Cardiovasc Surg. 2007;13(6):378-83.

[79] Gbadegesin R, Zhao S, Charpie J, Brophy PD, Smoyer WE, Lin JJ. Significance of hemolysis on extracorporeal life support after cardiac surgery in children. Pediatr Nephrol. 2009;24(3):589-95.

[80] Vermeulen Windsant IC, de Wit NC, Sertorio JT, van Bijnen AA, Ganushchak YM, Heijmans JH, et al. Hemolysis during cardiac surgery is associated with increased intravascular nitric oxide consumption and perioperative kidney and intestinal tissue damage. Front Physiol. 2014;5:340.

[81] Mateen FJ, Muralidharan R, Shinohara RT, Parisi JE, Schears GJ, Wijdicks EF. Neurological injury in adults treated with extracorporeal membrane oxygenation. Arch Neurol. 2011;68(12):1543-9.

[82] Graziani LJ, Gringlas M, Baumgart S. Cerebrovascular complications and neurodevelopmental sequelae of neonatal ECMO. Clin Perinatol. 1997;24(3):655-75.

[83] Risnes I, Wagner K, Nome T, Sundet K, Jensen J, Hynas IA, et al. Cerebral outcome in adult patients treated with extracorporeal membrane oxygenation. Ann Thorac Surg. 2006;81(4):1401-6.

[84] Nasr DM, Rabinstein AA. Neurologic Complications of Extracorporeal Membrane Oxygenation. J Clin Neurol. 2015;11(4):383-9.

[85] Bizzarro MJ, Conrad SA, Kaufman DA, Rycus P, Extracorporeal Life Support Organization Task Force on Infections EMO. Infections acquired during extracorporeal membrane oxygenation in neonates, children, and adults. Pediatr Crit Care Med. 2011;12(3):277-81.

[86] O'Horo JC, Cawcutt KA, De Moraes AG, Sampathkumar P, Schears GJ. The Evidence Base for Prophylactic Antibiotics in Patients Receiving Extracorporeal Membrane Oxygenation. ASAIO J. 2016;62(1):6-10.

[87] Gardner AH, Prodhan P, Stovall SH, Gossett JM, Stern JE, Wilson CD, et al. Fungal infections and antifungal prophylaxis in pediatric cardiac extracorporeal life support. J Thorac Cardiovasc Surg. 2012;143(3):689-95.

[88] Pellegrino V, Hockings LE, Davies A. Veno-arterial extracorporeal membrane oxygenation for adult cardiovascular failure. Curr Opin Crit Care. 2014;20(5):484-92.

[89] Aiyagari RM, Rocchini AP, Remenapp RT, Graziano JN. Decompression of the left atrium during extracorporeal membrane oxygenation using a transseptal cannula incorporated into the circuit. Crit Care Med. 2006;34(10):2603-6.

[90] Guirgis M, Kumar K, Menkis AH, Freed DH. Minimally invasive left-heart decompression during venoarterial extracorporeal membrane oxygenation: an alternative to a percutaneous approach. Interact Cardiovasc Thorac Surg. 2010;10(5):672-4.

[91] Vlasselaers D, Desmet M, Desmet L, Meyns B, Dens J. Ventricular unloading with a miniature axial flow pump in combination with extracorporeal membrane oxygenation. Intensive Care Med. 2006;32(2):329-33.

[92] Weymann A, Schmack B, Sabashnikov A, Bowles CT, Raake P, Arif R, et al. Central extracorporeal life support with left ventricular decompression for the treatment of refractory cardiogenic shock and lung failure. J Cardiothorac Surg. 2014;9:60.

[93] Chung M, Shiloh AL, Carlese A. Monitoring of the adult patient on venoarterial extracorporeal membrane oxygenation. Scientific World Journal. 2014;2014:393258.

[94] Aissaoui N, Luyt CE, Leprince P, Trouillet JL, Leger P, Pavie A, et al. Predictors of successful extracorporeal membrane oxygenation (ECMO) weaning after assistance for refractory cardiogenic shock. Intensive Care Med. 2011;37(11):1738-45.

[95] Schmidt M, Burrell A, Roberts L, Bailey M, Sheldrake J, Rycus PT, et al. Predicting survival after ECMO for refractory cardiogenic shock: the survival after veno-arterial-ECMO (SAVE)-score. Eur Heart J. 2015;36(33):2246-56.

[96] Muller G, Flecher E, Lebreton G, Luyt CE, Trouillet JL, Brechot N, et al. The ENCOURAGE mortality risk score and analysis of long-term outcomes after VA-ECMO for acute myocardial infarction with cardiogenic shock. Intensive Care Med. 2016;42(3):370-8.

[97] Riou B, Adnet F, Baud F, Cariou A, Carli P, Combes A, et al. Recommandations sur les indications de l'assistance circulatoire dans le traitement des arrêts cardiaques réfractaires. 2008;Annales Françaises d'Anesthésie et de Réanimation 28 (2009) 182–186.

[98] Abrams DC, Prager K, Blinderman CD, Burkart KM, Brodie D. Ethical dilemmas encountered with the use of extracorporeal membrane oxygenation in adults. Chest. 2014;145(4):876-82.

Extracorporeal Membrane Oxygenation Support as Treatment for Early Graft Failure After Heart Transplantation

Antonio Loforte, Giacomo Murana,
Mariano Cefarelli, Jacopo Alfonsi,
Giuliano Jafrancesco, Francesco Grigioni,
Lucio Careddu, Emanuela Angeli,
Gaetano Gargiulo and Giuseppe Marinelli

Abstract

Early graft failure (EGF) is a major risk factor for death after heart transplantation (Htx) accounting for >40% of deaths within 30 days postoperatively. According to the last International Society for Heart and Lung Transplantation (ISHLT) consensus statement, the graft dysfunction (GD) is to be classified into primary (PGD), in case of an unknown triggering factor or secondary (SGD) where there is a discernible cause such as acute rejection, pulmonary hypertension, or known surgical complications. The diagnosis of GD is to be made within 24 h after completion of Htx surgery and a severity scale for GD should include mild, moderate, or severe grades based on specified criteria. Mechanical circulatory support (MCS) for GD should be considered when medical management is not sufficient to support the newly transplanted graft. Currently, extracorporeal membrane oxygenation (ECMO) is widely accepted as treatment of severe EGF, given its easy and quick setup, the system versatility, the optimal end-organ perfusion provided, and the possibility of both biventricular and lung assistance by usage of a low-cost single pump.

Keywords: heart transplantation, early graft failure, cardiogenic shock, mechanical circulatory support, extracorporeal membrane oxygenation

1. Introduction

A recent examination of early mortality after heart transplantation (Htx), documented in the International Society for Heart and Lung Transplantation (ISHLT) Registry, reveals that >40% of deaths within 30 days post-operatively are due to early graft failure (EGF) [1, 2]. Results get even worst in the pediatric transplant population where an early mortality of 88% after diagnosis has been reported [3]. To better define the classification, diagnosis and management of this condition, a Consensus Conference was organized on April 23, 2013 during the 33rd Annual ISHLT meeting. There were 71 specialists on this field including cardiologists, immunologists, pathologists, and surgeons, representing 42 heart centers worldwide. According to the consensus statement [1], graft dysfunction (GD) has been classified into primary (PGD), in case of an unknown triggering factor or secondary (SGD) when a discernible cause such as hyper-acute rejection, pulmonary hypertension, or known surgical complications [1] can be identified. The diagnosis of GD is to be made within 24 h after completion of heart transplantation (Htx) surgery and a severity scale for GD should include mild, moderate, or severe grades based on specified criteria. Risks are often multifactorial and usually include donor, recipient, and surgical variables. Before the advent of short-term ventricular assist devices (VADs) and extra-corporeal membrane oxygenation (ECMO) support after transplant, severe EGF was likely considered to be fatal. Currently, the use of mechanical circulatory support (MCS) devices as treatment of GD is more widely well accepted and adopted whenever maximal medical management is not sufficient to support the newly transplanted graft. In this chapter, we will focus on actual indications, surgical strategies, and future perspectives of veno-arterial ECMO as a bridge to graft recovery in both pediatric and adult populations.

2. Clinical background and epidemiology

The exact incidence of PGD has been unknown until 2013 due to the lack of standardization of diagnostic criteria according to the historical observational studies as stated by the above mentioned ISHLT consensus paper [1]. However, the ISHLT registry data always offered specific information concerning epidemiology and clinical characteristics of PGD by time. The examination of early mortality after heart transplant documented in the registry shows that 66% of the death that occurs in the first 30 days after transplant are due to "graft failure" and "multi-organ dysfunction" [1]. Most of these events are probably the result of fatal PGD. An analysis of the United Network for Organ Sharing (UNOS) database was conducted for transplants occurring from 1999 to 2007 (n = 16,716) [3]. For this analysis, PGD was defined by "hard outcomes," meaning postoperative death or retransplant, where the incidence of PGD was 2.5%. In this PGD group, 85% were due to deaths and 15% were due to retransplants [3]. A closer look at early mortality from the ISHLT revealed that more than 100,000 patients who received Htx between 1982 and 2011 shows that approximately 10% of patients dies within 30 days of transplant, and this number increases to 14% after 90 days [1]. The risk of 30-day and 90-day mortality was the highest in retransplant (18% and 22%) and congenital heart disease (17% and 21%), intermediate in valvular cardiomyopathy (14% and 18%), and the lowest in ischemic (10% and 14%) and non-ischemic (8% and 12%) cardiomyopathy patients [1]. Increasing recipient age is a known risk factor associated with intermediate-term and long-term mortality after heart transplant; however, 30-day and 90-day mortality varies little in patients of different age groups, including patients older than 70 years. Sizable majority of early post-transplant deaths likely results from PGD. The recent reduction of early post-transplant mortality might have resulted from lower incidence and/or better treatment of PGD. There are considerable differences in early post-transplant mortality in patients who receive transplants for different heart disease etiologies, and early post-transplant mortality continues to represent a significant problem despite better survival. Concerning epidemiological data of Htx in children a retrospective review showing ECMO need in the early post-transplant period at Denver Children's Hospital, Aurora, Colorado. From 1990 to 2007, 310 children underwent Htx, and 28 children who underwent transplantation (9%) were placed on ECMO for postoperative primary graft failure [4]. They conclude that primary graft failure requiring mechanical circulatory support in the early period after transplantation is not uncommon in children (9%), and a long ischemic time is a major risk factor of graft dysfunction [4]. Pediatric cardiac allografts can be successfully salvaged by ECMO in a reasonable proportion of patients (54%) [4].

2.1. Pathogenesis

The transplant process may lead to donor heart graft several kinds of insults due to:

– Brain death and its sequelae in the donor.

– Hypothermic ischemia during transport.

– Warm ischemia during implant surgery.

– Reperfusion injury after release of the aortic cross-clamp in the recipient.

Systemic factors in the recipient determine a "hostile" environment that further compromises donor heart function after reperfusion. Associated with brain death in the donor, there is a series of events that result in impaired myocardial contractility and sensitize the heart to ischemia-reperfusion injury. An example is the intense release of myocardial norepinephrine immediately after brain death that causes cytosolic and mitochondrial calcium overload [5]. Mitochondrial calcium overload may activate autophagy, apoptosis, or necrosis [6]. During donor resuscitation, administration of exogenous catecholamines may determine a reduction of myocardial β-receptor sensitivity and an activation of multiple pro-inflammatory mediators, including complement [7–9]. Referring to hypothermic ischemia, during transport most donor hearts are stored in a cold preservation solution and transported on ice. Hypothermia slows but does not stop cellular metabolism, so progressive ischemic injury is an inevitable consequence of prolonged static storage. In addition, the absence of normal aerobic metabolism arrests the activity of transmembrane Na^+/K^+ adenosinetriphosphatase pump consequently the switch to anaerobic metabolism during cold storage causes a rapid decline in high-energy phosphates and development of lactic acidosis [10]. Na^+/H^+ exchanger is activated by intracellular acidosis and it exchanges H^+ for Na^+ across the cell membrane. The increasing of intracellular Na^+ determines an accu-

Donor risk factors	Recipient risk factors	Surgical procedural risk factors
• Age	• Age	• Ischemia time
• Cause of death	• Weight	• Donor-recipient mismatch
• Trauma	• Mechanical support	• Weight mismatch
• Cardiac dysfunction	• Congenital heart disease	• Experience of procurement team and center volume
• Inotropic support	• Multiple reoperation	• Cardioplegic solution
• Comorbidities: (diabetes, hypertension)	• LVAD explant	• Increased blood transfusion
	• Comorbidities: (renal/liver dysfunction)	• Elective vs. emergency transplant
• Drug abuse		
• LV hypertrophy	• Ventilator dependent	
• Valvular disease	• Multiorgan transplant	
• Hormone treatment	• Elevated PVR	
• CAD	• Allosensitization	
• Sepsis	• Infection	
• Troponin trend	• Retransplant	
• Hypernatremia		

Table 1. Risk factors for EGF.

mulation of intracellular Ca^{2+} by activation of the Na^+/Ca^+ exchanger [11]. Other factors, recipient related, contribute to early graft dysfunction. It is possible to find two clinical conditions. The first is the presence of a high pulmonary vascular resistance in the recipient [12, 13]. In this case, the graft failure is considered secondary (to a known recipient factor) rather than primary. However, even with recipient pulmonary pressures and resistances within the accepted ranges for heart transplantation, a lower degree of pulmonary hypertension correlates with a lower incidence of PGD. The second scenario is characterized by activation of the systemic inflammatory response in the recipient, which causes vasodilated systemic circulation that is not responsive to medical therapy [14]. This "vasoplegic" response is associated with risks factors such as mechanical circulatory support before transplantation, large transfusion requirements, and prolonged cross-clamp time. In this circumstance, the "hostile environment" of the recipient results in PGD. The pathophysiology of PGD in this setting is not so clear, but it could involve the multiple action of many pro-inflammatory cytokines leading to upregulation of inducible nitric oxide synthase or indoleamine dioxygenase, with overproduction of nitric oxide or other endogenous vasodilators [14, 15]. The multiple risk factors for PGD include not only donor and perioperative factors but also recipient characteristics, confirming the multifaceted nature of PGD. The risk factors (**Table 1**) for PGD related to recipient are: age, parameters reflecting pulmonary hypertension and more severe pre-transplant condition, including dependence on intravenous inotropic support, mechanical support and mechanical ventilation. Donor factors include age, female donor, and cause of brain death. Procedural factors are represented by ischemic time and donor-to-recipient weight mismatch. The RADIAL score (**Table 2**) is today the only validated scoring system for the prediction of PGD [16]. This predictive model was obtained after multivariate analysis of independent risk factors for PGD in a single-center derivation cohort of 621 heart transplants performed from 1984 to 2006. Six factors with similar influence were chosen to form the acronym RADIAL: four of these are related to the recipient: right atrial pressure (4–10 mmHg), age (4–60 years), diabetes and inotropic support dependence; and two are associated with the donor: age (4–30 years) and length of ischemia time (4–240 min). The presence of each of these factors in an individual patient adds one point to the final score. According to the RADIAL model, there are three groups with low (0–1 points), medium (2 points), and high (>3 points) risk for PGD.

R (recipient)	Right atrial pressure	>10 mmHg	1
A (recipient)	Age	>60 years	1
D (recipient)	Diabetes	Diagnosis/treatment	1
I (recipient)	Inotropic support dependence		1
A (recipient)	Age	>30 years	1
L (recipient)	Length of ischemia	>240 min	1
Low risk for PGD		**(0–1) points**	
Medium risk for PGD		(2) points	
High risk for PGD		(>3) points	

Table 2. Radial score.

2.2. Classification

According to the consensus statement [1], graft dysfunction should be classified into PGD or secondary graft dysfunction (SGD) where there is a discernible cause such as hyperacute rejection, pulmonary hypertension, or known surgical complications (e.g., uncontrolled bleeding; **Table 3**). It is necessary to made the diagnosis of PGD within 24 h after completion of the cardiac transplant surgery. There is an important difference between treatment of patients with RV failure and LV failure, so it was decided to divide PGD into two entities: PGD-LV, which includes LV and biventricular failure, and PGD-RV alone (**Table 3**). Finally, it was created a grading system for PGD-LV, which includes the descriptors of mild, moderate, and severe dysfunction. These were carefully defined with the use of hemodynamic variables, echocardiography results, level of inotropic support, and need for mechanical circulatory support. Because RV failure can often be more difficult to quantify, there are no grades for the severity of PGD-RV.

Primary graft dysfunction (PGD)		Secondary graft dysfunction
a. PGD-left ventricle (PGD-LV): includes [21] left and biventricular dysfunction b. PGD-right ventricle (PGD-RV): includes right ventricular dysfunction alone		Occurs when there is a discernible cause for graft dysfunction (e.g., hyperacute rejection, pulmonary hypertension, known surgical complication)
PGD-left ventricle (PGDLV):	*Mild PGD-LV: one of the following criteria must be met*	LVEF < 40% by echocardiography, or hemodynamics with RAP > 15 mmHg, PCWP > 20 mmHg, CI < 2.0 L/min/m^2 (lasting more than 1 h) requiring low-dose inotropes
	Moderate PGD-LV: must meet one criterion from I and another criterion from II:	I. One criteria from the following: left ventricular ejection fraction < 40%, or hemodynamic compromise with RAP > 15 mmHg, PCWP > 20 mmHg, CI < 2.0 L/min/m^2, hypotension with MAP < 70 mmHg (lasting more than 1 h). II. One criteria from the following: *High-dose inotropes—Inotrope score > 10[a] or **Newly placed IABP (regardless of inotropes)
	Severe PGD-LV	Dependence on left or biventricular mechanical support including ECMO, LVAD, BiVAD, or percutaneous LVAD. Excludes requirement for IABP
PGD-right ventricle (PGDRV):	*Diagnosis requires either both I and II, or III alone:*	I. Hemodynamics with RAP > 15 mmHg, PCWP < 15 mmHg, CI < 2.0 L/min/m^2 II. TPG < 15 mmHg and/or pulmonary artery systolic pressure < 50 mmHg, or III. Need for RVAD

BiVAD, biventricular assist device; CI, cardiac index; ECMO, extracorporeal membrane oxygenation; IABP, intra-aortic balloon pump; LVAD, left ventricular assist device; PCWP, pulmonary capillary wedge pressure; RAP, right atrial pressure; RVAD, right ventricular assist device; TPG, transpulmonary pressure gradient.

[a]Inotrope score = dopamine(x1) + dobutamine(x1) + amrinone(x1) + milrinone(x15) + epinephrine(x100) + norepinephrine(x100) with each drug dosed in μg/kg/min [k2].

Table 3. Classification of graft dysfunction.

2.3. Pharmacologic and mechanical management

Before the introduction of short-term VAD support and ECMO after Htx, PGD was frequently fatal except for that cases where emergency salvage retransplantation was possible. D'Alessandro et al. from La Pitié-Salpétrière in Paris retrospectively evaluated the use of ECMO temporary support as a treatment for PGD [17]. They studied 394 patients, who underwent cardiac transplant between 2000 and 2006. In 90 patients, PGD after transplant occurred. In this study, PGD was defined as the need for inotrope support with epinephrine and/or the necessity for mechanical circulatory support in the postoperative 48 h. Of these 90 patients, 54 received ECMO, 8 used other assist devices, and 28 were treated only with maximal inotropes [17]. Of those medically treated (i.e., on maximal inotropes only), survival was 46% compared with a survival of 50% for those on ECMO [17]. These data confirm that ECMO is becoming a safer and more effective technique to manage patients with PGD. A retrospective analysis of short-term VAD use after transplantation found that in 38 patients from 2003 to 2008 who have been implanted with the CentriMag device (Levitronix, Waltham, MA) for PGD survival was 50% at 30 days and 32% at 1 year [18]. Earlier implantation of the device after transplant seemed to correlate with improved survival, and all survivors were supported with the device for no more than 30 days [18]. In summary, medical treatment of PGD consists of inotrope and vasodilator support and these are considered the first line therapy for PGD and may be helpful for milder cases of PGD. ECMO and other mechanical circulatory support are the only effective options for more severe cases, appearing to reduce mortality compared with other treatments. From the data, early intervention and short-term support appears to be associated with improved survival.

3. Indication of ECMO in EGF

EGF is the main cause of early mortality after transplantation. Hemodynamic deterioration caused by cardiogenic shock due to the pump failure unresponsive to inotropes has a catastrophic progression if not corrected in time [2]. As the pathophysiology of EGF is often unclear, specific treatment remains still challenging and the choice of the most suitable support option (e.g., ventricular assist device [VAD] or extracorporeal membrane oxygenation [ECMO]) remains controversial. In particular, ECMO support, even if associated with mortality and a high rate of morbidity (such as bleeding, ischemic or thromboembolic events and infections), is considered a valid therapeutic route [19, 20].

3.1. Adult population

Actually, there is not a real or unique indication for ECMO implanting in case of EGF. What we can consider are the single centers experience. Routinely, after exclusion of surgical problems, the first line treatment starts using inotropic drags such as milrinone, epinephrine, and dopamine. In case of hard weaning from CPB machine because of unstable, hemodynamics should be considered the use of intra-aortic balloon pump (IABP) and prepare the patient for ECMO implantation (**Figure 1**). In the Cedars-Sinai Heart Institute, for example, they place on ECMO if cardiac index remains <2.5 L/min/m^2 with central venous pressure and left atrial pressure >12 mmHg and a mean arterial pressure <65 mmHg. The approach of the Columbia University at the management of PGD has evolved: most patients now receive BiVAD support, usually a C-Mag BiVAD with left apical cannulation. More recently ventricular-arterial ECMO has also become a more common mode of support. The median length of device support at their transplant center was 7 days, with an in-hospital mortality of 51%. Only 5.7% survived to re-transplantation [1].

3.2. Pediatric population

ECMO represents the most commonly used method of mechanical circulatory support in the post-transplantation period of pediatric patients [21]. In the same way of the adult, also for the pediatric population, the indications for the ECMO implantation are not clear. In almost all centers, the extracorporeal membrane oxygenation is started in the operating room because of the inability to wean from cardiopulmonary bypass, and only a few cases required ECMO in the first 48 h after transplantation requiring a cannulation in the cardiac intensive care unit [4]. In particular, as reported by Tissot et al. [4], the timing of ECMO cannulation is not predictive of outcome. In their population, in fact, the survival is not significantly different between patients started on ECMO in the operating room with those cannulated in the first 48 h after transplantation for hemodynamic instability or cardiac arrest in the cardiac intensive care unit. This is in contrast with Galantowicz et al. [22], who reported no chance of survival if the cardiac allograft could not support the patient after cardiopulmonary bypass.

4. Surgical approach

Mechanical circulatory support has evolved markedly over recent years even in terms of surgical techniques. In particular, ECMO support can be deployed peripherally or centrally, using a traditional or minimally-invasive approach. There is still a great debate about the cannulation site strategies (**Table 1**). The central cannulation has several advantages such as full antegrade outflow and avoidance of peripheral ischemic complications [23]. However, it

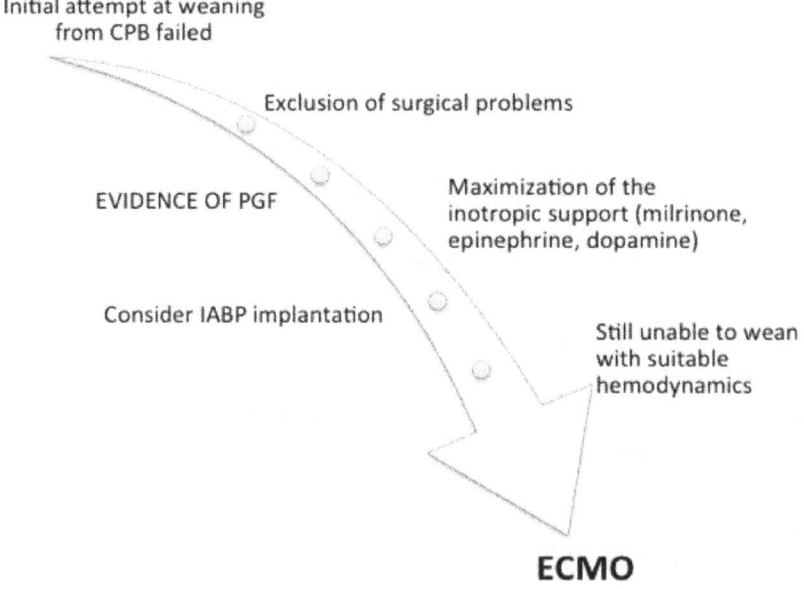

Figure 1. Decision algorithm for ECMO implantation for EGF.

leads to an high risk for bleeding, tamponade, and infection [24]. These are the main reasons why a lot of centers adopt a peripheral setting.

4.1. Peripheral cannulation

For veno-arterial ECMO installation, a femoral vein and a femoral artery are usually used for vascular access. The correct position of the venous cannula tip is the mid-right atrium to have an homogenous drainage of venous blood from both caval veins. The femoral arterial cannula should be fully introduced till its tip reaches the common iliac artery, in adults (**Figure 2**). Commonly, in our center, we use a DLP Biomedicus 15–19 Fr (Medtronic Inc., Minneapolis, MN) cannula for the femoral artery, and a DLP Biomedicus 17–23 Fr (Medtronic Inc.) cannula inserted into the femoral vein for the venous drainage [25]. Both insertions are performed using the Seldinger technique after anterior vessel wall exposure and secured with pledgeted, reinforced purse string prolene sutures. Combined IABP support is additionally adopted in the peripheral ECMO population to indirectly "vent" the left ventricle and avoids the pulmonary edema. For peripheral cannulation, a continuous-wave Doppler image of the tibial artery flow and pulsatility should be acquired every 2 days, in the presence of a consultant vascular surgeon, to evaluate and provide a correct distal leg perfusion.

Although, as described above, the peripheral cannulation reduces the risk of bleeding and of infection, it can lead to important lower limb ischemia and the so-called "watershed phenomenon." The "native" flow meet the retrograde blood flow from the arterial cannula somewhere between the ascending aorta and the renal arteries at a point called the "watershed." All areas distal to this zone received blood oxygenated by the ECMO; meanwhile, the upper part receives blood from the left ventricle depending on respiratory function of the lung which can be severely compromised [26]. In an effort to minimize these matters, some centers reported on the use of a side graft sutured on the axillary artery as arterial return for ECMO peripheral setting. The advantages include: a low grade of atherosclerosis vessel disease, an antegrade flow into the aorta, and a preferential delivery of oxygenated blood into the heart and brain [27].

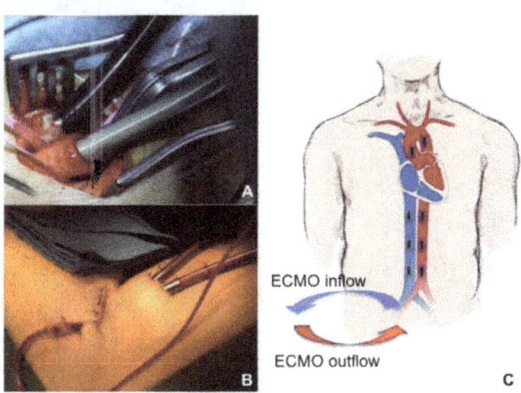

Figure 2. Peripheral ECMO setting (A: intra-operative direct cannulation; B: intra-operative percutaneous approach; C: setting).

4.2. Central cannulation

The easiest way to perform a central approach for ECMO implantation after Htx is to re-utilize the cannulas adopted for aortic arterial return and atrial venous drainage during the cardio-pulmonary bypass (CPB). Usually, the aortic cannula is left in situ to avoid new aortic puncturing, while the venous cannula is placed into the right atrium through its lateral wall. At our center, the central cannulation is performed using the right atrium, through its lateral wall as access, and the left atrium, between the right pulmonary veins as access, for venous drainage [25]. The employed cannulae are two 28-Fr wire-reinforced angled veno-atrial cannula (Jostra Venous Catheter OD; Maquet Cardiopulmonary AG, Hirrlingen, Germany) for both atria. The outflow cannula is always positioned into the ascending aorta [straight aortic perfusion cannula (22 or 24 Fr); Edwards Lifesciences LLC, Irvine, CA]. All cannulas are secured with pledgeted, reinforced purse string prolene sutures, tunneled through sub-costal incisions to allow chest closure, and then connected to the circuit, avoiding air in the system. In case of graft isolated right ventricular failure (RVF) and pre-transplant recipient severe pulmonary hypertension, the extracorporeal right-to-left atrium bypass (ECRLAB) ECMO setting may be adopted (**Figure 3**) [25]. Briefly, the cannulation is performed centrally, using the right atrium for venous drainage and the left atrium, between the right pulmonary veins, for arterial return. The cannulae are two 28-Fr wire-reinforced angled veno-atrial cannula (Maquet) for both atria. The conventional circuits, with the inflow cannula in the right atrium and the outflow cannula in the pulmonary artery, could not completely decompress the right heart in case of high pulmonary arterial pressures, presumably because no blood entering the chamber can be ejected across the pulmonary valve. ECRLAB improves the right-sided pressures, showing that the component of the right ventricular afterload is "reversible" [25]. ECRLAB appears as well, by increasing both cardiac output and return to the left atrium and ventricle, to improve end organ function avoiding any eventual multiple organ failure syndrome (MOF).

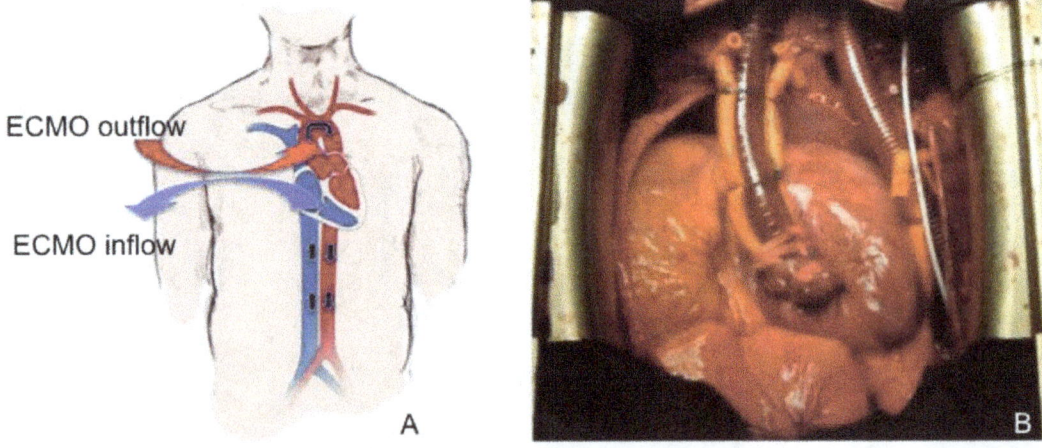

Figure 3. Central ECMO setting (A: setting; B: intra-operative picture).

4.3. Minimally invasive

A challenging option to reduce the ECMO-related risk of complications is the adoption of minimally invasive surgical approaches. There are few reports in the literature. In a recent paper, Weymann et al. describe their technique [28]. After a small right-sided thoracotomy at the eighth intercostal space, flexible arterial and venous cannulas are tunneled. A sewing ring is secured to the right atrium and a tube graft is anastomosed to the ascending aorta. Following full-dose heparinization, the arterial cannula is inserted with the tip into the vascular graft for the ascending aorta and the venous cannula via the ring into the right atrium. After de-airing, the central extracorporeal life support is set at full flow. So far, this surgical approach has not been described in patients who underwent ECMO implantation as treatment of early graft failure, but it might be considered a valid idea for future implantations.

5. Weaning protocol

There are no standardized methods or techniques with regards to weaning ECMO. Usually, the factors indicating cardiac recovery, and so the possibility of weaning from the ECMO, are: increasing blood pressure, falling central venous and/or pulmonary pressures, and improving of cardiac contraction [23]. It is so useful reassess the myocardial function every 24/48 h with TTE, trans-thoracic echocardiography / TEE, trans-esophageal echocardiography in addition to daily hemodynamics. It would be reasonable to reduce pump flows in 0.5 L decrements to 2 L/min over 36–48 h checking the above mentioned variables. The weaning protocols change from center to center according to the personal experience. Lima et al. [29], for example, routinely use the intra-aortic balloon pump for ECMO weaning. At our institution, full ECMO flow is instituted for at least 72 h [25]. Criteria for weaning include an $SvO_2 \geq 70\%$, a hematocrit of 28–30%, the absence of bleeding or tamponade, the absence of left heart distension, improvement in contraction of both ventricles, normal blood lactate levels (<1.5 mmol/L), and a normal urine output (>80 mL/h). A gradual weaning by reducing the ECMO flow by 10% every ~12 h is our main strategy, together with close TEE and Swan-Ganz catheter examinations. Once an ECMO flow of 1.5 L/min/m² is reached, in the presence of two or more consultant surgeons, the pump flow is radically reduced at 0.5 L/min/m² for ~30 min. If the hemodynamics in terms of systemic arterial pressure (mean pressure >60 mmHg), LV contractility (EF >40%), aortic blood flow time-velocity integral >10 cm, central venous pressure (10–12 mmHg), wedge pressure (10–12 mmHg) and SvO_2 (>70%) show no significant changes without the addition of new inotropes, the heparin is stopped, and ECMO support is removed in the operating room within the next 3 h [25].

6. Outcomes

In case of primary graft failure, when all pharmacological options fail, ECMO system represents surely a good option in cardiac surgeon's hands to secure a valid circulatory support. Outcomes in both subtypes, adult and pediatric population, vary among the different centers (**Table 4**). This may be related to several aspects such as the time of implantation and surgical techniques.

Transplantation center	Year	ECMO in PGF/ total cardiac transplants	Surgical approach
Cedars-Sinai Heart Institute [1]	2005–2012	8/555	—Central cannulation: 100% —Peripheral cannulation: 0
Instituto de Cardiologia do Distrito Federal, Brasília [29]	2007–2013	11/71	—Central cannulation: 81.8% —Peripheral cannulation: 18.2%
Heart Center Leipzig [35]	1997–2011	28/298	—Central cannulation: 0 —Peripheral cannulation: 100%
Cardiac surgery and Heart Transplant Unit (ISMETT), Palermo [30]	2006–2013	18/114	—Central cannulation: 77.8% —Peripheral cannulation: 16.7% —Central arterial cannulation and peripheral venous cannulation: 5.5%
Cleveland Clinic [36]	1990–2009	43/1417	—Central cannulation: 0 —Peripheral cannulation: 100%
The Alfred Hospital, Melbourne [37]	2000–2009	39/239	—Central cannulation: 66.6% —Peripheral cannulation: 41%
Groupe hospitalier Pitié-Salpétrière [17]	2000–2006	54/394	—Central cannulation: 48.1% —Peripheral cannulation: 51.9%
S. Orsola-Malpighi Hospital [38]	2002–2007	11/188	—Central cannulation: 54.6% —Peripheral cannulation: 45.4%

Table 4. Outcomes of ECMO support as treatment of EGF.

6.1. Adult

In literature, the successful ECMO weaning rate ranges from 68% to 82% and corresponds to a hospital mortality rate of 50%. In the experience reported by Santise et al. [30], 13 patients (72.2%—13/18) were weaned from the mechanical circulatory support, and eight of them (44%) were discharged home. The causes of death of the patients weaned from ECMO were multi-organ failure, sepsis and acute mycotic rupture of pulmonary artery. Also the group of La Pitié-Salpétrière [17], in an older paper, report good results after ECMO implantation. Among the 54 patients supported with ECMO, 36 were weaned from the assistance and 27 were discharged. In this study, patients treated with ECMO had the same 1-year conditional survival as patients not having suffered EGF: 94% at 3 years.

6.2. Pediatric

Early primary graft failure after Htx in children is associated with significant rates of mortality and morbidity. Extracorporeal membrane oxygenation is widely used and is well established to support circulatory function in children with post-cardiotomy low cardiac output syndrome [31]. The manuscript with the largest series on pediatric heart transplantation is that of Tissot from Denver Children's Hospital, Aurora, Colorado [4]. They retrospectively analyzed the indications and outcome of extracorporeal membrane oxygenation for early primary graft failure and determined its impact on long-term graft function and rejection risk. From 1990 to 2007, 28 (9%) of 310 children who underwent transplantation for cardiomyopathy or congenital heart disease required ECMO support. Fifteen children were successfully weaned off ECMO and discharged alive (54%). This is comparable to what has been previously reported in the pediatric population [21, 32, 33].

Mean duration of ECMO was 2.8 days for survivors (median 3 days) compared with 4.8 days for non-survivors (median 5 days). The duration of cannulation was so important in this series, with no child surviving ECMO support for >4 days. The long-term outcome in those patients supported by ECMO for primary graft failure and surviving to hospital discharge was excellent. There was, in fact, 100% 3-year survival in the ECMO survivor group, with 13 patients (46%) currently alive at a mean follow-up of 8.1 ± 3.8 years.

7. Conclusions and perspectives

PGD is the main cause of early mortality after Htx. Hemodynamic deterioration caused by cardiogenic shock due to pump failure unresponsive to inotropes has a catastrophic progression if not solved in time. Early institution of ECMO allows myocardial graft function recovery despite multifactorial insults and prevents the development of an eventual multisystem organ failure which would otherwise occur in case of a prolonged period of uncorrected cardiogenic shock [34]. In addition to the short-term effects, it has been observed that ECMO implantation, as a bridge to graft recovery after transplantation, can be used without influencing the long-term outcome of this high-risk postoperative cohort of patients. Currently, we take advantage from a wide available range of surgical options for ECMO setting. However, we are still too far from the ideal mechanical support device as routine and well-accepted treatment strategy.

Author details

Antonio Loforte[1*], Giacomo Murana[1], Mariano Cefarelli[1], Jacopo Alfonsi[1],
Giuliano Jafrancesco[1], Francesco Grigioni[2], Lucio Careddu[3], Emanuela Angeli[3],
Gaetano Gargiulo[3] and Giuseppe Marinelli[1]

*Address all correspondence to: antonioloforte@yahoo.it

1 Department of Cardiovascular Surgery and Transplantation, S. Orsola-Malpighi Hospital,
Bologna University, Bologna, Italy

2 Department of Cardiology and Transplantation, S. Orsola-Malpighi Hospital, Bologna
University, Bologna, Italy

3 Department of Pediatric Cardiac Surgery and Transplantation, S. Orsola-Malpighi Hospital, Bologna University, Bologna, Italy

References

[1] Kobashigawa J, Zuckermann A, Macdonald P, et al. Consensus conference participants.
Report from a consensus conference on primary graft dysfunction after cardiac
transplantation. J Heart Lung Transplant 2014;33(4):327–340.

[2] Stehlik J, Edwards LB, Kucheryavaya AY, et al. The registry of the international society
for heart and lung transplantation: 29th official adult heart transplant report — 2012. J
Heart Lung Transplant 2012;31(10):1052–64.

[3] Russo MJ, Iribarne A, Hong KN, et al. Factors associated with primary graft failure after
heart transplantation. Transplantation 2010;90:444–50.

[4] Tissot C, Buckvold S, Phelps CM et al. Outcome of extracorporeal membrane oxygenation for early primary graft failure after pediatric heart transplantation. J Am Coll
Cardiol 2009;54:730–7

[5] Shivalkar B, Van Loon J, Wieland W, et al. Variable effects of explosive or gradual
increase of intracranial pressure on myocardial structure and function. Circulation
1993;87:230–9.

[6] Yen WL, Klionsky DJ. How to live long and prosper: autophagy, mitochondria, and
aging. Physiology (Bethesda) 2008;23:248–62.

[7] D'Amico TA, Meyers CH, Koutlas TC, et al. Desensitization of myocardial beta-adrenergic receptors and deterioration of left ventricular function after brain death. J
Thorac Cardiovasc Surg 1995;110:746–51. 22.

[8] Pratschke J, Wilhelm MJ, Kusaka M, Hancock WW, Tilney NL. Activation of proin-flammatory genes in somatic organs as a consequence of brain death. Transplant Proc 1999;31:1003–5. 23.

[9] Atkinson C, Floerchinger B, Qiao F, et al. Donor brain death exacerbates complement-dependent ischemia/reperfusion injury in transplanted hearts. Circulation 2013;127:1290–9.

[10] Hicks M, Hing A, Gao L, Ryan J, Macdonald PS. Organ preservation. Methods Mol Biol 2006;333:331–74.

[11] Karmazyn M. NHE-1: still a viable therapeutic target. J Mol Cell Cardiol 2013;61:77–82.

[12] Gorlitzer M, Ankersmit J, Fiegl N, et al. Is the transpulmonary pressure gradient a predictor for mortality after orthotopic cardiac transplantation? Transpl Int 2005;18:390–5.

[13] Butler J, Stankewicz MA, Wu J, et al. Pre-transplant reversible pulmonary hypertension predicts higher risk for mortality after cardiac transplantation. J Heart Lung Transplant 2005;24:170–7.

[14] Patarroyo M, Simbaqueba C, Shrestha K, et al. Pre-operative risk factors and clinical outcomes associated with vasoplegia in recipients of orthotopic heart transplantation in the contemporary era. J Heart Lung Transplant 2012;31:282–7.

[15] Wang Y, Liu H, McKenzie G, et al. Kynurenine is an endothelium-derived relaxing factor produced during inflammation. Nat Med 2010;16:279–85.

[16] Segovia J, Cosio MD, Barcelo JM, et al. RADIAL: a novel primary graft failure risk score in heart transplantation. J Heart Lung Transplant 2011;30:644–51.

[17] D'Alessandro C, Aubert S, Golmard JL, et al. Extra-corporeal membrane oxygenation temporary support for early graft failure after cardiac transplantation. Eur J Cardio-thorac Surg 2010;37:343–9.

[18] Thomas HL, Dronavalli VB, Parameshwar J, Bonser RS, Banner NR. Steering Group of the UK Cardiothoracic Transplant Audit. Incidence and outcome of Levitronix CentriMag support as rescue therapy for early cardiac allograft failure: a United Kingdom national study. Eur J Cardiothorac Surg 2011;40:1348–54.

[19] Holman WL, Park SJ, Long JW et al. Infection in permanent circulatory support: experience from the rematch trial. J Heart Lung Transplant 2004;23:1359.

[20] Lazar RM, Shapiro PA, Jaski BE et al. Neurological events during long-term mechanical circulatory support for heart failure: the randomized evaluation of mechanical assis-tance for the treatment of congestive heart failure (rematch) experience. Circulation 2004;109:2423.

[21] Mitchell MB, Campbell DN, Bielefeld MR, Doremus T. Utility of extracorporeal membrane oxygenation for early graft failure following heart transplantation in infancy. J Heart Lung Transplant. 2000;19(9):834–839.

[22] Galantowicz ME, Stolar CJ. Extracorporeal membrane oxygenation for perioperative support in pediatric heart transplantation. J Thorac Cardiovasc Surg 1991;102:148–51, discussion 151–2.

[23] Marasco SF, Lukas G, McDonald M, McMillan J, Ihle B. Review of ECMO (Extra Corporeal Membrane Oxygenation) support in critically ill adult patients. Heart Lung Circ. 2008;17(Suppl. 4):S41–7.

[24] Zangrillo A, Landoni G, Biondi-Zoccai G, Greco M, Greco T, Frati G, Patroniti N, Antonelli M, Pesenti A, Pappalardo F. A meta-analysis of complications and mortality of extracorporeal membrane oxygenation. Crit Care Resusc 2013;15:172–178.

[25] Loforte A, Marinelli G, Musumeci F, et al. Extracorporeal membrane oxygenation support in refractory cardiogenic shock: treatment strategies and analysis of risk factors. Artif Organs 2014, 38(7):E129–E141.

[26] Hoeper MM, Tudorache I, Kühn C, et al. Extracorporeal membrane oxygenation watershed. Circulation 2014;130(10):864–5.

[27] Navia JL, Atik FA, Beyer EA, Ruda VP. Extracorporeal membrane oxygenation with right axillary artery perfusion. Ann Thorac Surg 2005;79:2163–5.

[28] Weymann A, Sabashnikov A, Patil NP, et al. Minimally invasive access for central extracorporeal life support: how we do it. Artif Organs 2015;39(2):179–81.

[29] Lima EB, da Cunha CR, Barzilai VS et al. Experience of ECMO in primary graft dysfunction after orthotopic heart transplantation. Arq Bras Cardiol 2015;105(3):285–91.

[30] Santise G, Panarello G, Ruperto C, et al. Extracorporeal membrane oxygenation for graft failure after heart transplantation: a multidisciplinary approach to maximize weaning rate. Int J Artif Organs 2014;37(9):706–14.

[31] Kanter KR, Pennington G, Weber TR, Zambie MA, Braun P, Martychenko V. Extracorporeal membrane oxygenation for postoperative cardiac support in children. J Thorac Cardiovasc Surg. 1987;93(1):27–35.

[32] Bae JO, Frischer JS, Waich M, Addonizio LJ, Lazar EL, Stolar CJ. Extracorporeal membrane oxygenation in pediatric cardiac transplantation. J Pediatr Surg 2005;40:1051–6, discussion 1056–7.

[33] Fenton KN, Webber SA, Danford DA, Gandhi SK, Periera J, Pigula FA. Long-term survival after pediatric cardiac transplantation and postoperative ECMO support. Ann Thorac Surg 2003;76:843–6, discussion 847.

[34] Kittleson M, Patel J, Moriguchi J, Kawano M, Davis S, Hage A, et al. Heart transplant recipients supported with extracorporeal membrane oxygenation: outcomes from a single-center experience. J Heart Lung Transplant 2011;30(11):1250–6.

[35] Lehmann, Uhlemann M, Etz CD. Extracorporeal membrane oxygenation: experience in acute graft failure after heart transplantation. Clin Transplant. 2014;28(7):789–96.

[36] Mihaljevic T, Jarrett CM, Gonzalez-Stawinski G. Mechanical circulatory support after heart transplantation. Eur J Cardiothorac Surg. 2012;41(1):200–6; discussion 206.

[37] Marasco SF, Vale M, Pellegrino V et al. Extracorporeal membrane oxygenation in primary graft failure after heart transplantation. Ann Thorac Surg 2010;90(5):1541–6.

[38] Arpesella G, Loforte A, Mikus E, Mikus PM. Extracorporeal membrane oxygenation for primary allograft failure. Transplant Proc. 2008;40(10):3596–7.

3

Cardiac Catheterisation and Intervention on ECMO

Christopher Duke, Chris J. Harvey,
Vikram Kudumula, Elved B. Roberts and
Suhair O. Shebani

Abstract

Cardiac catheterisation is an essential tool to evaluate patients who require ECMO support for severe haemodynamic impairment. In the first part of this chapter, we describe the equipment, teamwork, expertise, techniques and precautions that are necessary to carry out safe and effective cardiac catheterisation on ECMO. We have moved on from an early pioneering era to a stage where the multidisciplinary team approach has been worked out in detail, using operational procedures that deal with the technical challenges and minimise the risks of ECMO catheterisation and intervention. In the second part of the chapter, we explain in detail how cardiac catheterisation and intervention on ECMO contribute to the management of (1) post-operative congenital heart disease patients, (2) cardiac patients who suffer sudden haemodynamic deterioration, (3) patients with low cardiac output who require left heart decompression because of extracorporeal support, (4) patients with haemodynamically unstable arrhythmias and (5) haemodynamically unstable patients who require percutaneous coronary intervention. We also provide state-of-the-art information on the elective use of ECMO to support congenital and structural catheter interventions. Acute survival and long-term outcome are now related to the underlying conditions rather than complications of the catheterisation procedure itself.

Keywords: ECMO, cardiac catheterisation, catheter intervention, congenital heart disease, myocarditis, cardiomyopathy, balloon septostomy, atrial septal stent, arrhythmia, radiofrequency ablation, percutaneous coronary intervention, structural intervention

1. Introduction

Since cardiac catheterisation and transcatheter intervention in patients on ECMO was pioneered in the late 1980s, interventional cardiologists and ECMO teams have learned to work together to provide rapid accurate diagnosis and safe interventional solutions for patients with the most challenging anatomical problems and the most fragile physiologies. In the current era, experienced teams provide excellent results. The aim of this chapter was to describe state-of-the-art practice in this area.

Catheterisation is most commonly required in the setting of extracorporeal support in the following scenarios:

a. Following surgery for congenital heart disease

b. When acute haemodynamic collapse occurs in a cardiac patient unrelated to surgery

c. To decompress the left heart in patients with poor left ventricular function

d. Patients with haemodynamically unstable refractory arrhythmias

e. Percutaneous coronary intervention in patients with severe haemodynamic instability

f. Elective ECMO support for high-risk congenital and structural transcatheter interventional procedures

The first part of this chapter will address the practical issues related to carrying out cardiac catheterisation in patients on ECMO. The second part of the chapter will focus on up-to-date knowledge and practice in each of the clinical scenarios listed above.

2. Practical tips for ECMO catheterisation

2.1. Staffing

To maximise the safety of ECMO support, the entire team should be familiar with all local ECMO protocols and experienced in moving patients on ECMO. When out of the intensive care unit, the patient is accompanied by the bedside ECMO specialist, ECMO coordinator and a perfusionist. Surgical expertise is available in the event of a cannulation issue, and an anaesthetist or intensive care specialist always accompanies the patient. The circuit is maintained as if it were in the intensive care unit with the same routine circuit checks and monitoring of anticoagulation. The ECMO specialist needs to ensure that there is an adequate supply of syringes and ACT cartridges close by and that the ECMO emergency box containing spare connectors and pigtails accompanies the patient at all times. Each member of the team is tasked with surveillance of a different part of the circuit or patient during the transport.

2.2. Transport between intensive care and the catheter laboratory

The ECMO system should be mounted on a mobile cart. As most modern ECMO systems are capable of operating on battery power for extended periods, the patient and circuit can be transferred in a slow and steady manner to the catheter suite. The patient must be fully monitored and sufficient gas supply must be carried to provide oxygen both to the ECMO circuit, as sweep gas, and to the ventilator. All drug infusions should be continued. The ECMO circuit often represents the safest and most reliable access point as pre-existing central lines may need to be rewired and upsized to permit the procedure. It is, however, recommended that at least one well-functioning peripheral cannula is available in case there is a circuit-related complication. As with most critical care transfers, the ECMO patient should be appropriately sedated or anaesthetised prior to leaving the unit. All studies that have assessed the process of patient transport have described excellent outcomes with no cannula displacement, morbidity or mortality [1–3].

2.3. Cannulation

The exact method of ECMO cannulation is largely dictated by patient factors, mainly the weight and age of the patient, but consideration needs to be given to any anatomical variation or loss of vessels either secondary to prolonged ITU stay, surgery or previous catheter interventions. In children below 10 kg in weight, the carotid artery and the jugular vein are the vessels of choice. For most patients, a right-sided cut-down centred on the medial border of the sternocleidomastoid muscle approximately 1.5–2 cm above the clavicle provides excellent access to both of these vessels. Cannulas between 8 and 14 Fr may be inserted depending on the size of the patient and vessels and the amount of support required. In children over 10 kg, cannulation of a femoral vein and artery are preferred. This approach avoids damage to the carotid artery and alterations to flow of blood to the brain. It must be remembered that the femoral artery is an end vessel and the distal perfusion of the leg needs careful consideration in order to prevent limb ischaemia. An additional small cannula either placed antegradely into the superficial femoral artery or retrogradely into the posterior tibial artery can be used satisfactorily to prevent critical limb ischaemia. Once inserted, the cannulas should be firmly secured with at least two sutures.

Occasionally, a patient who is cannulated centrally through an open chest may need treatment in the catheter laboratory. This is almost exclusively in the post-operative patient and although possible carries a significantly higher risk than the patient cannulated peripherally. Centrally placed cannulas are usually shorter and therefore much more prone to being dislodged on patient movement or during the procedure. For such patients, a surgeon capable of reinserting the cannula is essential and additional caution must be exercised by the entire team.

2.4. In the catheter laboratory

A briefing is essential so that the cardiologist understands the ECMO set-up but also so that the ECMO team may fully appreciate what the diagnostic or interventional procedure involves. It is relatively straight forward to position the ECMO circuit to the side of the patient if the catheter procedure can be achieved utilising simple antero-posterior imaging. However, for more complex procedures, requiring imaging through a wide range of planes, we have found it preferential to position both the ECMO pump and the oxygenator on the catheter table, away from the traditional ECMO cart (**Figure 1**). By securing the circuit on the table, the cardiologist can move the patient and position the C-arm without fear of inadvertent decannulation or damage to the circuit components. It is essential to ensure that the circuit is connected to a main's power supply and that the ECMO heater unit is running to prevent unwanted cooling of the patient throughout the procedure. When possible, oxygen should be connected to the wall supply.

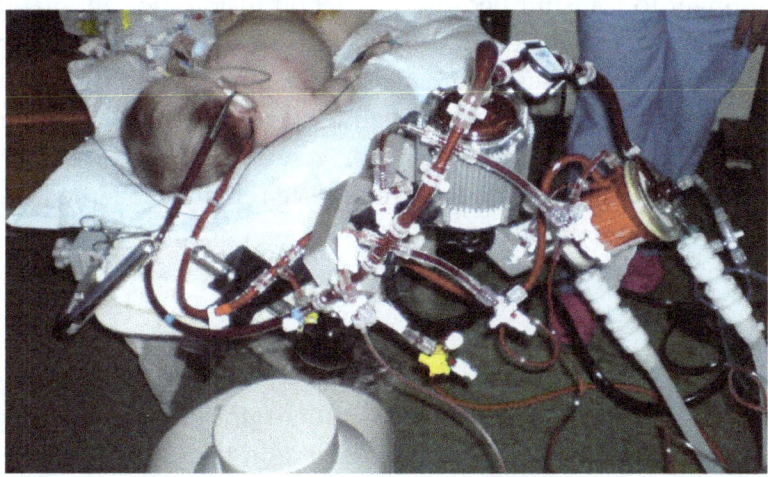

Figure 1. The ECMO circuit secured to the catheter table.

2.5. Vascular access

As the patient is heparinised, it is preferable to avoid new punctures. Existing central venous lines or arterial pressure monitoring lines are therefore exchanged over a wire for a sheath whenever possible. However, new punctures are required in the majority of procedures and complications are surprisingly rare [2, 4, 5]. Only one study described complications, in 13% patients, including venous thrombosis, lower extremity oedema without thrombosis, transient loss of peripheral pulses and lower extremity compartment syndrome requiring fasciotomy [3]. Patients often have a history of previous operations, interventions and prolonged intensive care. It is therefore important to check in advance whether any vessels are known to be occluded and to confirm vessel patency with vascular ultrasound before attempting new access. It is preferable to use vascular ultrasound during puncture attempts to minimise complications [2].

Draping the patient and maintaining sterility can be challenging, as old lines are being exchanged for sterile sheaths, requiring extra care to lift the line that is being removed away from the patient without contaminating the sterile field. Changing gloves after removing the old line and a second pair of hands to assist the exchange are advisable.

To avoid the morbidity of additional vascular access, angiography can be carried out by injecting contrast directly via the ECMO cannula, using a three-way adaptor in the connector [2]. This manoeuvre requires a coordinated sequence of transient flow cessation, contrast injection, saline flush, image acquisition and recommencement of flow [2]. With this technique, it is possible to get good images of the aortic root and coronary arteries, particularly if the aorta distal to the cannula is transiently occluded in patients with an open chest [2]. It is also possible to cut a Y-connector into the arterial limb of the ECMO circuit, through which catheters can be inserted [6–9]. The blind end of the Y-connector is closed with a haemostatic valve (Check-Flo Performer accessory adapter, Cook Medical, USA). Although this allows direct access to the heart, without the need for further punctures, catheters are more difficult to manipulate and torque takes longer to transmit because of friction inside the cannula and Y-connector. This loss of feel may hamper the procedure. For this reason, we reserve this approach for simple diagnostic procedures and for cases where vessels are absent or thrombosed or attempts to gain alternative access have failed. When the catheter is completed, the Y-connector must be removed. One study describes similarly placing a Y-connector in the venous limb of the ECMO circuit to obviate the need for venous puncture [2]. We remain concerned that this approach has the potential to rapidly entrain air into the venous circulation because of the negative pressure generated by the centrifugal pump.

2.6. Angiography

The ECMO circuit will normally be positioned to the right of the patient's head with neck cannulation. This usually makes it impossible to bring in the lateral camera C-arm, so most ECMO catheters are carried out with single plane fluoroscopy and angiography. Before starting the case, the image intensifier should be moved through a full range of right and left

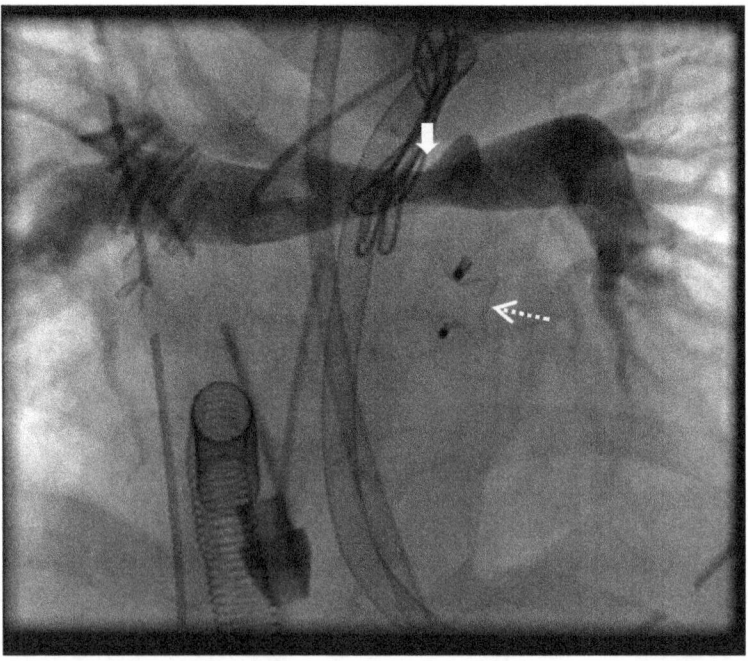

Figure 2. Clutter in the X-ray field. Legend—The image includes ECMO cannulas, chest drains, surgical clips, swabs, a nasogastric tube, a cardiac catheter and a vascular occlusion device (dashed arrow). There is a significant stenosis at the pulmonary artery bifurcation (solid arrow) following cardiac surgery (superior cavopulmonary shunt).

anterior oblique angles, to check whether any equipment is impeding the movement of the C-arm. The ECMO circuit and ancillary equipment should be positioned to maximise the range of camera angles. Test screening is carried out to check that equipment does not encroach on the field of view in the camera angles that are likely to be used during the case. ECG leads and electrodes that are not radiolucent may need to be removed, saturation probes repositioned, chest drain tubing moved and bundles of epicardial pacing wires taped over the abdomen rather than the chest. If it is anticipated that angles approaching the lateral plane may be required, the arms should be lifted up and supported either side of the head, taking care not to displace the ECMO cannulas. Sometimes items of equipment that cannot be moved, for example ECMO cannulas, chest drains, pacing leads, swabs with radio-opaque markers, chest spreaders and clamps, clutter the X-ray field and overlie the area of interest (**Figure 2**). Unusual camera angles may therefore be needed to properly visualise the area without hardware encroaching on the image. For angiography, 1 ml/kg contrast, or even lower volumes for low flow states, gives good image quality [2].

2.7. Catheter technique

Catheter manipulation is not usually any more difficult because of the extracorporeal support, though appreciation of catheter position is sometimes limited by single plane fluoroscopy. ECMO flow may need to be diminished or temporarily discontinued to document cardiac haemodynamics. ECMO can actually facilitate intervention, as it offers a stable haemodynamic platform to carry out interventions that might otherwise cause significant haemodynamic derangement. Furthermore, if the chest is open and a surgeon is close at hand, it is justifiable to accept a greater risk of vessel rupture during balloon angioplasty or stenting as the area is rapidly accessible for surgical repair. Complications during catheterisation are rare. One study reported myocardial perforation in 2 patients (3%), dealt with by inserting a pericardial drain without the need for surgery [5]. Another study reported retroperitoneal haematoma secondary to arterial trauma when removing an embolised coil [4]. Even in the earliest study, transseptal puncture was carried out in a fully anticoagulated state without complication [10]. The safety of transseptal puncture can now be enhanced by intraprocedural transoesophageal echocardiography, even in small children, using a micro-TOE probe.

2.8. Return to the intensive care unit

On completing the catheter, the circuit is resecured to the ECMO trolley if needed and the patient is returned to the intensive care unit. If additional vascular access was utilised for the procedure, this should be left in place until the patient returns to ICU. In this way, the clotting status of the patient can assessed prior to line removal. Although some have recommended that sheaths should be left in place until the patient is weaned from ECMO, most sheaths can be safely removed and bleeding controlled by manual compression [2, 4]. The ongoing need for anticoagulation and inherent platelet dysfunction mean that pressure needs to be applied for longer than would be expected for non-ECMO patients. Alternatively, venous sheaths can be exchanged for a central line of equal outer diameter, venous puncture sites can be closed with a Z-suture or the vessels can be repaired surgically.

3. Clinical scenarios where catheterisation on ECMO is required

3.1. ECMO catheterisation following surgery for congenital heart disease

3.1.1. Why is ECMO required following surgery?

ECMO support may be required following surgery for congenital heart disease in the following circumstances: (a) failure to separate from cardiopulmonary bypass; (b) ventricular dysfunction with low cardiac output in the immediate post-operative period; (c) unexpected cardiac arrest requiring extracorporeal CPR; (d) lung disease; (e) pulmonary hypertension; and (f) refractory arrhythmias [11]. In such cases, it is important to quickly assess the integrity of the surgical repair and establish whether there are any residual anatomical problems that require correction, as studies have shown between 6% and 28% of post-operative patients requiring ECMO have residual lesions [11–14].

3.1.2. Why is cardiac catheterisation required following surgery?

In the majority of cases, echocardiography does not provide complete information because ventilation, dressings, pacing wires, chest drains, air in the anterior mediastinum and an open chest restrict the available echocardiographic windows. In one study, where ECMO was established using central cannulation with the chest open, only 17% of residual lesions were identified by echocardiography [11]. Other studies confirm that echocardiography has clear limitations in this context, with residual problems detected in at best 41% and at worst 19% of patients [1, 5]. Echocardiography is particularly poor at identifying problems with branch pulmonary arteries and systemic to pulmonary artery shunts. In contrast, in one of the largest studies on post-operative ECMO, cardiac catheterisation identified 78% of residual lesions. About 91% of cardiac catheterisation procedures yielded unexpected diagnostic information of clinical importance [11]. Both surgeon and cardiologist therefore need to remain open to the fact that something may have been missed. In 70–83% of cases, management is altered by the results of cardiac catheterisation [1, 2, 4, 5, 11]. The findings may result in redo surgery, cardiac intervention or elective withdrawal of ECMO in patients with severe neurological impairment or lack of myocardial recovery. Cardiac catheterisation is therefore mandated whenever there is any doubt about the cause of the patient's poor haemodynamic status.

3.1.3. Survival after catheterisation on ECMO

Table 1 shows how outcomes for patients who require cardiac catheterisation on ECMO have improved over time. The studies listed describe a mixed group of paediatric cardiac ECMO patients, not just patients who required ECMO in the post-operative period. Nevertheless, the trend towards improved survival is impressive.

Outcome	1990–1995 Desjardins et al. (1999) [4]	1984–2001 Booth et al. (2002) [5]	2009–2012 Panda et al. (2014) [2]	2004–2013 Callahan et al. (2015) [3]
Weaned from ECMO	53%	72%	82%	86%
Discharged from hospital	29%	48%	68%	72%
Survival on follow-up	14%	43%	64%	69%

Table 1. Outcomes in patients who have cardiac catheterisation on ECMO.

In a study that included only children on ECMO following paediatric cardiac surgery, children with residual lesions had 87% survival to decannulation when lesions were detected within 3 days of the operation, compared with 36% survival when the lesions were detected later. Most lesions were detected by cardiac catheterisation. Survival to discharge was 58% and 18%, respectively, in the two groups [11]. These findings reinforce the 2011 recommendations of the American Heart Association that cardiac catheterisation with potential for intervention is indicated early in the post-operative period in any patient who requires mechanical cardio-pulmonary support without a clear cause [15].

3.1.4. The timing of cardiac catheterisation

Although there is a natural tendency to attribute the need for extracorporeal support to myocardial stun following cardiopulmonary bypass and cross-clamping, if patients fail to wean from ECMO within 3 days, cardiac catheterisation is strongly advised. Catheterisation should be carried out earlier if haemodynamic measurements made on PICU or echocardiog-raphy suggest a residual problem. In cases where the surgeon suspects a residual problem or coronary artery issues could result in permanent myocardial damage, it is preferable to proceed straight from theatre to the cardiac catheterisation laboratory. In our centre, it is routine to carry out a detailed assessment of every surgical repair in theatre either by TOE or by epicardial echocardiography. Intracardiac problems are therefore usually identified early and repaired immediately. In view of this, when a patient fails to wean from ECMO on PICU, it is likely that any residual lesion will be beyond the reach of echocardiographic imaging. Branch pulmonary artery problems, aortic problems and distortion, stenosis and thrombosis of cavopulmonary and aortopulmonary shunts remain a blind spot for the echocardiographer.

3.1.5. Types of catheter procedures required in the post-operative period

Indications for catheterisation include the evaluation of coronary arteries (**Figure 3**), pulmo-nary arteries (**Figure 4**), pulmonary venous obstruction, aortic obstruction, shunts and aortopulmonary collaterals. The surgeon who carried out the operation is usually present in the catheter laboratory at the time of the study. If a residual lesion is identified, our practice is to convene a short meeting in the catheter laboratory control room with surgeons, cardiologists and intensivists represented. An immediate decision is made whether the patient should return to the operating theatre or should proceed to have catheter intervention. About 20–50% of residual lesions can be dealt with in the catheter laboratory [2, 11, 16]. Interventions include duct stenting (**Figure 5**), shunt angioplasty or stenting, branch pulmonary artery angioplasty or stenting, coronary stenting, stent fenestration of Fontan circulation, balloon atrial septostomy, ASD device closure, VSD device closure, coil occlusion of collaterals and catheter-directed thrombolysis [3, 5, 11, 17]. Complications are rare [2–5, 11, 16]. As the circulation is fully supported, hybrid procedures are possible, particularly when the chest is open. For example, branch pulmonary artery stenting can be carried out with a sheath introduced through the anterior wall of the main pulmonary artery or right ventricular outflow tract. A greater risk of vessel rupture during angioplasty or stenting can be accepted when the chest is open, the patient is draped for a surgical procedure and the whole theatre team are scrubbed and on standby in the catheter laboratory, as the surgeon can quickly control bleeding and repair even major damage to blood vessels (**Figure 4**).

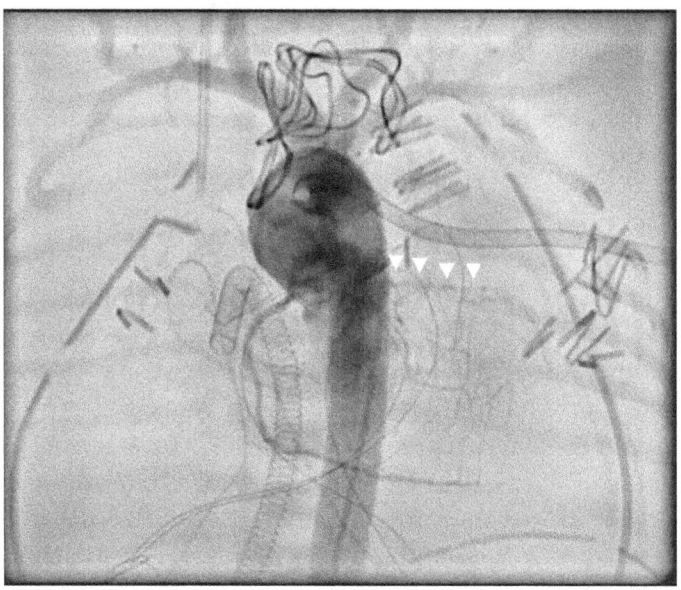

Figure 3. Partial occlusion of the left coronary artery post-repair of common arterial trunk. Legend—The arrowheads show weak opacification of the left coronary artery.

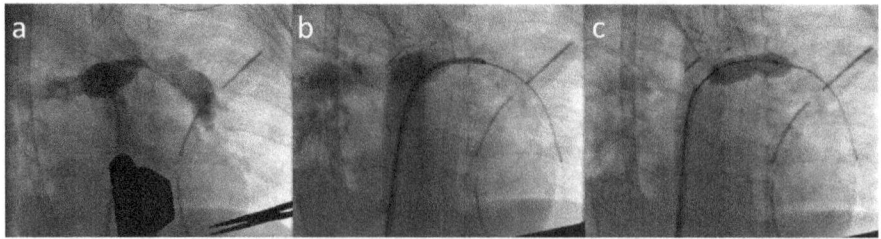

Figure 4. (a) Torsion of the left pulmonary artery following unifocalisation surgery for pulmonary atresia with VSD and MAPCAS (major aortopulmonary collateral arteries); (b) A premounted stent is positioned across the site of stenosis; (c) The stent is deployed but has a residual waist. As the balloon is inflated to higher pressure, the pulmonary artery ruptures at the stenotic anastomotic site and has to be repaired immediately by the surgeon who is on standby.

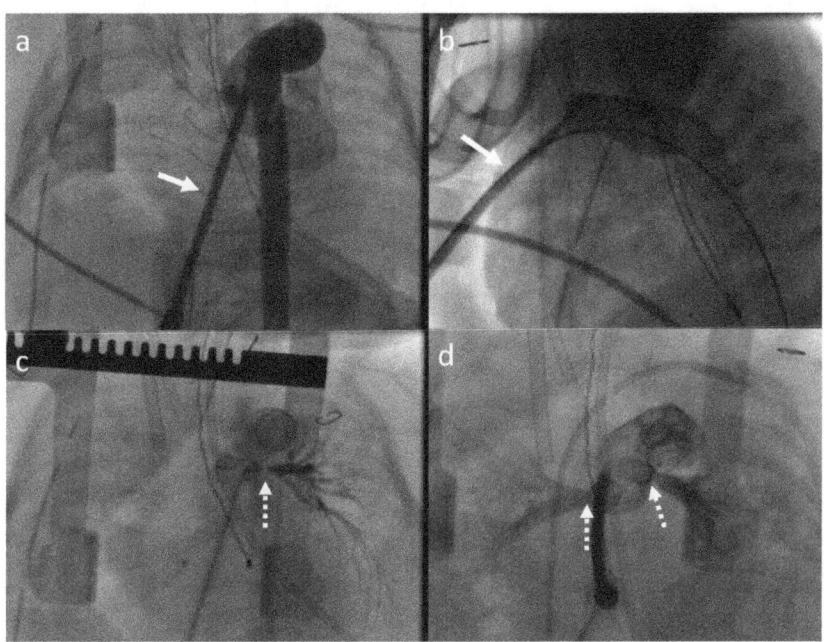

Figure 5. Stenting the arterial duct and altering pulmonary artery bands in a hybrid Norwood procedure. (a) Angiography is carried out via a sheath introduced through the anterior wall of the pulmonary artery (solid arrow). The pulmonary arteries are not opacified as the bands are too tight; (b) Lateral view showing flow into the aorta after stenting the arterial duct; (c) Very tight left pulmonary artery band (dashed arrow); (d) Good flow into the pulmonary arteries with mild proximal narrowing (dashed arrows) after loosening the pulmonary artery bands.

3.2. The cardiac patient with acute haemodynamic collapse unrelated to surgery

3.2.1. When is diagnostic catheterisation indicated?

Neonates who present moribund with shock or profound cyanosis may require urgent extracorporeal support before a full cardiac evaluation can be carried out. When congenital heart disease is present, a full diagnosis is usually then secured with transthoracic echocardiography alone. However, it may be difficult to diagnose obstructed total anomalous pulmonary venous drainage, as its clinical presentation mimics lung disease and pulmonary venous drainage can be hard to define once VA ECMO has been commenced, even when ECMO flows are reduced to encourage flow through the pulmonary circulation. In view of this, ECMO patients have sometimes required cardiac catheterisation to establish or exclude TAPVD [18, 19]. However, in the current era, every effort is made to establish pulmonary venous drainage echocardiographically before sick neonates are placed on ECMO. When this is not possible, contrast CT may offers a less invasive alternative.

3.2.2. Catheter intervention in children on ECMO

When ECMO is initiated to treat shock or cyanosis in cardiac patients, cardiac catheterisation is normally only necessary when intervention is planned. A wide array of interventions have been described following emergency ECMO in paediatric patients, including balloon angio-plasty of critical aortic stenosis [1, 20], balloon angioplasty of a restrictive cor triatriatum membrane [21], balloon atrial septostomy in the context of hypoplastic left heart syndrome with a restrictive atrial septum [4] and radiofrequency ablation of incessant tachycardia [22, 23].

3.2.3. ECMO salvage as an alternative to balloon atrial septostomy for moribund patients with transposition of the great arteries

Patients with transposition of the great arteries deserve special mention. When such patients present profoundly hypoxic and acidotic, the team is under great pressure to perform balloon atrial septostomy quickly. However, it may sometimes be difficult and time-consuming to gain vascular access. In such circumstances, it is occasionally easier and quicker to cannulate the neck vessels for ECMO. Once the patient is on ECMO, balloon atrial septostomy can be undertaken or the patient can proceed to theatre for an arterial switch procedure after a period of stabilisation [24].

3.2.4. Catheter intervention in adults on ECMO

Adult patients may also require emergency ECMO support followed by catheter intervention. Patients with massive pulmonary embolism may need to be resuscitated using extracorporeal support, following which catheter-directed thrombolytic therapy, catheter embolus fragmen-tation or percutaneous thrombectomy can be carried under stable conditions [25–27]. As structural intervention gains momentum, patients who need ECMO support because of shock or cardiac failure caused by severe valvar stenosis or regurgitation may increasingly be treated using transcatheter therapy on extracorporeal support. TAVI has already been carried out following emergency ECMO [28] and one patient with severe mitral regurgitation requiring ECMO has been successfully treated with a MitraClip [29]. However, results are likely to better if ECMO is used to electively support interventional procedures in high-risk patients, before acute haemodynamic decompensation occurs [28].

3.3. Left heart decompression in patients with poor ventricular function

3.3.1. Why is left heart decompression necessary?

When VA ECMO is commenced to support patients with severe myocardial dysfunction, the heart may stop ejecting completely because of the increased afterload caused by the extracor-poreal circulation. In these circumstances, left ventricular end-diastolic pressure rises sharply because of acute left heart distension, and the increased wall stress, reduced myocardial perfusion and subendocardial ischaemia that occur as a consequence compromise recovery of ventricular function. Left atrial pressure increases, causing pulmonary venous hypertension, pulmonary oedema and in severe cases pulmonary haemorrhage. Left heart decompression is necessary to decrease pulmonary oedema, avoid pulmonary haemorrhage and allow myo-cardial recovery [30–32].

3.3.2. Making the decision to decompress the left heart

Approximately 10–20% patients who require ECMO for poor left ventricular function will require left heart decompression [31–33]. The decision to decompress the left atrium is usually made within 24 h of commencing ECMO, on the basis of left heart dilation on echocardiography and pulmonary oedema on chest X-ray [32]. Direct surgical left atrial cannulation is possible in post-operative patients [31, 32]. However, a non-surgical approach is preferable in patients with myocarditis and post-operative patients where there is a plan to switch to neck cannulation in order to close the chest.

3.3.3. Percutaneous decompression using drains incorporated into the ECMO circuit

Percutaneous decompression may be achieved by introducing a transseptal left atrial drain from a femoral venous approach [32, 34–37] or passing a pigtail catheter into the left ventricle from a femoral artery approach [38, 39]. The return from these drains is incorporated into the venous limb of the ECMO circuit. However, there are concerns about systemic thromboembolism when hardware remains in the left heart for a prolonged period of time. Also, transseptal drains have become less popular in recent years because of problems with kinking, poor flow and drain movement with patient care [32].

3.3.4. Percutaneous left atrial decompression by opening the atrial septum

In the majority of patients, left atrial decompression is achieved by balloon atrial septostomy [30, 32, 40]. If prolonged extracorporeal support is anticipated or balloon septostomy fails to achieve an adequate interatrial communication, atrial septal stenting is carried out [32, 41]. Transseptal puncture is required as a first step in approximately 90% of patients, as only about 10% have a pre-existing interatrial communication [30, 32]. Most transseptal punctures are carried out using a Brockenbrough needle. Accidental left atrial perforation is a particular concern as the patient is fully anticoagulated. However, the largest series reported only one left atrial perforation, which closed without requiring pericardial drainage [32]. Needle position may be guided by transthoracic or transoesophageal echocardiography to minimise complications [40, 42]. Radiofrequency transseptal perforation is an alternative and may be preferable when the septum is very thick, but there is some concern that an accidental burn hole in the atrial wall may be less likely to close spontaneously. In young infants, it is possible to perform a Rashkind balloon atrial septostomy, rapidly jerking a septostomy balloon from the left to the right atrium in order to tear a hole in the atrial septum. Older patients require a static balloon septostomy, as the septum is too thick for the Rashkind technique to be effective.

3.3.5. Static balloon septostomy

To perform a static balloon septostomy, a long sheath is advanced over the transseptal needle into the left atrium. A catheter is then advanced through the transseptal sheath and directed into the left upper pulmonary vein. A wire is passed through the catheter into the pulmonary vein and the catheter and sheath are withdrawn. A balloon is advanced over the wire until it is centred across the atrial septum. Balloons are usually in the 12–18 mm range, but smaller and larger diameters may be required, depending on patient size [32, 33]. The balloon is then inflated to tear a hole in the septum (**Figure 6**). Historically, blade atrial septostomy was carried out after transseptal puncture to ensure that a large hole could be created, but blade septostomy has now almost disappeared from practice. If the hole is not big enough to reduce left atrial pressure to less than about 20 mmHg, a larger balloon can be used, a second hole can be created by a separate transseptal puncture, a cutting balloon (Boston Scientific, Natick, USA) can be used to create blade cuts in the margins of the defect to allow more effective balloon dilation, or atrial septal stenting can be carried out.

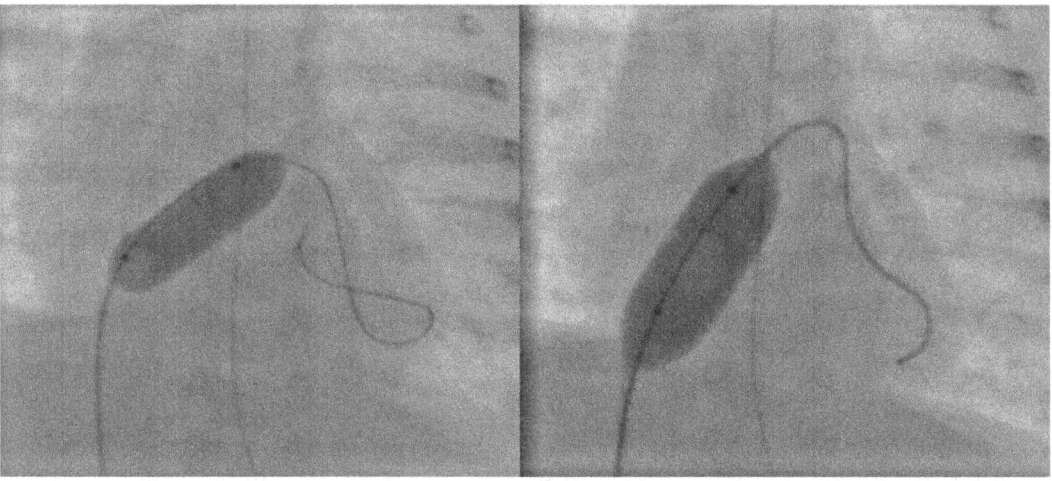

Figure 6. Static balloon dilation of the atrial septum with progressively larger balloons.

3.3.6. Stenting the atrial septum

Stenting can be carried out using the 'dog-bone' technique described by Stumper et al. (**Figure 7**) [43] or simply by implanting a straight stent across the septum (**Figure 8**) [42]. Echocardiography is used to measure the distance from the inferior vena cava to the atrial septum and from the septum to the pulmonary veins to guide what length of stent should be chosen. The stent should not project more than about halfway across the atrial cavity, to avoid the risk of puncturing the atrial wall, particularly when the heart size reduces as the patient recovers. Transoesophageal echocardiography can be used to check that the stent is accurately centred on the septum before the balloon is inflated. A hole with a diameter of about 4–5 mm is usually adequate [33]. To achieve this, when a straight stent is implanted, it is usually mounted on an 8- to 10-mm-diameter balloon, which is inflated at low pressure to leave a waist at the septum. In the current era, premounted stents are often used [42]. When the dog-bone technique is used, a 15-mm balloon should be used with a 4- to 5-mm constraining loop that prevents the centre of the balloon expanding. If a larger communication is required, the stent can be post-dilated. If the communication is too large, the centre of the stent can be constricted with a gooseneck snare [43].

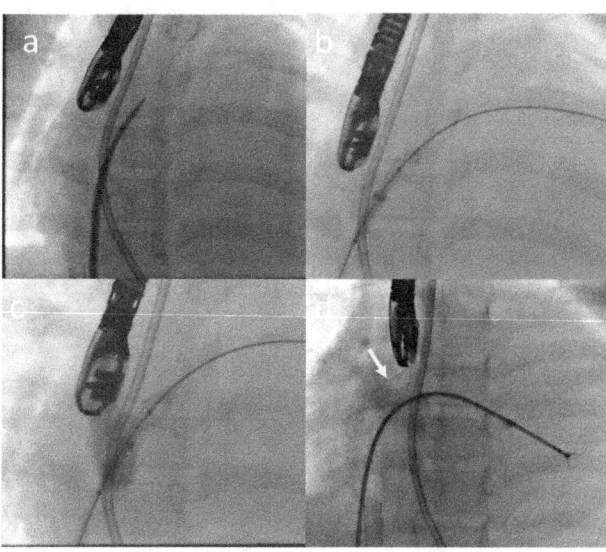

Figure 7. 'Dog-bone' stenting the atrial septum. (a) Brockenbrough needle transseptal puncture; (b) A wire is introduced into the left pulmonary vein, and a stent mounted on a balloon is advanced through a long sheath. The stent balloon assembly is half-unsheathed so that the distal half of the stent can be inflated and pulled back against the atrial septum; (c) As the sheath is pulled back to the right atrium to expose the whole stent, contrast injected through the side arm of the sheath defines the plane of the atrial septum and shows the stent is well centred; (d) The stent has been deployed across the atrial septum (arrow). There is a central waist which stabilises the stent on the septum. The waist was produced by tying a loop of prolene around the middle of the balloon before the stent was mounted. Myocardial biopsy is also shown.

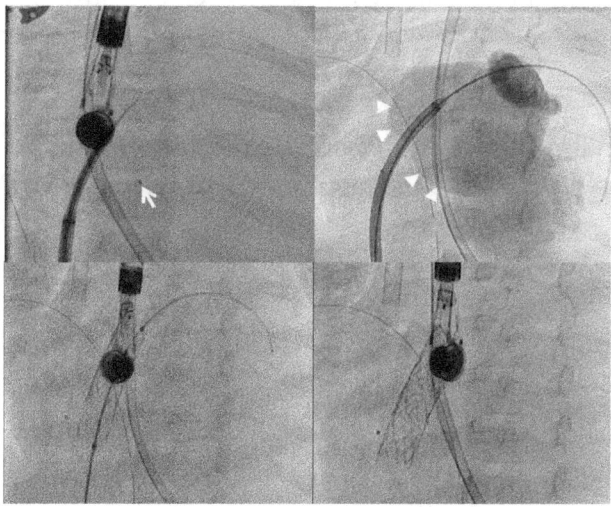

Figure 8. Implanting a straight stent across the atrial septum. (a) Brockenbrough needle transseptal puncture. The arrow highlights the small radio-opaque marker at the tip of the ECMO cannula. Most of the distal cannula is radiolucent; (b) The tip of the transseptal sheath is in the left atrium. Contrast injected into the left atrium defines the plane of the atrial septum (arrow heads); (c) A balloon mounted stent was deployed, but was not well centred on the septum. A second stent was therefore implanted overlapping the first stent to prevent embolisation; (d) The balloon and wire have been removed, leaving the 2 overlapping stents in a stable position.

3.3.7. Does the atrial communication need to be closed after the patient recovers?

Patients who survive ECMO after left atrial decompression should have routine follow-up echocardiography to check whether the atrial septal defect has closed. One study found that 80% of such patients had a residual defect and 44% required either transcatheter or surgical closure [33]. However, this may be an overestimate, as less than 20% of patients in another series had residual defects, and only one of those patients needed device closure [32].

3.4. Patients with haemodynamically unstable refractory arrhythmias

3.4.1. Why is ECMO required in arrhythmia patients?

Patients with haemodynamically unstable arrhythmias fall into two main categories:

(1) Adults with ventricular arrhythmias; (2) infants with tachycardia mediated cardiomyopathy secondary to incessant supraventricular tachycardia [44]. Such patients may require ECMO because (a) there is an abrupt haemodynamic deterioration; (b) there is no therapeutic window for drug treatment, because antiarrhythmic drugs have caused an unacceptable deterioration in the patient's haemodynamics; (c) catheter ablation is indicated but cannot proceed without extracorporeal support, either because the patient cannot maintain cardiac output in tachycardia or because the patient's haemodynamics are so precarious that there is a significant risk of cardiac arrest during the procedure.

3.4.2. ECMO support of VT ablation in adult patients

It is debatable whether adult patients with haemodynamically unstable VT benefit from ablation with ECMO support. ECMO certainly provides a stable platform to carry out activation mapping of VT where the arrhythmia is not haemodynamically tolerated [45]. However, VT ablation can now be carried out by substrate mapping, which does not require the patient to remain in the unstable tachycardia. The authors of a leading article in 2009 that advocated VT ablation with ECMO support have now retreated from that position [45]. They point out that greater experience with substrate mapping and the widespread availability of three-dimensional mapping systems have allowed the vast majority of haemodynamically unstable VTs to be successfully treated during sinus rhythm with very reasonable long-term success rates and very low morbidity. Their use of ECMO support for VT ablation therefore fell from 9% (2003–2007) to 0.5% (2007–2012) [46]. There will inevitably be cases where patients with VT require extracorporeal CPR or urgent ECMO for critically compromised haemodynamics. In such patients, who are small in number, it is sensible to proceed to ablate the VT whilst on mechanical support [47]. However, the era of elective ECMO support to allow activation mapping seems to have passed.

3.4.3. When is radiofrequency ablation on ECMO necessary in infancy?

In infants with tachycardia-related cardiomyopathy, ECMO is commenced when drug refractory incessant tachycardia causes progressive deterioration in haemodynamics or when antiarrhythmic drugs cause cardiovascular collapse requiring extracorporeal CPR [23, 48].

Once the patient is receiving extracorporeal support, approximately 2/3 should be treatable with antiarrhythmic drug therapy alone. However, catheter ablation may be required in about 1/3 patients [44]. Ablation may be necessary because the tachyarrhythmia is truly drug resistant. However, ablation is also reasonable when the tachycardia is very difficult to control on ECMO, requiring high-dose or multiple antiarrhythmic medications, as invasive treatment can shorten the duration of ECMO support and minimise the risk of tachycardia recurrence [23, 48]. It is important to avoid tachycardia recurrence following decannulation as it is may be very difficult to recannulate the neck vessels if the child becomes unstable again.

3.4.4. Elective use of ECMO to support paediatric ablation procedures

ECMO can be used to electively support paediatric ablation procedures when patients cannot maintain an adequate cardiac output in tachycardia, either because of congenital heart disease or poor ventricular function, and mapping in tachycardia is an essential part of the procedure [49]. In such procedures, the length of time the patient will need to spend in tachycardia, the degree of haemodynamic impairment this will cause, the size of the patient, the technical difficulty of the ablation and the possibility of extracorporeal CPR being required all factor into the decision to use ECMO pre-emptively.

3.4.5. Technical aspects

Very few publications focus on catheter ablation of arrhythmias in children on ECMO. Although some of the larger series dealing with paediatric cardiac catheterisation on ECMO include a few patients who had ablation, only basic information is provided [2, 5]. The sum total of published information consists of 13 patients described in a multicentre review [44] and 16 patients described in various case reports and case series [2, 5, 22, 23, 48–54], with possible overlap between these sources.

Atrial septostomy may be needed at the same time as ablation when left heart distension has developed on ECMO, as ventricular function and cardiac output may take several days to improve after the tachycardia is successfully ablated [22, 23, 44, 51]. Left atrial decompression may speed up resolution of pulmonary oedema, improve function and shorten the time to decannulation.

Most infant ablation procedures on ECMO are carried out with 2 vascular access points. A single diagnostic catheter and a 5 Fr 4-mm tip ablation catheter are usually used [44]. An oesophageal bipolar electrode can be added for atrial sensing and stimulation [48]. The largest study described an average of two ablation substrates per patient. Right-sided accessory pathways and left-sided ventricular tachycardia were the most common ablation targets. About 69% were successfully treated with radiofrequency ablation alone. In 29% cases, there were problems with convective cooling of the catheter tip, resulting in inadequate lesion formation. Energy delivery and thermodynamics were not improved by reducing ECMO flow to increase blood flow through the heart. After converting to cryoablation, the tachycardias were successfully ablated. Although this series described a procedural success rate of 100%, the complication rate was 15%, with one patient suffering transient heart block and one mitral valve damage that ultimately required valve replacement [44]. The desire to produce effective lesions to avoid tachycardia recurrence must be tempered by caution. Lesion depth should be kept at a minimum to reduce the risk of perforation and damage to adjacent cardiac structures, such as valves or coronary arteries, which are particularly close to the endocardium of the atrioventricular junction in infants. There are no robust data to suggest how much energy should be delivered to achieve this balance. Although successful ablation has been described with energy as low as 5 W [23], we recommend initially setting up the ablator to deliver 20 s lesions at a power of 10 W with a temperature limit of 50° when treating infants. Where convective cooling does not allow delivery of an effective lesion, successful ablation can also be achieved with a cooled tip ablation catheter [23].

3.5. Percutaneous coronary intervention on ECMO in critically ill patients

3.5.1. Types of mechanical support available for percutaneous coronary intervention

There are occasions when percutaneous coronary intervention (PCI) cannot be carried out without additional haemodynamic support. The characteristic scenarios are cardiac arrest, cardiogenic shock and global critical coronary perfusion status. In these circumstances, various types of mechanical circulatory support are available, including VA ECMO, intra-aortic balloon pump, Impella (Abiomed, Danvers, MA) and Tandem Heart (Cardiac Assist, Inc., Pittsburgh, PA). Impella uses an axial flow pump to propel blood from the left ventricle to the aorta. Tandem Heart pumps blood extracorporeally from the left atrium to the femoral artery via a transseptally placed left atrial cannula. Current evidence on the utility of these devices is summarised in the 2015 SCAI/ACC/HFSA/STS consensus statement on mechanical circulatory support [55]. Choice between these various modalities is dictated by the patients' haemodynamic status, availability of equipment and local expertise. In our centre, where there is a large ECMO programme and considerable experience with emergent use of ECMO,

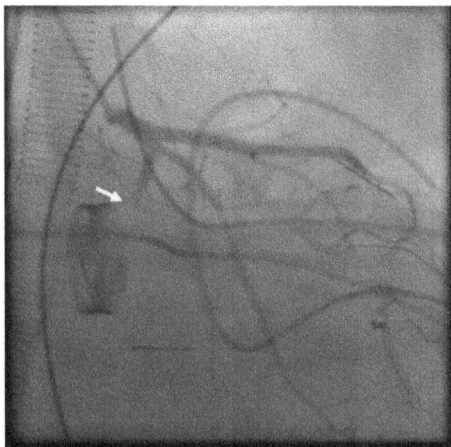

Figure 9. Circumflex occlusion (arrow) following mitral valve replacement. Stent implantation successfully opened the occluded segment.

patients are more likely to receive ECMO support when their haemodynamic status is critically compromised. ECMO should be chosen in preference to other ventricular assist devices when there is impaired oxygenation or right ventricular failure. Post-operative patients on ECMO may occasionally require PCI when there is an unexpected coronary lesion (**Figure 9**).

3.5.2. PCI on ECMO in patients who have a cardiac arrest

Patients who have cardiac arrest before or during PCI present the greatest challenge to the interventional team. To carry out PCI while there is no spontaneous cardiac output is extremely difficult. Manual CPR in this setting, even if performed to perfection, requires pauses for X-ray imaging and soon becomes ineffective in most cases. When extracorporeal CPR is instituted soon after cardiac arrest, it provides a haemodynamically stable platform for PCI that allows the operator to focus on the technique itself, rather than dealing with volatile haemodynamics and a jerky, mobile X-ray view of the target vessel. There are reports of excellent outcomes from PCI in patients on ECMO following cardiac arrest [56–61]. However, Kagawa et al. described only 29% 30-day survival in 61 patients with acute coronary syndrome who received emergency ECMO coupled with PCI to treat cardiac arrest unresponsive to manual CPR [62]. Arlt et al. described 40% survival to hospital discharge in a cohort of patients who received PCI coupled with extracorporeal CPR using a miniaturised ECMO system [63]. Better results were described in the CHEER trial, which included 26 patients with resistant cardiac arrest who were treated with emergency ECMO, combined with 30 ml/kg of intravenous ice-cold saline to induce therapeutic hypothermia. Eleven of these patients proceeded to have PCI on ECMO. Six patients survived with full neurological recovery [64]. A well-organised extracorporeal CPR service is important to achieve the best outcomes in this context. Patients should be established on ECMO quickly by an expert team, following high-quality CPR without severe metabolic disturbance or tissue hypoxia, to maximise their chance of survival with intact neurology.

3.5.3. PCI on ECMO in patients with profound cardiogenic shock

When patients who require PCI present with severe cardiogenic shock (usually defined as systolic blood pressure less than 75 mmHg on high-dose inotropic support), extracorporeal support can be used to offload the left ventricle and boost cardiac output during revascularisation. Recent studies have suggested that survival is improved when ECMO is used as an adjunct to PCI in this patient group. Esper et al. [65] showed an impressive 67% survival to discharge in patients with severe shock who received ECMO in the cardiac catheter laboratory. Good outcome has also been demonstrated following left main stem PCI in patients with cardiogenic shock supported by ECMO [66]. Data from true randomised comparison of outcomes with and without ECMO are absent. However, comparison between present and historic cohorts provides some insight. Sheu et al. [67] demonstrated a statistically significant reduction in 30-day mortality in PCI patients with profound shock, from 72% to 39%, following introduction of ECMO support in 2002. Tsao et al. [68] demonstrated a significant difference in 30-day (32% vs 67%) and 1-year (24% vs 64%) survival in PCI patients with severe shock when they compared cohorts treated without ECMO (2004–2006) and with ECMO (2007–2009), respectively. Unai et al. [69] found similar results after introducing ECMO support for PCI patients with profound shock in 2010. Existing evidence therefore supports early ECMO intervention in this patient group, particularly to avoid the peak in mortality that normally occurs in the first few days after revascularisation [67]. A recent meta-analysis suggests that this positive effect on in-hospital mortality is found only in patients treated with ECMO and that treatment with percutaneous left ventricular assist devices, such as the Impella or Tandem Heart, does not confer a survival benefit [70].

3.5.4. Elective use of ECMO to support high-risk PCI

Percutaneous coronary intervention is regarded as high risk when there is moderate-to-severe left ventricular dysfunction, a large amount of myocardium is subtended by the stenosed vessels and, in addition, the procedure involves technical difficulties, such as the presence of bifurcation lesions, triple vessel disease, left main stenosis or chronic total occlusion. In such cases, where there is a significant risk that the intervention will precipitate haemodynamic decompensation, it is intuitive to suppose that elective extracorporeal support will reduce mortality. Yet, better outcomes have not been convincingly demonstrated in high-risk PCI procedures supported by intra-aortic balloon pump or Impella [71–73]. In contrast to this, a recent study using elective Tandem Heart support yielded promising results, with 30-day and 6-month survival rates of 90% and 87%, respectively [73]. From this study, it is tempting to extrapolate that elective ECMO may improve outcome in this patient group, where the safety margin is very small. Case reports have certainly described success in high-risk PCI using ECMO to produce a stable haemodynamic platform [74, 75]. One single-centre prospective study reported 100% PCI success with no in-hospital major adverse cardiac events in 12 consecutive patients who underwent high-risk PCI with ECMO support. At 6-month follow-up, neither death nor myocardial infarction were noted [76]. Notwithstanding this, there are at present no large volume conclusive multicentre trials of these techniques. It is possible that other means of haemodynamic support may be just as effective as ECMO in these situations. Technological advances in usability and further attempts at generating good scientific evidence for the role of ECMO in PCI will go hand in hand and hopefully provide strong evidence for guideline development in the longer term.

3.6. ECMO support for high-risk elective congenital and structural catheter intervention procedures

3.6.1. When has elective ECMO support been used for high-risk procedures?

Elective use of ECMO to support high-risk intervention is a new area of practice. There is little published information. The larger series that deal with paediatric catheterisation on ECMO do not include data on ECMO use in this context [2–5, 11]. One series dealing with extracorporeal CPR in the paediatric catheter laboratory included two patients with critically low cardiac output and one with severe hypoxaemia who had elective ECMO support before catheterisation [77]. The patients survived with no neurological damage. A handful of case reports have also shown that elective ECMO before catheterisation allows procedures to be undertaken safely in patients with extremely fragile haemodynamics. Interventions included branch pulmonary artery stenting [78, 79], radiofrequency ablation of a Mahaim pathway [49], radiofrequency ablation of VT [52] and tricuspid valve implantation [80]. In adult patients, 100% procedural success and 0% mortality were described in a small very high-risk TAVI cohort where ECMO was instituted electively before the procedure. These results were clearly superior to those cases where high-risk TAVI patients were rescued by emergency ECMO during the procedure [28]. Such 'ECMO hybrid procedures' allow us to deal with increasingly complex interventional problems in sicker patients without increasing mortality.

3.6.2. The team approach to using ECMO in high-risk catheter procedures

In our catheter laboratory, the risks of procedures that could potentially have catastrophic complications are mitigated by collaboration with the ECMO team. Whenever there is a significant possibility of lethal complications, the case is discussed with the interventional team, the ECMO team, cardiac intensivists and cardiac surgeons. A joint plan is made in advance at a multidisciplinary team meeting. A detailed team briefing then takes place on the morning of the procedure, with all disciplines represented. Participants are encouraged to raise any potential issues in advance. It is important to plan as much as possible before the procedure, anticipating difficulties rather than reacting to them as they occur [81].

3.6.3. Our local 3 level strategy to support high-risk catheter procedures

Depending on the perceived level of risk, we have three different levels of ECMO support:

3.6.3.1. Level 1

The first level of support is used for cases where serious complications are possible but unlikely. We include duct stenting or right ventricular outflow tract stenting in this category, as it is possible that the patient's only source of pulmonary blood supply can be compromised by the intervention. In such cases, the ECMO team and surgical team are made aware that the procedure is taking place, but no special precautions are taken. Sharing information cuts down the response time, should extracorporeal CPR become necessary.

3.6.3.2. Level 2

The second level of support is used for cases where there is a significant possibility of a lethal complication. In this category, we include patients undergoing stenting and high-pressure balloon dilation of a calcific right ventricle to pulmonary artery conduit, particularly where aggressive dilation is planned at a site where rupture would be difficult to control with a covered stent, for example at the pulmonary artery bifurcation. If there is a massive rupture, the only possible rescue strategy may be to occlude the entire conduit with a balloon and place the patient on VA ECMO while preparations are made for cardiac surgery. In such cases, in addition to the vascular access that is required to perform the intervention, we place an extra sheath in the contralateral femoral artery and vein. These sheaths can be rewired and used for percutaneous ECMO cannulation in an emergency. An ECMO circuit is assembled and kept in the catheter laboratory. Blood and products are prepared in advance as if the patient were going for cardiac surgery. The ECMO team, a cardiac surgeon and a theatre team remain in the catheter laboratory during the procedure, and a cardiac theatre is kept free. When the risk is particularly high and the response needs to be immediate, the ECMO circuit is primed with blood before the procedure starts. High-risk neonatal interventions in this category involve preparing the neck for cannulation rather than the groin. This may consist of prepping and draping the neck area and inserting a sheath that can be easily rewired into the jugular vein or may extend to cut down and exposure of the neck vessels for cannulation in very high-risk cases.

3.6.3.3. Level 3

The third level of support is reserved for patients with poor ventricular function and low cardiac output, where there is a high risk of cardiac arrest or acute haemodynamic decompensation during the catheter procedure (**Figure 10**). Also in this category are patients who have critically low oxygen saturation because of narrowed shunts or branch pulmonary arteries, where pulmonary blood flow will be further compromised during the intervention. In these patients, ECMO is electively instituted in advance of the case while the patient is on the intensive care unit. We have used this approach to carry out conduit stenting in an adult patient with gross right heart failure secondary to severe chronic right ventricle to pulmonary artery conduit stenosis. The patient, who had an excellent result, was decannulated on the

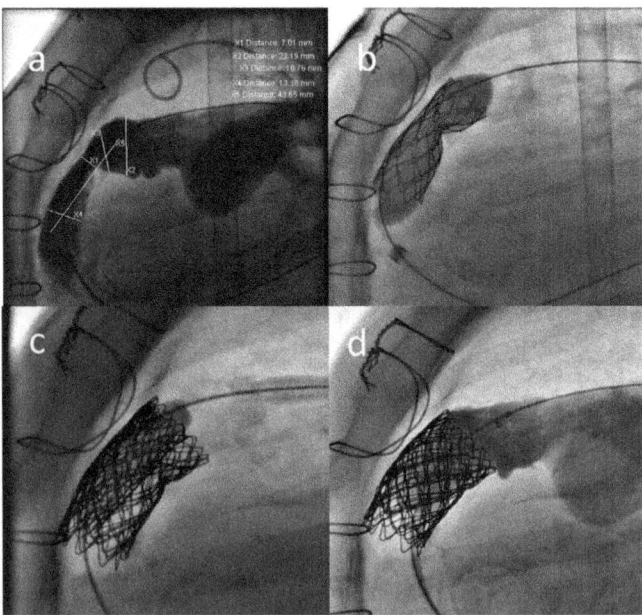

Figure 10. Elective ECMO support of right ventricle to pulmonary artery conduit stenting. (a) Angiography shows a tight stenosis in the right ventricle to pulmonary artery conduit; (b) A covered stent is implanted in the conduit. Further stents were subsequently implanted and dilated with a high-pressure balloon; (c) A Melody (Medtronic, Minneapolis, MN) percutaneous pulmonary valve is implanted in the prestented conduit at a second procedure 5 months later; (d) A well-expanded conduit with a competent pulmonary valve is ultimately achieved.

same day as the procedure and ultimately had successful percutaneous pulmonary valve implantation.

Author details

Christopher Duke[1*], Chris J. Harvey[2], Vikram Kudumula[3], Elved B. Roberts[4] and Suhair O. Shebani[3]

*Address all correspondence to: akd11@le.ac.uk

1 Department of Paediatric Cardiology, King Faisal Cardiac Centre, National Guard Health Affairs, Jeddah, Saudi Arabia and East Midlands Congenital Heart Disease Centre, Glenfield Hospital, Leicester, UK

2 Department of Cardiothoracic Surgery, Glenfield Hospital, Leicester, UK

3 East Midlands Congenital Heart Disease Centre, Glenfield Hospital, Leicester, UK

4 Department of Cardiology, Glenfield Hospital, Leicester, UK

References

[1] Prodhan P, Fiser RT, Cenac S, Bhutta AT, Fontenot E, Moss M, et al. Intrahospital transport of children on extracorporeal membrane oxygenation: indications, process, interventions, and effectiveness. Pediatr Crit Care Med. 2010;11(2):227–33. doi:10.1097/ PCC.0b013e3181b063b2

[2] Panda BR, Alphonso N, Govindasamy M, Anderson B, Stocker C, Karl TR. Cardiac catheter procedures during extracorporeal life support: a risk-benefit analysis. World J Pediatr Congenit Heart Surg. 2014;5(1):31–7. doi:10.1177/2150135113505297

[3] Callahan R, Trucco SM, Wearden PD, Beerman LB, Arora G, Kreutzer J. Outcomes of pediatric patients undergoing cardiac catheterization while on extracorporeal membrane oxygenation. Pediatr Cardiol. 2015;36(3):625–32. doi:10.1007/s00246-014-1057-5

[4] desJardins SE, Crowley DC, Beekman RH, Lloyd TR. Utility of cardiac catheterization in pediatric cardiac patients on ECMO. Catheter Cardiovasc Interv. 1999;46(1):62–7. doi:10.1002/(SICI)1522-726X(199901)46:1<62::AID-CCD17>3.0.CO;2-9

[5] Booth KL, Roth SJ, Perry SB, del Nido PJ, Wessel DL, Laussen PC. Cardiac catheterization of patients supported by extracorporeal membrane oxygenation. J Am Coll Cardiol. 2002;40(9):1681–6.

[6] Endemann DH, Philipp A, Hengstenberg C, Luchner A, Puhler T, Hilker M, et al. A simple method of vascular access to perform emergency coronary angiography in patients with veno-arterial extracorporeal membrane oxygenation. Intensive Care Med. 2011;37(12):2046–9. doi:10.1007/s00134-011-2383-1

[7] Ucer E, Fredersdorf S, Jungbauer C, Debl K, Philipp A, Amann M, et al. A unique access for the ablation catheter to treat electrical storm in a patient with extracorporeal life support. Europace: European pacing, arrhythmias, and cardiac electrophysiology: journal of the working groups on cardiac pacing, arrhythmias, and cardiac cellular electrophysiology of the European Society of Cardiology. 2014;16(2):299–302. doi: 10.1093/europace/eut165

[8] Kogon B, Villari C, Shah N, Kirshbom P, Kanter K, Kim D, et al. Occlusion of the modified Blalock-Taussig shunt: unique methods of treatment and review of catheter-based intervention. Congenit Heart Dis. 2007;2(3):185–90. doi:10.1111/j. 1747-0803.2007.00095.x

[9] Thuys C, MacLaren G, d'Udekem Y, Eastaugh L. Vascular access for pediatric coronary angiography on extracorporeal membrane oxygenation. World J Pediatr Congenit Heart Surg. 2015;6(1):126–9. doi:10.1177/2150135114554303

[10] Ettedgui JA FF, Park SC, Fischer DR, Siewers RD, del Nido, PJ. Cardiac catheterization in children on extracorporeal membrane oxygenation. Cardiol Young. 1996;6:59–61.

[11] Agarwal HS, Hardison DC, Saville BR, Donahue BS, Lamb FS, Bichell DP, et al. Residual lesions in post-operative pediatric cardiac surgery patients receiving extracorporeal membrane oxygenation support. J Thorac Cardiovasc Surg. 2014;147(1):434–41. doi: 10.1016/j.jtcvs.2013.03.021

[12] Kulik TJ, Moler FW, Palmisano JM, Custer JR, Mosca RS, Bove EL, et al. Outcome-associated factors in pediatric patients treated with extracorporeal membrane oxygenator after cardiac surgery. Circulation. 1996;94(9 Suppl):II63-8.

[13] Alsoufi B, Al-Radi OO, Gruenwald C, Lean L, Williams WG, McCrindle BW, et al. Extracorporeal life support following cardiac surgery in children: analysis of risk factors and survival in a single institution. Eur J Cardiothorac Surg. 2009;35(6):1004–11; discussion 11. doi:10.1016/j.ejcts.2009.02.015

[14] Chaturvedi RR, Macrae D, Brown KL, Schindler M, Smith EC, Davis KB, et al. Cardiac ECMO for biventricular hearts after paediatric open heart surgery. Heart. 2004;90(5): 545–51.

[15] Feltes TF, Bacha E, Beekman RH, 3rd, Cheatham JP, Feinstein JA, Gomes AS, et al. Indications for cardiac catheterization and intervention in pediatric cardiac disease: a scientific statement from the American Heart Association. Circulation. 2011;123(22): 2607–52. doi:10.1161/CIR.0b013e31821b1f10

[16] Zahn EM, Dobrolet NC, Nykanen DG, Ojito J, Hannan RL, Burke RP. Interventional catheterization performed in the early post-operative period after congenital heart surgery in children. J Am Coll Cardiol. 2004;43(7):1264–9. doi: 10.1016/j.jacc.2003.10.051

[17] Anderson BW, Barron DJ, Jones TJ, Edwards L, Brawn W, Stumper O. Catheter takedown in the management of the acutely failing Fontan circulation. Ann Thorac Surg. 2011;92(1):346–8. doi:10.1016/j.athoracsur.2011.01.040

[18] Zylberberg R, Cook L, Roberts J, Edmonds D, Reese A, Groff D. Total anomalous pulmonary venous return: report of a case diagnosed on ECMO. J Perinatol. 1987;7(3): 185–8.

[19] Faulkner SC, Chipman CW, Moss MM, Frazier EA, Love JC, Harrell JE, et al. Extracorporeal life support of neonates with congenital cardiac defects: techniques used during cardiac catheterization and surgery. J Extra Corpor Technol. 1994;26(1):28–33.

[20] Butler TJ, Yoder BA, Seib P, Lally KP, Smith VC. ECMO for left ventricular assist in a newborn with critical aortic stenosis. Pediatr Cardiol. 1994;15(1):38–40. doi:10.1007/BF00797005

[21] Schiller O, Burns KM, Sinha P, Cummings SD. Cor triatriatum with partial anomalous pulmonary venous return: a rare case of parallel obstruction and successful staged treatment. Pediatr Cardiol. 2012;33(2):363–5. doi:10.1007/s00246-011-0148-9

[22] Khan M, Gauri A, Grifka R, Elmouchi D. Radiofrequency Ablation of a Left Atrial Appendage Tachycardia on ECMO Support. Case Rep Pediatr. 2013;2013:203241. doi: 10.1155/2013/203241

[23] Shebani SO, Ng GA, Stafford P, Duke C. Radiofrequency ablation on veno-arterial extracorporeal life support in treatment of very sick infants with incessant tachymyopathy. Europace: European pacing, arrhythmias, and cardiac electrophysiology: journal of the working groups on cardiac pacing, arrhythmias, and cardiac cellular electrophysiology of the European Society of Cardiology. 2015;17(4):622–7. doi:10.1093/europace/euu365

[24] O'Connor TA, Downing GJ, Ewing LL, Gowdamarajan R. Echocardiographically guided balloon atrial septostomy during extracorporeal membrane oxygenation (ECMO). Pediatr Cardiol. 1993;14(3):167–8. doi:10.1007/BF00795647

[25] Griffith KE, Jenkins E, Haft J. Treatment of massive pulmonary embolism utilizing a multidisciplinary approach: a case study. Perfusion. 2009;24(3):169–72. doi: 10.1177/0267659109346663

[26] Munakata R, Yamamoto T, Hosokawa Y, Tokita Y, Akutsu K, Sato N, et al. Massive pulmonary embolism requiring extracorporeal life support treated with catheter-based interventions. Int Heart J. 2012;53(6):370–4.

[27] Nakamura M, Sunagawa O, Tsuchiya H, Miyara T, Taba Y, Touma T, et al. Rescue balloon pulmonary angioplasty under veno-arterial extracorporeal membrane oxygenation in a patient with acute exacerbation of chronic thromboembolic pulmonary hypertension. Int Heart J. 2015;56(1):116–20. doi:10.1536/ihj.14-257

[28] Husser O, Holzamer A, Philipp A, Nunez J, Bodi V, Muller T, et al. Emergency and prophylactic use of miniaturized veno-arterial extracorporeal membrane oxygenation in transcatheter aortic valve implantation. Catheter Cardiovasc Interv. 2013;82(4):E542–51. doi:10.1002/ccd.24806

[29] Staudacher DL, Bode C, Wengenmayer T. Severe mitral regurgitation requiring ECMO therapy treated by interventional valve reconstruction using the MitraClip. Catheter Cardiovasc Interv. 2015;85(1):170–5. doi:10.1002/ccd.25332

[30] Seib PM, Faulkner SC, Erickson CC, Van Devanter SH, Harrell JE, Fasules JW, et al. Blade and balloon atrial septostomy for left heart decompression in patients with severe ventricular dysfunction on extracorporeal membrane oxygenation. Catheter Cardiovasc Interv. 1999;46(2):179–86. doi:10.1002/(SICI)1522-726X(199902)46:2<179::AID-CCD13>3.0.CO;2-W

[31] Kotani Y, Chetan D, Rodrigues W, Sivarajan VB, Gruenwald C, Guerguerian AM, et al. Left atrial decompression during venoarterial extracorporeal membrane oxygenation for left ventricular failure in children: current strategy and clinical outcomes. Artif Organs. 2013;37(1):29–36. doi:10.1111/j.1525-1594.2012.01534.x

[32] Eastaugh LJ, Thiagarajan RR, Darst JR, McElhinney DB, Lock JE, Marshall AC. Percutaneous left atrial decompression in patients supported with extracorporeal membrane oxygenation for cardiac disease. Pediatr Crit Care Med. 2015;16(1):59–65. doi:10.1097/PCC.0000000000000276

[33] O'Byrne ML, Glatz AC, Rossano JW, Schiavo KL, Dori Y, Rome JJ, et al. Middle-term results of trans-catheter creation of atrial communication in patients receiving mechanical circulatory support. Catheter Cardiovasc Interv. 2015;85(7):1189–95. doi:10.1002/ccd.25824

[34] Aiyagari RM, Rocchini AP, Remenapp RT, Graziano JN. Decompression of the left atrium during extracorporeal membrane oxygenation using a transseptal cannula incorporated into the circuit. Crit Care Med. 2006;34(10):2603–6. doi:10.1097/01.CCM.0000239113.02836.F1

[35] Ward KE, Tuggle DW, Gessouroun MR, Overholt ED, Mantor PC. Transseptal decompression of the left heart during ECMO for severe myocarditis. Ann Thorac Surg. 1995;59(3):749–51. doi:10.1016/0003-4975(94)00579-6

[36] Hlavacek AM, Atz AM, Bradley SM, Bandisode VM. Left atrial decompression by percutaneous cannula placement while on extracorporeal membrane oxygenation. J Thorac Cardiovasc Surg. 2005;130(2):595–6. doi:10.1016/j.jtcvs.2004.12.029

[37] Swartz MF, Smith F, Byrum CJ, Alfieris GM. Transseptal catheter decompression of the left ventricle during extracorporeal membrane oxygenation. Pediatr Cardiol. 2012;33(1):185–7. doi:10.1007/s00246-011-0113-7

[38] Fumagalli R, Bombino M, Borelli M, Rossi F, Colombo V, Osculati G, et al. Percutaneous bridge to heart transplantation by venoarterial ECMO and transaortic left ventricular venting. Int J Artif Organs. 2004;27(5):410–3.

[39] Barbone A, Malvindi PG, Ferrara P, Tarelli G. Left ventricle unloading by percutaneous pigtail during extracorporeal membrane oxygenation. Interact Cardiovasc Thorac Surg. 2011;13(3):293–5. doi:10.1510/icvts.2011.269795

[40] Johnston TA, Jaggers J, McGovern JJ, O'Laughlin MP. Bedside transseptal balloon dilation atrial septostomy for decompression of the left heart during extracorporeal membrane oxygenation. Catheter Cardiovasc Interv. 1999;46(2):197–9. doi:10.1002/(SICI)1522-726X(199902)46:2<197::AID-CCD17>3.0.CO;2-G

[41] Haynes S, Kerber RE, Johnson FL, Lynch WR, Divekar A. Left heart decompression by atrial stenting during extracorporeal membrane oxygenation. Int J Artif Organs. 2009;32(4):240–2.

[42] Sivakumar K. Atrial septal stenting—How I do it? Ann Pediatr Cardiol. 2015;8(1):37–43. doi:10.4103/0974-2069.149516

[43] Stumper O, Gewillig M, Vettukattil J, Budts W, Chessa M, Chaudhari M, et al. Modified technique of stent fenestration of the atrial septum. Heart. 2003;89(10):1227–30.

[44] Silva JN, Erickson CC, Carter CD, Greene EA, Kantoch M, Collins KK, et al. Management of pediatric tachyarrhythmias on mechanical support. Circulation Arrhythmia and electrophysiology. 2014;7(4):658–63. doi:10.1161/CIRCEP.113.000973

[45] Carbucicchio C, Della Bella P, Fassini G, Trevisi N, Riva S, Giraldi F, et al. Percutaneous cardiopulmonary support for catheter ablation of unstable ventricular arrhythmias in high-risk patients. Herz. 2009;34(7):545–52. doi:10.1007/s00059-009-3289-3

[46] Bella PD, Maccabelli G. Temporary percutaneous left ventricular support for ablation of untolerated ventricular tachycardias: is it worth the trouble? Circ Arrhythm Electrophysiol. 2012;5(6):1056–8. doi:10.1161/CIRCEP.112.979013

[47] Rizkallah J, Shen S, Tischenko A, Zieroth S, Freed DH, Khadem A. Successful ablation of idiopathic left ventricular tachycardia in an adult patient during extracorporeal membrane oxygenation treatment. Can J Cardiol. 2013;29(12):1741 e17-9. doi:10.1016/j.cjca.2013.08.015

[48] Walker GM, McLeod K, Brown KL, Franklin O, Goldman AP, Davis C. Extracorporeal life support as a treatment of supraventricular tachycardia in infants. Pediatr Crit Care Med. 2003;4(1):52–4. doi:10.1097/01.PCC.0000043916.45503.34

[49] Carmichael TB, Walsh EP, Roth SJ. Anticipatory use of venoarterial extracorporeal membrane oxygenation for a high-risk interventional cardiac procedure. Respir Care. 2002;47(9):1002-6.

[50] Thomas V, Lawrence D, Kogon B, Frias P. Epicardial ablation of ventricular tachycardia in a child on venoarterial extracorporeal membrane oxygenation. Pediatr Cardiol. 2010;31(6):901–4. doi:10.1007/s00246-010-9734-5

[51] Cisco MJ, Asija R, Dubin AM, Perry SB, Hanley FL, Roth SJ. Survival after extreme left atrial hypertension and pulmonary haemorrhage in an infant supported with extracorporeal membrane oxygenation for refractory atrial flutter. Pediatr Crit Care Med. 2011;12(3):e149–52. doi:10.1097/PCC.0b013e3181e8b3e5

[52] Arya SO, Karpawich PP, Gupta P, Buddhe S, Singh HR, Hussein Y, et al. Primary endocardial fibroelastosis presenting in a young child as incessant ventricular tachycardia and dilated cardiomyopathy. Tex Heart Inst J. 2012;39(5):714–8.

[53] Dyamenahalli U, Tuzcu V, Fontenot E, Papagiannis J, Jaquiss RD, Bhutta A, et al. Extracorporeal membrane oxygenation support for intractable primary arrhythmias and complete congenital heart block in newborns and infants: short-term and medium-term outcomes. Pediatr Crit Care Med. 2012;13(1):47–52. doi:10.1097/PCC.0b013e3182196cb1

[54] Koutbi L, Chenu C, Mace L, Franceschi F. Ablation of idiopathic ventricular tachycardia arising from posterior mitral annulus in an 11-month-old infant by transapical left ventricular access via median sternotomy. Heart Rhythm: The Official Journal of the Heart Rhythm Soc. 2015;12(2):430–2. doi:10.1016/j.hrthm.2014.10.030

[55] Rihal CS, Naidu SS, Givertz MM, Szeto WY, Burke JA, Kapur NK, et al. 2015 SCAI/ACC/HFSA/STS clinical expert consensus statement on the use of percutaneous mechanical circulatory support devices in cardiovascular care (Endorsed by the American heart association, the cardiological society of India, and sociedad latino Americana de cardiologia intervencion; Affirmation of value by the canadian association of interventional cardiology-association canadienne de cardiologie d'intervention). Catheter Cardiovasc Interv. 2015;85(7):E175–96. doi:10.1002/ccd.25720

[56] Dahdouh Z, Roule V, Sabatier R, Lognone T, Labombarda F, Pellissier A, et al. Extracorporeal life support, transradial thrombus aspiration and stenting, percutaneous blade and balloon atrioseptostomy, all as a bridge to heart transplantation to save one life. Cardiovasc Revasc Med. 2012;13(4):241–5. doi:10.1016/j.carrev.2012.02.007

[57] Galassi AR, Ganyukov V, Tomasello SD, Haes B, Leonid B. Successful antegrade revascularization by the innovation of composite core dual coil in a three-vessel total occlusive disease for cardiac arrest patient using extracorporeal membrane oxygenation. Eur Heart J. 2014;35(30):2009. doi:10.1093/eurheartj/ehu070

[58] Lazzeri C, Sori A, Bernardo P, Picariello C, Gensini GF, Valente S. In-hospital refractory cardiac arrest treated with extracorporeal membrane oxygenation: a tertiary single

center experience. Acute Card Care. 2013;15(3):47–51. doi: 10.3109/17482941.2013.796385

[59] Lee MS, Pessegueiro A, Tobis J. The role of extracorporeal membrane oxygenation in emergent percutaneous coronary intervention for myocardial infarction complicated by cardiogenic shock and cardiac arrest. J Invasive Cardiol. 2008;20(9):E269–72.

[60] Magovern GJ Jr, Simpson KA. Extracorporeal membrane oxygenation for adult cardiac support: the Allegheny experience. Ann Thorac Surg. 1999;68(2):655–61.

[61] Ricciardi MJ, Moscucci M, Knight BP, Zivin A, Bartlett RH, Bates ER. Emergency extracorporeal membrane oxygenation (ECMO)-supported percutaneous coronary interventions in the fibrillating heart. Catheter Cardiovasc Interv. 1999;48(4):402–5.

[62] Kagawa E, Dote K, Kato M, Sasaki S, Nakano Y, Kajikawa M, et al. Should we emergently revascularize occluded coronaries for cardiac arrest?: rapid-response extracorporeal membrane oxygenation and intra-arrest percutaneous coronary intervention. Circulation. 2012;126(13):1605–13. doi:10.1161/CIRCULATIONAHA.111.067538

[63] Arlt M, Philipp A, Voelkel S, Schopka S, Husser O, Hengstenberg C, et al. Early experiences with miniaturized extracorporeal life-support in the catheterization laboratory. Eur J Cardiothorac Surg. 2012;42(5):858–63. doi:10.1093/ejcts/ezs176

[64] Stub D, Bernard S, Pellegrino V, Smith K, Walker T, Sheldrake J, et al. Refractory cardiac arrest treated with mechanical CPR, hypothermia, ECMO and early reperfusion (the CHEER trial). Resuscitation. 2015;86:88–94. doi:10.1016/j.resuscitation.2014.09.010

[65] Esper SA, Bermudez C, Dueweke EJ, Kormos R, Subramaniam K, Mulukutla S, et al. Extracorporeal membrane oxygenation support in acute coronary syndromes complicated by cardiogenic shock. Catheter Cardiovasc Interv. 2015;86 Suppl 1:S45–50. doi: 10.1002/ccd.25871

[66] Lee WC, Tsai TH, Chen YL, Yang CH, Chen SM, Chen CJ, et al. Safety and feasibility of coronary stenting in unprotected left main coronary artery disease in the real world clinical practice—a single center experience. PloS one. 2014;9(10):e109281. doi:10.1371/journal.pone.0109281

[67] Sheu JJ, Tsai TH, Lee FY, Fang HY, Sun CK, Leu S, et al. Early extracorporeal membrane oxygenator-assisted primary percutaneous coronary intervention improved 30-day clinical outcomes in patients with ST-segment elevation myocardial infarction complicated with profound cardiogenic shock. Crit Care Med. 2010;38(9):1810–7. doi:10.1097/CCM.0b013e3181e8acf7

[68] Tsao NW, Shih CM, Yeh JS, Kao YT, Hsieh MH, Ou KL, et al. Extracorporeal membrane oxygenation-assisted primary percutaneous coronary intervention may improve survival of patients with acute myocardial infarction complicated by profound cardiogenic shock. J Crit Care. 2012;27(5):530 e1–11. doi:10.1016/j.jcrc.2012.02.012

[69] Unai S, Tanaka D, Ruggiero N, Hirose H, Cavarocchi NC. Acute myocardial infarction complicated by cardiogenic shock: an algorithm-based extracorporeal membrane

oxygenation program can improve clinical outcomes. artif organs. 2015. doi:10.1111/aor.12538

[70] Romeo F, Acconcia MC, Sergi D, Romeo A, Francioni S, Chiarotti F, et al. Percutaneous assist devices in acute myocardial infarction with cardiogenic shock: review, meta-analysis. World J Cardiol. 2016;8(1):98–111. doi:10.4330/wjc.v8.i1.98

[71] Perera D, Stables R, Thomas M, Booth J, Pitt M, Blackman D, et al. Elective intra-aortic balloon counterpulsation during high-risk percutaneous coronary intervention: a randomized controlled trial. JAMA. 2010;304(8):867–74. doi:10.1001/jama.2010.1190

[72] Romeo F, Acconcia MC, Sergi D, Romeo A, Gensini GF, Chiarotti F, et al. Lack of intra-aortic balloon pump effectiveness in high-risk percutaneous coronary interventions without cardiogenic shock: a comprehensive meta-analysis of randomised trials and observational studies. Int J Cardiol. 2013;167(5):1783–93. doi:10.1016/j.ijcard.2012.12.027

[73] O'Neill WW, Kleiman NS, Moses J, Henriques JP, Dixon S, Massaro J, et al. A prospective, randomized clinical trial of haemodynamic support with Impella 2.5 versus intra-aortic balloon pump in patients undergoing high-risk percutaneous coronary intervention: the PROTECT II study. Circulation. 2012;126(14):1717–27. doi:10.1161/CIRCULATIONAHA.112.098194

[74] Kass M, Moon M, Vo M, Singal R, Ravandi A. Awake extracorporeal membrane oxygenation for very high-risk coronary angioplasty. Can J Cardiol. 2015;31(2):227 e11–3. doi:10.1016/j.cjca.2014.11.004

[75] Spina R, Forrest AP, Adams MR, Wilson MK, Ng MK, Vallely MP. Veno-arterial extracorporeal membrane oxygenation for high-risk cardiac catheterisation procedures. Heart Lung Circ. 2010;19(12):736–41. doi:10.1016/j.hlc.2010.08.015

[76] Tomasello SD, Boukhris M, Ganyukov V, Galassi AR, Shukevich D, Haes B, et al. Outcome of extracorporeal membrane oxygenation support for complex high-risk elective percutaneous coronary interventions: a single-center experience. Heart Lung. 2015;44(4):309–13. doi:10.1016/j.hrtlng.2015.03.005

[77] Allan CK, Thiagarajan RR, Armsby LR, del Nido PJ, Laussen PC. Emergent use of extracorporeal membrane oxygenation during pediatric cardiac catheterization. Pediatr Crit Care Med. 2006;7(3):212–9. doi:10.1097/01.PCC.0000200964.88206.B0

[78] Zampi JD, Rocchini A, Hirsch-Romano JC. Elective ECMO support for pulmonary artery stent placement in a 4.9-kg shunt-dependent patient. World J Pediatr Congenit Heart Surg. 2015;6(1):101–4. doi:10.1177/2150135114549077

[79] Ward CJ, Mullins CE, Barron LJ, Grifka RG, Gomez MR, Cuellar-Gomez MR. Use of extracorporeal membrane oxygenation to maintain oxygenation during pediatric interventional cardiac catheterization. Am Heart J. 1995;130(3 Pt 1):619–20. doi:

[80] Kefer J, Sluysmans T, Vanoverschelde JL. Transcatheter Sapien valve implantation in a native tricuspid valve after failed surgical repair. Catheter Cardiovasc Interv. 2014;83(5):841–5. doi:10.1002/ccd.25330

[81] Dalton HJ. Planning for the unexpected: extracorporeal membrane oxygenation in the catheterization laboratory and beyond. Pediatr Crit Care Med. 2006;7(3):279–81. doi: 10.1097/01.PCC.0000216673.97153.D9

4

Extracorporeal Membrane Oxygenation in Traumatic Injury

Ronson Hughes, James Cipolla, Peter G. Thomas and
Stanislaw P. Stawicki

Abstract

Severe respiratory failure may develop in the trauma patient as a consequence of direct lung injury, in response to trauma-associated systemic inflammatory response syndrome (SIRS), as a result of infection, or at times as an unintended consequence of the life-saving management of the acute traumatic injury. Approximately 0.5% of all adult trauma patients develop some form of pulmonary dysfunction along the acute lung injury (ALI) – acute respiratory distress (ARDS) spectrum, with the incidence of severe respiratory failure reaching 10–20% in multisystem trauma victims. Of concern, mortality in patients with acute respiratory failure who go on to develop severe pulmonary dysfunction can be as high as 37–50% with the use of conventional therapeutic modalities. Extracorporeal membrane oxygenation (ECMO) has been proposed as a rescue strategy when less invasive primary or adjunctive attempts fail. Numerous case reports and single-center studies demonstrate potential benefits of early implementation of veno-venous (VV)-ECMO for the treatment of severe respiratory failure associated with trauma or sequelae of trauma. In this clinical context, VV-ECMO can be employed to correct for both ventilatory and oxygenation failure while allowing the treating physician to provide much needed rest to the patient's lungs and permit healing to take place. The use of ECMO (mainly veno-venous, with limited use of veno-arterial circuits for cardiac indications) has been described in patients with severe chest injuries, traumatic pneumonectomy, bronchopleural fistulas, and various forms of respiratory failure refractory to conventional therapies.

Keywords: VV-ECMO, VA-ECMO, ALI, ARDS, acute respiratory failure, trauma, indications, contraindications

1. Introduction

Approximately 0.5% of all adult trauma patients develop some form of pulmonary dysfunction, with the incidence of severe respiratory failure reaching 10–20% in multisystem trauma victims [1]. Mortality may be as high as 50% in trauma patients with acute respiratory failure who go on to develop severe pulmonary dysfunction [2]. Novel approaches to mechanical ventilation and adjunctive strategies may help improve outcomes, but continue to fall short of the desired paradigm change [3–6]. Extracorporeal membrane oxygenation (ECMO) has been proposed as a rescue strategy when less invasive primary or adjunctive attempts fail [7–9]. Due to ample case-based literature on the topic of ECMO use in the trauma patient, the goal of this chapter is to provide the reader with a high-level overview of trauma-specific considerations, controversies, pitfalls, indications, and potential avenues for future development in the use of ECMO in the trauma patient.

2. ECMO: a synopsis

There are four major types of short-term mechanical circulatory assist devices used for cardiopulmonary support: (1) intra-aortic balloon pumps, (2) percutaneous ventricular assist devices, (3) extracorporeal membrane oxygenators (ECMO), and (4) non-percutaneous centrifugal pumps [10, 11]. The use of ECMO is limited largely to non-trauma applications, including respiratory (veno-venous or VV-ECMO) and mixed cardiac and respiratory support (veno-arterial or VA-ECMO) in pathophysiologic states considered refractory to maximal standard therapies [12–14]. Circuit characteristics, technical considerations, and other fundamentals of ECMO have been discussed elsewhere in this book. This chapter including the use of ECMO in trauma patients, including indications, contraindications, competing priorities, and practical clinical considerations.

Key considerations must first be addressed before continuing the discussion of ECMO in trauma. Cardiopulmonary support was initially introduced to facilitate and assist cardiac surgical interventions [12, 15]. Subsequent evolution of this technology included device miniaturization and clinical translation to environments outside of the operating room, such as the intensive care units (ICU) [12, 15, 16]. Consequently, it became much easier to deliver ECMO-based therapies, in the setting of acute, refractory respiratory failure, for extended periods of time [17]. Prolonged cardiopulmonary support based on ECMO is now considered a viable option in risk-appropriate, carefully selected non-cardiac surgery patients [18, 19]. At the same time, other non-interventional treatment options and adjuncts are being refined and potential new indications proposed which are actively and dynamically changing the landscape of clinical utilization of ECMO [20–25]. Finally, financial aspects of ECMO therapy must be recognized as well, with significant barriers to wider implementation due to healthcare institutions being increasingly focused on cost containment and value [26–28].

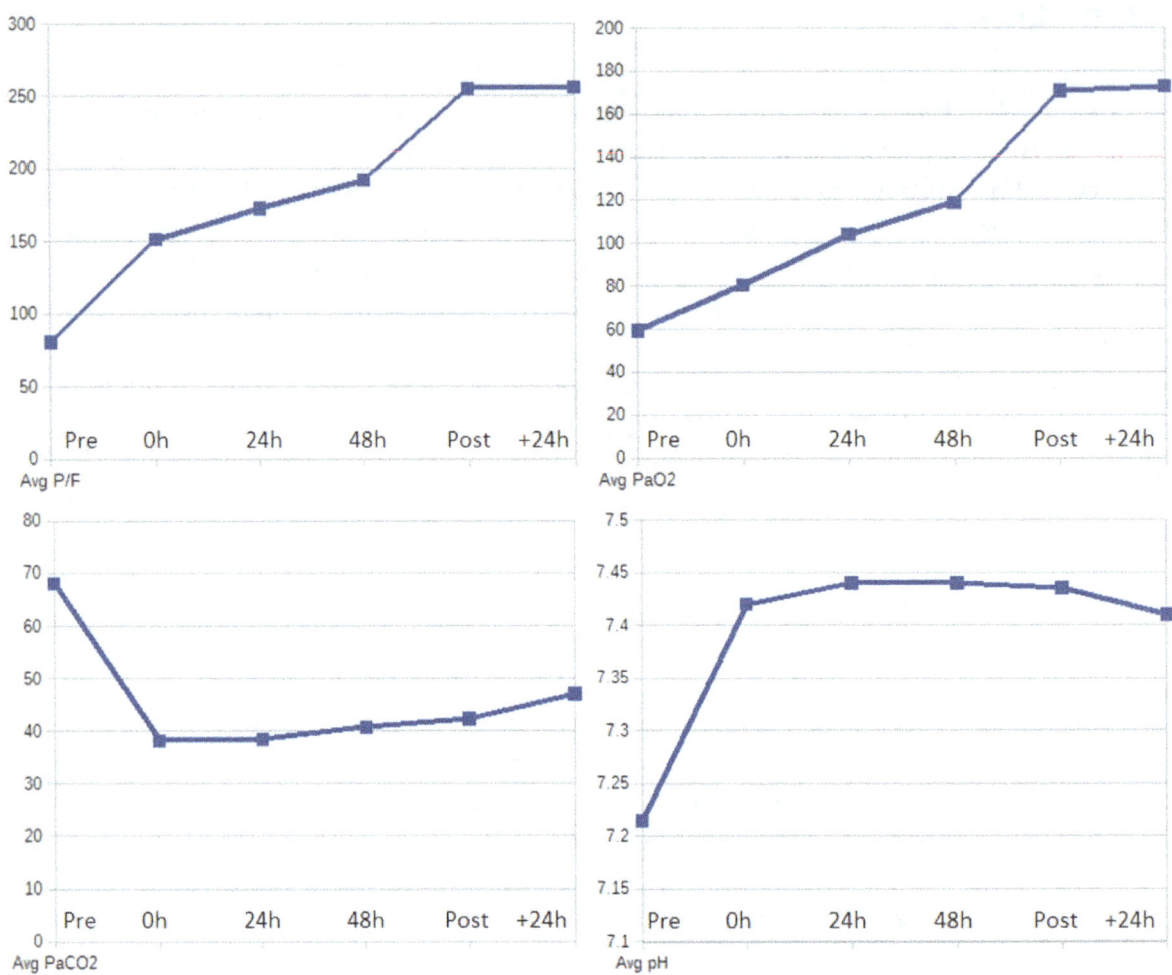

Figure 1. Simplified demonstration of the behavior of key physiologic parameters modifiable with the use of ECMO. Each graph above shows the baseline parameter value, followed by the initial post-ECMO, 24- and 48-h, and then immediate post-weaning measurements. The final value for each parameter represents average measurement for each corresponding variable at 24 h post-ECMO. (**Top left**) Average PaO_2/FiO_2 values; (**top right**) average PaO_2 values (mmHg); (**bottom left**) average $PaCO_2$ values (mmHg); (**bottom right**) average pH values. Data compiled from: Arlt et al. [33], Bonacchi et al. [110], Muellenbach et al. [89], Ried et al. [111], Wu et al. [45].

During ECMO, blood is drained from the patient's native vascular system, propagated by a mechanical pump device, and then re-introduced back into circulation [17, 29]. There are two major types of ECMO: (a) VV-ECMO and (b) VA-ECMO [30]. Both provide a support framework that is capable of essentially correcting systemic abnormalities related to catastrophic failure of pulmonary oxygenation and/or ventilation (**Figure 1**), with the main difference being the ability for VA-ECMO to actively augment systemic perfusion [30, 31]. As outlined above, systems capable of providing full pulmonary (but not cardiac) support in patients with severe hypoxemic respiratory failure are termed VV-ECMO devices [32]. Modern VV-ECMO systems take advantage of high flow rates in order to both maximize gas exchange capacity and decrease the risk of thrombotic complications, thus creating an additional potential benefit for patients with contraindications to heparin use [30, 33]. Because VV-ECMO accounts for the majority of ECMO applications in trauma, we briefly discuss basic principles of venous cannulation required for the deployment of veno-venous ECMO circuits. Cannulation for VA-ECMO is beyond the scope of the current discussion and has been described in other parts of this text.

As outlined elsewhere in this book, the VV-ECMO "inflow catheter" is typically placed in the superior vena cava (SVC) by way of right internal jugular (IJ) central venous access [12, 34]. The "outflow catheter" is typically placed in the inferior vena cava (IVC) by way of femoral central venous access [35, 36]. At the bedside, the distinction between the two can be determined visually in most cases, as the "inflow catheter" blood is generally bright red and the "outflow catheter" blood is usually darker in appearance [37]. The care of the complex trauma patient is characterized by the presence of multiple competing clinical priorities [38, 39]. Thus, providers may need to be flexible in terms of vascular access options for ECMO. For example, cervical spine injury in the trauma patient may preclude internal jugular cannulation [40]. Moreover, significant pelvic or lower extremity fractures may preclude accessing the femoral vessels [41]. Finally, significant complications have been reported during and following ECMO catheter placement, highlighting the need for providers with appropriate level of expertise to be present throughout the entire ECMO delivery process [42, 43]. Image-guided approaches may provide an added degree of procedural safety during the cannula placement process [35, 44].

During its earliest applications, ECMO in trauma required the use of substantial amounts of heparin for anticoagulation due to the risk of clot formation and circuit occlusion [29]. This, in turn, limited ECMO's use due to the potential for hemorrhagic complications in patients with traumatic brain injury, solid organ injuries, or major vascular disruption related to trauma. ECMO circuits of the past were large, bulky, difficult to transport, and not as biocompatible as systems of today [29]. However, since then, ECMO circuits have evolved into essentially portable pump-driven devices that are compact, easy to transport, and carry a much lower risk of circuit clotting due to the synergies between device miniaturization, optimization of flow rates, and heparin-bonded circuits that are more biocompatible [29, 33]. Even when systemic heparinization is required during active ECMO therapy, mortality figures continue to be better than those for comparable non-ECMO trauma patients with equivalent injury severity [45]. In one study, 67.8% of trauma patients receiving ECMO with systemic heparinization survived [45]—a number comparable to non-heparinized trauma patients [46]. Later in the chapter, we discuss the application of ECMO *without* the use of anticoagulation, including important preconditions, indications, contraindications, and risks associated with such approaches.

When full cardiopulmonary support is required for patients in circulatory failure and/or cardiogenic shock, the VA-ECMO approach is utilized [12, 32]. Because the vast majority of trauma-related ECMO applications involve severe respiratory failure (e.g., VV-ECMO) and do not involve or require the need to augment systemic perfusion (e.g., VA-ECMO), we refer the reader to portions of this book that refer to VA-ECMO applications for specialized guidance regarding the patient with refractory cardiac failure. However, when applicable, VA-ECMO use in trauma will be outlined in the context of general ECMO applicability and clinically relevant aspects central to the current discussion.

3. ECMO in trauma: general considerations, indications, and contraindications

Broadly speaking, ECMO provides the ICU team with an opportunity to ameliorate a broad range of cardiorespiratory maladies, from cardiogenic shock to refractory pulmonary failure [47–50]. In fact, ECMO may be the only clinical "bridge" for patients who otherwise would not be expected to survive the acute phase of their critical illness [47–50]. The degree to which ECMO is able to facilitate various clinical objectives depends on the principal patient diagnosis (e.g., the primary reason for extracorporeal circuit support) and the type of ECMO circuit used [12, 51–53]. In addition to improvement in key oxygenation and circulatory parameters, the vicious cycle of metabolic acidosis, coagulopathy, and hypothermia (e.g., "the lethal triad") in the polytrauma patient can be limited and even reversed with early and aggressive use of ECMO [33, 54]. In the past, ECMO was utilized as a "last resort" or a salvage therapy when all other modes of intervention had failed. However, evidence is now emerging that early ECMO implementation can limit, or even reverse, the extent of multisystem organ failure resulting from trauma-related sequelae traditionally associated with high mortality, especially in the setting of severe chest injuries [29].

In terms of specific indications and contraindications, the literature pertaining to trauma in this evolving area of cardiopulmonary circulatory support remains scant. It has been proposed that indications for ECMO in the setting of trauma should generally mirror indications in non-trauma settings, as outlined in the Extracorporeal Life Support Organization (ELSO) guidelines (**Table 1**) [55, 56]. Typically, ECMO is indicated in the setting of severe hypoxemia and/ or hypercarbia with anticipated mortality in excess of 80% using conventional ventilation strategies [56]. Consequently, patient eligibility should be determined utilizing a case-by-case, highly individualized selection process [57]. The overall risk–benefit equation must be taken into careful consideration, with general contraindications to ECMO being advanced age, the presence of significant comorbid conditions, and recent intracranial hemorrhage [56]. This selection process must also consider initiation of therapy prior to irreversible pulmonary damage and the emergence of non-preventable mortality. A delay in therapy due to stringent inclusion criteria may make any attempt at salvage moot [58]. Additional potential contraindications include the prospect of irreversible end-organ failure despite timely initiation of ECMO support, pre-ECMO ventilator support duration of >7 days, uncorrected coagulopathy, contraindication to anticoagulation, active systemic infection, recent stroke, severe peripheral arterial disease, inability to cannulate due to patient factors, and severe aortic regurgitation [57, 59, 60]. Because many of the above contraindications are viewed as being "relative" as opposed to "absolute," each patient's case must be considered individually. Perhaps more importantly, outcomes appear to be better in centers that support dedicated, highly experienced ECMO and perfusion teams (optimally able to support at least six ECMO cases per year) [56].

Inclusion criteria

Anderson et al. [46]

- Total static lung compliance <0.5 mL/cm H_2O/kg.

- Transpulmonary shunt <30% on FiO_2 >60%

- Reversible respiratory failure

- Time on mechanical ventilation ≤5 days (10 day absolute maximum)

Biderman et al. [8]

- Injury severity score (ISS) >16

- Conventional mechanical ventilation failed to control:

  ○ Hypoxemia

  ○ Hypercapnia/respiratory acidosis

Cordell-Smith et al. [75]

- Severe, but potentially reversible, respiratory failure

- Murray lung injury score >3.0 or uncompensated hypercapnia with pH <7.20

Gothner et al. [40], p. 1–6

- Hypoxemia, with PaO_2/FiO_2 of <200; FiO_2 between 0.8 and 1.0; and ventilation time >8 h

- Tidal volume >4–6 mL/kg ideal body weight

- Inspiratory pressure (P_{insp}) >32–34 mmHg

- Respiratory acidosis (pH <7.25) and/or

- Arterial oxygen saturation <90%

Michaels et al. [108]

- Potentially reversible respiratory failure

- Mechanical ventilation <7–10 days

- PaO_2/FiO_2 of <100

- Shunt fraction >30%

- Static lung compliance <0.5 mL/cm H_2O/kg or <30 mL/cm H_2O at tidal volume 10 mL/kg

- Failure to resolve the above indicators despite aggressive conventional management

Muellenbach et al. [89]

- Optimization/maximization of lung-protective ventilation strategy (tidal volume 6 mL/kg and high PEEP prior to ECMO)

- PaO_2/FiO_2 of <80, and FiO_2 >90%

Wu et al. [112]

Inclusion criteria

Anderson et al. [46]

- Severe hypoxemia, with PaO_2/FiO_2 of <60, and PEEP >10 cm H_2O despite maximal ventilator support

- Initial PaO_2/FiO_2 of <60, with rapidly deteriorating pulmonary and hemodynamic status despite maximal ventilator support

- Irreversible CO_2 retention in the presence of hemodynamic instability

Exclusion criteria

Anderson et al. [46]

- Potential for severe bleeding

- Duration of mechanical ventilation >10 days ("11 days or greater")

- Necrotizing pneumonia

- Poor quality of life (e.g., patients with metastatic malignancy, major central nervous system injury, or quadriplegia)

- Age >60 years

Biderman et al. [8]

- Age >60 years

- Prolonged mechanical ventilation (>7 days) with

  ○ Peak airway pressures >30 cm H_2O and/or

  ○ FiO_2 >80%

- Septic shock and multi-organ failure

- Non-commitment of staff/family to full treatment

Michaels et al. [108]

- Mechanical ventilation >7–10 days

- Age >60 years

- Excessive risk of central nervous system bleeding with heparinization

- Septic shock

- Advanced multi-organ failure

- Severe pulmonary hypertension (mean pulmonary artery pressure >45 mmHg or >75% systemic pressure)

- Pre-existing terminal disease

Table 1. Compilation of parameters used during the determination of ECMO suitability in various literature reports pertaining to trauma population.

After an indication for ECMO has been met, the decision regarding percutaneous cannulation versus open central cannulation has to be made [61, 62]. In addition, the provider team needs to determine whether to use anticoagulation or to proceed without anticoagulation [63–65]. This decision must consider issues not only related to initiation and maintenance but also weaning of ECMO support (e.g., ability to maintain clot-free circuit with lower flow rates) [65]. The choice of anticoagulation is also important, with alternative options available (e.g., argatroban, bivalirudin) for patients with a contraindication to heparin use (e.g., heparin-induced thrombocytopenia) [64, 66]. Some additional considerations include potential/relative contraindications to ECMO, such as severe aortic regurgitation, severe peripheral arterial disease, uncontrolled sepsis, bleeding diathesis, recent cerebrovascular accident (CVA), or an irreversible cause for the end-organ failure being treated [59]. Previous studies show short-term survival rates between 35% and 83% among patients who appropriately receive ECMO, depending on patient population and primary disease characteristics [67–71]. Additionally, the Conventional Ventilation or ECMO for Severe Acute Respiratory Failure (CESAR) trial showed that patients referred to an ECMO center had a significant increase in survival without disability at 6 months compared to conventional management (63% versus 47%, respectively) [72]. Of note, the CESAR study included a small subset of trauma patients [72]. From this point forward, this chapter focuses on the use of ECMO as a supportive therapy in critically ill trauma patients with respiratory failure.

4. ECMO for refractory respiratory failure in trauma

Approximately 0.5% of all adult trauma patients may be at risk of developing severe respiratory failure or ARDS, with the incidence increasing to 10–20% in multiply injured, high-risk patients [1]. The list of potential causes for trauma-related respiratory distress is heterogeneous and includes pulmonary contusions, fat emboli from long bone/pelvic fractures, thermal injuries, massive transfusion, traumatic brain injury, infection/sepsis, and severe pancreatic trauma, among other etiologies [73–77]. Veno-venous ECMO can be employed to improve systemic physiologic parameters while facilitating pulmonary rest and promoting healing of the lung in patients with the most severe chest injuries and worsening/refractory respiratory failure. Among some of the reported clinical scenarios where VV-ECMO has been successfully utilized are post-traumatic pneumonectomy, bronchopleural fistulas, tracheal injury, and severe/refractory respiratory failure associated with various primary causes [29, 54, 78–81]. For more cardiac-specific indications, including traumatic cardiac injury, VA-ECMO has been utilized [54, 82–84].

As suggested in previous sections of this chapter, early use of ECMO in trauma-related severe respiratory failure may improve outcomes and limit the extent of the post-injury "lethal triad" of acidosis, hypothermia, and coagulopathy that ultimately leads to multisystem organ failure and mortality [29, 46, 58, 85]. In order for VV-ECMO to produce optimal outcomes, a high degree of clinical vigilance, early diagnosis, and prompt management of refractory respiratory failure are required. Clinicians must be familiar with, and recognize the "vulnerable phase" of lung injury. The typical time frame during which pulmonary injury peaks in severity is between 48 and 96 h [86]. Thus, it is logical that pre-ECMO mechanical ventilatory support of >7 days portends poor outcome [46, 57].

The majority of traumatic pulmonary contusions improve with conservative treatment alone; however, patients with involvement of >20% of the lung volume have been shown to progress to more severe respiratory failure in as many as 80% of cases [87]. Moreover, severe pulmonary contusions may be associated with findings of blood-filled pneumatoceles, lung lacerations, and multiple fractured ribs; the presence of which may further increase the already elevated mortality of the polytrauma patient [29, 88, 89].

Another special consideration is the clinical scenario of traumatic pneumonectomy, with the potential to cause severe acute right heart failure, potentially leading to refractory hypoxemia and very high mortality rates [29, 78]. In this setting, VV-ECMO may be considered as a life-saving therapy that helps minimize various post-trauma pneumonectomy physiologic derangements [29]. In other reports, ECMO was used to facilitate successful repair of ruptured mitral papillary muscle [90], resection of post-traumatic ruptured lung abscess with empyema [91], and postoperative cardiorespiratory support following repair of traumatic aorto-right atrial fistula and tricuspid valve rupture [92].

5. ECMO in the setting of neurologic (brain and spinal cord) injury

Ensuring adequate tissue oxygenation remains a basic tenet of neurologic injury management. The ability to maintain adequate arterial oxygen saturation can prevent secondary brain injury and mitigate against poor outcomes [93]. Due to the simultaneous presence of significant pulmonary injury and brain trauma, the risk of mortality and morbidity may be greater than that of each individual organ system failure in isolation. The need for systemic anticoagulation with ECMO has historically precluded the use of this modality in patients with traumatic brain injury. However, advances in the circuit flow characteristics and oxygenator technology now allow for heparin bonding of the circuit [94]. This in turn reduces the need for anticoagulation during VV-ECMO therapy, thus decreasing the odds of hemorrhagic complications such as cavitary or intracranial bleeding [89].

Firstenberg et al. [95] published a case report of a 27-year-old male involved in a motor vehicle collision. The patient was intubated at the scene and upon hospital arrival was hypothermic with severe mixed respiratory and metabolic acidosis. Due to refractory nature of the patient's respiratory failure, salvage VV-ECMO was utilized as a life-saving "bridge" to pulmonary recovery. Of note, the patient had massive pulmonary contusions, multifocal intraparenchymal brain hemorrhages, as well as intraventricular and subdural blood on computed tomography (CT) imaging [95]. Repeat head CT scans on post-trauma days 1 and 5 showed no significant intracranial changes following the initiation of VV-ECMO [95]. It should be pointed out that due to the concerns for intracranial hemorrhagic complications, the patient received only 10,000 units of heparin systemically before percutaneous femoral-femoral VV-ECMO cannulation and no heparin for 48 h thereafter. Because the lack of heparin anticoagulation posed concerns for clotting of the circuit, frequent evaluations of the VV-ECMO circuit (e.g., every 6–8 h) were instituted, with no evidence found of clot formation within the circuit. There were no apparent inefficiencies of gas exchange noted [95]. Following a 96-h course of VV-ECMO, the patient underwent decannulation. On post-trauma day 23, he was transferred to an inpatient rehabilitation facility [95]. Muelenbach et al. likewise reported successful application of VV-ECMO without continuous anticoagulation and only heparin-coated cannulas and circuits for up to 5 days in patients with ARDS and traumatic brain injuries [89].

In another report, a 31-year-old male suffered severe bilateral pulmonary contusions, a right pneumothorax, traumatic frontal brain contusions, subdural hemorrhage, and right main bronchus disruption [96]. Definitive repair of bronchial disruption was feasible utilizing ECMO as "bridge" therapy. Although VV-ECMO was the preferred "bridge" to bronchial repair, due to concerns for right heart failure, VA-ECMO was chosen in this particular case. Because the cannulation catheter used was not heparin coated, low-dose heparin was used during pre-cannulation and VA-ECMO, without worsening of the patient's traumatic brain injuries [96].

Veno-venous ECMO has also been used in a patient with spinal cord injury [44]. An 18-year-old victim of a vehicular crash sustained multiple traumatic injuries, including left hemothorax, intracerebral bleeding, and complete paraplegia. After developing severe respiratory failure, the patient was placed on VV-ECMO "rescue" therapy. Interestingly, the cannulation was performed using fluoroscopy, without anticoagulation, and involved a double-lumen catheter inserted via the right IJ vein. The patient subsequently improved, was successfully weaned from VV-ECMO after 1 week, and was eventually transferred to a rehabilitation facility [44]. In another report, a small subset of patients with spinal cord injury underwent VV-ECMO for post-traumatic ARDS, without reported neurologic sequelae [40].

6. ECMO in polytrauma: managing the risk of traumatic hemorrhage

The use of ECMO has been reported in trauma patients with a range of severe blunt and penetrating injuries [14, 97]. Polytrauma, in turn, presents the treating physician with a number of competing priorities [38, 39]. Wen et al. [98] reported on successful use of VV-ECMO in a 19-year-old motorcyclist with severe hypoxia on presentation. His subsequent trauma evaluation showed significant right-sided lung contusions, pulmonary aspiration, as well as a grade IV liver laceration (without evidence of active bleeding) [98]. A non-heparinized VV-ECMO circuit was used for 5 days without major complications [98].

Fortenberry et al. [97] described five children and three adults with median duration of pre-ECMO mechanical ventilation of 6 days. Reported injuries included four liver lacerations, three pulmonary contusions, as well as renal trauma. Four patients underwent pre-ECMO laparotomies, including three splenectomies. Of note, the majority of patients (seven of eight) in that series underwent VV-ECMO, and significant bleeding was reported in seven patients while on ECMO [97]. The authors classified hemorrhagic complications of ECMO as "manageable." Survival in the pediatric subset of patients was 80% [97]. Similarly, Madershahian et al. [54] described successful ECMO use in patients with severe blunt injuries including pulmonary contusions, bronchial rupture, multiple fractures, and abdominal trauma. The authors encourage prompt institution of ECMO for the temporary management of gas exchange in trauma patients with refractory respiratory failure [54].

In another report, a patient with grade III liver laceration and blunt chest trauma complicated by endobronchial hemorrhage was treated with VV-ECMO [99]. The patient was maintained on low-dose heparin to maintain the activated partial thromboplastin time (aPTT) around 1.5–2.0 times normal, with no complications noted. The reported duration of VV-ECMO therapy in this case was 10 days [99]. Diffuse pulmonary hemorrhage may result from massive pulmonary contusions. In such cases, hemostasis may be difficult to achieve, even with surgical resection. Employment of single lung ventilation may be used, coupled with VV-ECMO and frequent bronchoscopic lavage [95]. Skarda et al. [14] reported on ECMO use in children with severe traumatic injuries, including open reduction and internal fixation and endoscopic procedures while on active extracorporeal support.

7. ECMO as bridge to definitive surgical management

Across various scenarios outlined in previous sections of this chapter, ECMO was believed to be the main factor contributing to patient survival in potentially futile situations. At times, patient survival is possible without the use of ECMO; however, definitive surgical repair may not be possible without extracorporeal support. Finally, ECMO may be necessary for both survival and definitive repair of injuries.

Gatti et al [9] published a case of a 27-year-old man who sustained a 4-cm-wide stab wound to the fifth left intercostal space, resulting in cardiac injury evidenced by a massive left hemothorax and a pericardial effusion. The patient experienced acute clinical decompensation, developed pulseless electrical activity (PEA) arrest, and underwent an emergency department implementation of VA-ECMO (using left internal jugular vein inflow and right femoral artery outflow) at flow rates between 4.5 and 5.0 L/min [9]. A median sternotomy was then performed, with drainage of a pericardial effusion, repair of a right ventricular injury and repair of an injured branch of the right coronary artery. This was followed by return of adequate cardiac function [9]. Overall, the patient underwent >40 minutes of cardiopulmonary resuscitation and was cannulated on VA-ECMO for approximately 120 minutes, with 350 units/kg of heparin administered during the duration of extracorporeal support [9]. Other than a mild postpericardiotomy syndrome, the patient recovered from his injury without neurological sequelae [9]. Other scenarios where ECMO was instrumental to satisfactory clinical outcomes following major cardiac trauma includ repair of ruptured mitral papillary muscle [90] and postoperative cardiorespiratory support following repair of traumatic aorto-right atrial fistula and tricuspid valve rupture [92].

Major airway trauma, including bronchopleural fistulae, has an associated mortality in excess of 30% [100]. In one case, VV-ECMO was used in the setting of severe hypoxemia as a bridge to surgical management of major bronchial injury [101]. A 31-year-old male sustained multiple injuries following an automobile collision, including a right-sided hemopneumothorax, cerebral contusion, subarachnoid and subdural hemorrhages, bilateral pulmonary contusions, and a right main stem bronchial tear that was immediately repaired operatively. On postoperative day 5, the patient developed complete occlusion of the right main stem bronchus, with severe respiratory failure and hemodynamic instability. Consequently, the patient was placed on a VA-ECMO circuit utilizing low-dose heparin to help facilitate the definitive surgical airway repair. The authors reported that they would have considered VV-ECMO if the patient was hemodynamically stable [101].

Ballouhey et al. [102] utilized ECMO in a 32-month-old girl who sustained major tracheobronchial trauma after being struck by a vehicle. Initial diagnostic imaging showed the endotracheal tube to be outside of the trachea. Due to the presence of hemodynamic instability, VA-ECMO was selected for the surgical repair. Of note, the authors did point out that in the presence of hemodynamic stability, VV-ECMO can be used to support patients in need of surgical correction of major tracheobronchial disruptions [102]. In some cases of unilateral pulmonary or bronchial trauma, either single-lung (e.g., selective ventilation of only one lung) or differential-lung (e.g., each lung managed independently via separate ventilator-tracheal tube circuits) ventilation can be coupled with ECMO to ensure adequate oxygenation while the healing of contralateral traumatic injury is taking place [103]. Following surgical repair of the airway, postoperative continuation of ECMO may be deemed appropriate because (a) healing of operatively repaired tissue may be otherwise affected or compromised [29] or (b) the patient may not be able to immediately wean off the extracorporeal support [92].

8. ECMO: summary of single-center experiences

A number of valuable single-center experiences have been reported, demonstrating successful use of VV-ECMO in trauma. Key findings from these studies are presented in **Table 2** and **Figure 2**. The subsequent discussion focuses on the most important "take-home" messages from this cumulative body of literature. In addition to supporting the notion that in carefully selected trauma patients ECMO can improve survival, there is emerging evidence that the performance of surgical procedures on extracorporeal support is safe, including repeated damage control operations [104–106].

Back in mid-1990s, Anderson et al. [46] presented a single-institution experience with 24 multiply injured patients treated with ECMO for refractory respiratory failure. Both VV-ECMO and VA-ECMO was utilized, with all patients receiving systemic heparinization. Hemorrhagic complications were reported in 75% of patients. The overall survival to hospital discharge was 63%, with early initiation of ECMO (<5 days) being associated with better outcomes [46]. In another early experience, Senunas et al. [107] reported on 14 multiply injured patients who sustained severe skeletal trauma and progressed to refractory respiratory failure. Consistent with data provided by others [46, 108], this study also showed improved survival when ECMO was initiated early (87% survival for <6 pre-ECMO ventilator days versus 16.7% survival for >6 pre-ECMO ventilator days) [107]. Michaels et al. further quantify the importance of early ECMO initiation in a series of 30 trauma patients, with associated odds ratio of 7.2 for patient survival when the duration of pre-ECMO ventilator support was ≤5 days [108].

Study	Patient data	ELS data	Complications	Mortality/survival	Comment
Anderson et al. [46]	N = 24. Mixed pediatric and adult population	Duration of ELS: 287 ± 43 h (12 ± 1.8 day); Heparinization: All patients; Circuit-related complications: Oxygenator failure: 8.3%; Raceway/tubing rupture: 8.3%; Pump failure: 4.2%; Circuit change: 25%	Hemorrhage: 75%; Renal failure: 21%; Cardiac: 12.5%; Stroke or intracranial bleeding: 21%; Pneumothorax: 8.3%	Survival to discharge from hospital: 63%; Time to ELS: Survivors 3.8 ± 0.8 days; Deceased 10 ± 1.4 days	Both VV-ECMO and VA-ECMO was utilized; Early intervention (e.g., ≤5 days to ECMO) was associated with better outcomes; Reduced anticoagulation levels were utilized in a patient with closed head injury and depressed skull fracture
Serunas et al. [107]	N = 14 (4 male; 10 female); Survivors: Mean ISS 19 (9–34); Mean GCS 14.5 (12–15); Non-survivors: Mean ISS 18 (11–29); Mean GCS 13.3 (6–15)	MV prior to ECMO: 6 days (1–19 days); Duration of ECMO: 240 h (50–624 h)	Hemorrhage: 57.1%	Overall survival: 57.1%; Survival for patients with <6 pre-ECMO ventilator days: 87.5%; Survival for patients with >6 pre-ECMO ventilator days: 16.7%	The study involved 14 multiply injured patients with major orthopedic trauma; 5 of 14 patients underwent surgical procedures while on ECMO; Consistent with experience reported by Anderson, et al., early initiation of ECMO was associated with better survival
Michaels et al. [108]	N = 30 (15 male; 15 female); Age 26.3 ± 2.1 years (15.59 years); Mean ISS 19.8 ± 2.2; Mean PaO_2/FiO_2 56.9 ± 5.4	Duration of ECMO: 237.8 ± 36.9; Circuit-related problems: Oxygenator change: 24%; Pump complication: 7%; Tubing change: 21%	Acute renal failure: 55%; Hemorrhage: 59%; Infection: 28% (positive cultures); Pneumothorax: 31%; Neurologic: 14%	Survival to discharge: 50%; Early use of ECMO (≤5 vent days) was associated with odds ratio of 7.2 for survival	Fewer ventilator days and more normal SvO_2 were associated with survival; Numerous patients underwent surgical procedures while on ECMO, including tracheostomy (50%), laparotomy (13%), thoracotomy (3%), femoral artery repair (3%), and open reduction of lower extremity fracture (3%)
Cordell-Smith et al. [75]	N = 28; Age 27 years; Mean ISS 18; Mean PaO_2/FiO_2 62; Lung injury score 3.1 (Murray)	Pre-ECMO MV: 69 h; Duration of ECMO: 141 h; Heparinization: All patients received systemic heparin, with activated clotting time targets between 180 and 220 s	Complication data not provided	Overall survival: 71.4%; Of interest, survivors had higher mean ISS (19) than non-survivors (14)	Mean time to ECMO was 61 h for survivors versus 87 h for non-survivors
Huang et al. [109]	N = 9; Age 35.1 ± 9.7 years (18–47 years); Mean ISS 44.56 ± 4.93 (35–50); Mean SOFA 12.1 ± 3.67 (7–16); Mean PaO_2 49.04 ± 9.82 mmHg (31–64); Mean $PaCO_2$ 66.4 ± 15.72 mmHg (45–86)	Time from injury to ECMO: 33 h (4–384 h); Duration of ECMO: 145 h (69–456 h)	Colonic rupture with sepsis: 1 patient (11%); Liver failure: 11%	Survival to discharge: 77.8%	VA-ECMO: 2 patients; VV-ECMO: 7 patients; 6 patients (66.7%) received additional surgeries while on ECMO
Arlt et al. [33]	N = 10 (8 male; 2 female); Age 34.8 years (21–62 years); Mean ISS 73 ± 4; $PaCO_2$ 67 (36–89); Median norepinephrine demand 3 mg/h (1.0–13.5)	Duration of ECMO: 5 days (0.5–11 days); The authors report on the use of a new miniaturized ECMO device, with initial therapy performed without heparinization	Sepsis/ Multi-organ failure: 30%	Overall hospital survival: 60%	VV-ECMO:7 patients; VA-ECMO: 3 patients; The study describes the use of ECMO in actively hemorrhaging patients
Biderman et al. [8]	N = 10 (6 male; 4 female); Age 29.8 ± 7.7 years (19–42); Mean ISS 50.3 ± 10.5 (29–57); PaO_2/FiO_2: ECMO 62 (35–82); iLA 92 (78–140); $PaCO_2$: ECMO 62 (48–95); iLA 85 (65–150); (+) Traumatic brain injury	Time to ECMO: 3 days (1–7 days); Time to iLA: 5 days (3–8 days); Duration of ECMO: 9.5 ± 4.5 days	Cannula related: Bleeding: 10%; Accidental removal: 10%; Pressure ulcer: 30%; Sepsis: 20%; Cardiogenic shock: 10%	ECMO survival: 60%; iLA survival: 80%	iLA Circuit: 5 patients; ECMO: 5 patients; iLA is a pumpless extrapulmonary gas exchange system (http://www.novalung.com/en/home)

Study	Patient data	ELS data	Complications	Mortality/survival	Comment
Bonacchi et al. [110]	N = 14 (10 male; 4 female); Age 47 ± 17.6 years; Mean ISS 46.5 ± 16.3; (+) Damage control surgery	Time from trauma to ECMO: 351.8 ± 242 min (145–950 min); Duration of ECMO: 128.7 ± 113 h (24–384 h); Heparin-free time on ECMO: 20.7 ± 19.8 h; Blood transfusion: 11.9 ± 5.3 units; rFVIIa administration during ECMO: 50%; Heparinization: ECMO circuit used was heparin-coated; systemic heparin was held in cases of bleeding (mean delay of 16.7 ± 19 h, range 2.5–72 h); Titration to mean aPTT of 40–50 s / activated clotting time of 160–180 s; Initially, 18 patients were considered for ECMO; however, due to inability to maintain adequate circuit flow and perfusion on VA-ECMO, only 14 patients were successfully treated	Renal failure requiring VV hemofiltration: 50%; Hepatic insufficiency: 14.2%; Sepsis: 21.4%; Leg ischemia: 7.1%; Oxygenator failure: 7.1%	ECMO survival: 35.7%; Organ donation: 42.9%; Death (w/o organ donation): 21.4%; All cases ($n = 4$) with inability to establish or maintain circuit flow/perfusion died	VV-ECMO: 4 patients; VA-ECMO: 10 patients; Cardiac index, mean arterial pressure, blood lactate, PaO_2, $PaCO_2$, and pH normalized within 3.5 ± 1.5 h of ECMO initiation; Intra-aortic balloon pump was used in 2 patients
Ried et al. [111]	N = 52 (49 male; 3 female); Age 32 ± 14 years (16–72 years); Mean BMI 28.2 ± 6.1; Mean ISS 58.9 ± 10.5; Mean LIS 3.3 ± 0.60; Mean SOFA 10.5 ± 3.0; PaO_2/FiO_2 63 (49–101); $PaCO_2$ 67 (50–87); Lactate 28 (14–49) mg/dL	Pre-ELS MV: 3.2 ± 4.1 day (0–21 days); Time to ELS: 5.2 ± 7.7 days (0–38 days); Duration of ELS: 6.9 ± 3.6 days (<1–19 days); ELS flow rate (L/min): 2.3 ± 0.9 (0.7–4.6); Duration of MV: 18.4 ± 10.6 days (1–51 days); ICU/ hospital stay: 22 days (14–32)/ 25 days (16–41); Surgical procedure: 86.5%; Thoracic procedure: 15.4%; Surgery with ELS: 30.8%	Cannula-related: PECLA 19% VV-ECMO 12%; RRT: 30.8%	8 (15.4%) during ELS support 3 (6%) after ELS weaning; Hospital mortality: 21%; Overall survival: 79%	VV-ECMO: 26 patients; pECLA: 26 patients; pECLA: Pumpless extracorporeal lung assist
Tseng et al. [104]	N = 9 (8 male; 1 female); Age 37 years (IQR 26.5–46 years); Median ISS 34 (IQR 15.5–41); (+) Damage control surgery	Median time to VA-ECMO: 6 h (IQR 4–47.5); Median duration of ECMO: 91 h (IQR 43–187)	Hemorrhage: 22%	Survival to discharge: 33%	VA-ECMO: 9 patients
Wu et al. [45]	N = 20; Age 38 years (22–61 years); Median ISS 35 (19–75); (+) Intracranial hemorrhage; (+) Damage control surgery	Time from trauma to ECMO: 64 h (IQR 12–230); Median duration of pre-ECMO ventilation: 45 h (IQR 8–148); Median ECMO duration: Survivors: 144 h (74–196 h) Deceased: 232 h (36–575 h); Post- ECMO intubation: 231 h (61–476 h); Hospital days: Survivors: 69 days (27–81 days) Deceased: 32 days (4–46 days)	Hemorrhage: 35%; CVVH: 35%; Tracheostomy: 40%	Overall survival: 70%; Age (survivors): 41 years (29–57); Age (non-survivors): 30 years (22–61 years); ISS (survivors): 29 (19–43); ISS (non-survivors): 63 (26–75); Mortality from sepsis: 15%	VV-ECMO: 20 patients; "Heparin-minimized" strategy was utilized in 55% of patients
Wu et al. [112]	N = 19 (17 male; 2 female); Age 38 years (25–58 years); Median ISS 29 (25–34); Median APACHE II 25 (21–36); PaO_2/FiO_2 60 (48–65); (+) Brain hemorrhage	Median blood transfusion: 5500 mL (3,500–13,000); Heparinization: 16 patients (84.2%); ICU duration: 16.8 ± 9.37 days	Pneumonia: 15.8%; Coagulopathy: 10.5%; Need for CVVH: 37%	Overall survival: 68.4%; Age (survivors): 30 years (21–39); Age (non- survivors): 53 years (48–63 years)	VV-ECMO: 9 patients; VA-ECMO: 10 patients; Five patients had pre-ECMO traumatic brain hemorrhage (3/5 or 60% survived); Mortality in heparin group was 5/16 (31.3%) Gothner et al. [40]
Gothner et al. [40]	N = 6 (all male); Age 45 years (31–54 years); Mean ISS 31 (20–48); (+) Spinal cord injury; (+) Minor brain injury	Time to ELS: 3 ± 5 days (0–13 days); Duration of ELS: 7 ± 5 days (6–18 days); ICU stay: 21 ± 7 days (13–30 days); Hospital stay: 60 ± 34 days (21–105 days); Blood transfusion: 8 Units (2–20 U) PRBC	Cannula related: 17% (thrombosis); Urethral bleeding: 17%; Acute renal failure: 17%; VAP: 83%	Overall survival: 100%	VV-ECMO: 6 patients; Authors describe the use of double lumen cannula placed via right IJ approach

Table 2. Important characteristics of major clinical studies of ECMO in trauma (1994–2015).

Cordell et al. [75] treated 28 multiply injured patients suffering from severe respiratory failure with VV-ECMO. In that series, patients received "limited anticoagulation" using intravenous heparin, with activated clotting times between 180 and 220 s [75]. The overall survival was 71.4%, with shorter "time to ECMO" associated with better survival (e.g., 61 h for survivors versus 87 h for non-survivors) [75]. Huang et al. describe 78% survival in nine trauma patients undergoing ECMO [109]. In that series, two-thirds of patients underwent additional surgeries while on extracorporeal support [109]. Arlt et al. [33] treated 10 multiply injured patients with hemorrhagic shock using a miniaturized ECMO circuit, without initial systemic heparinization. The 60% reported survival is very impressive given the mean ISS of 73 for the study cohort [33]. Others have found that independent predictors of mortality in trauma patients undergoing ECMO include ISS >63, pH <7.01 (mean of last three evaluations), and blood lactate of >14.4 mmol/L (mean of last three evaluations) [110].

Gothner et al. [40] published clinical experience based on six patients with major trauma (mean injury severity score [ISS], 31) and post-traumatic severe respiratory failure who were supported with VV-ECMO using a double lumen cannula. The authors reported mean pre-ECMO hospitalization of 3 days, mean ECMO run times of 7 days, mean hospital stays of 60 days, and 100% survival for the 6 study patients [40]. It was noted that the double lumen cannula utilized was not heparin coated and thus heparin dosages had to be adjusted to maintain the prothrombin time (PTT) in the range of 50–60. As such, this approach in patients

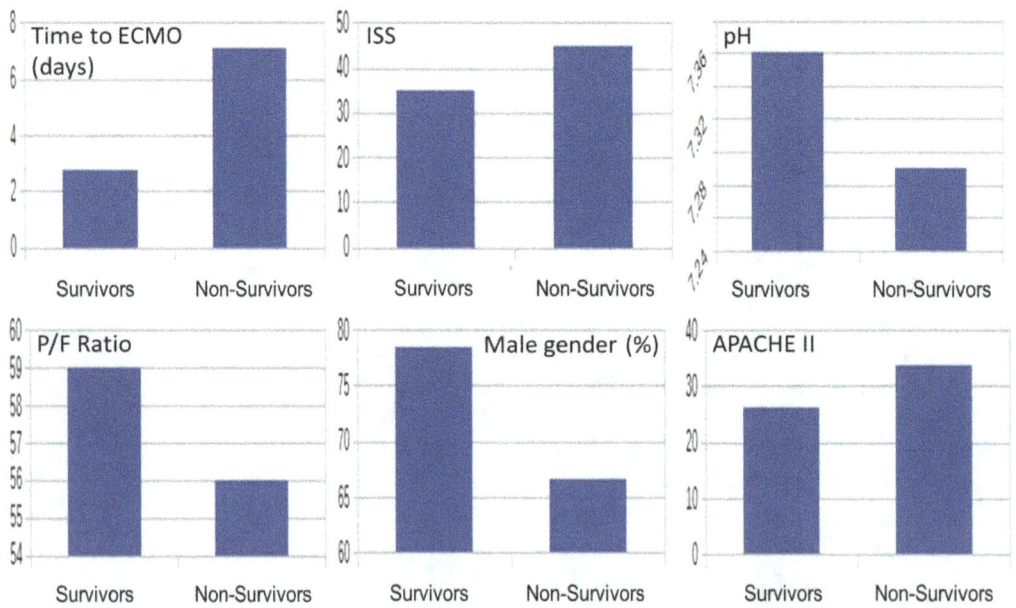

Figure 2. Comparison of important baseline parameters for trauma survivors and non-survivors, compiled from key single-center ECMO experiences. (**Top left**) Time from injury to ECMO (days); (**top middle**) injury severity score (ISS); (**top right**) pH values; (**bottom left**) PaO₂/FiO₂ ratio; (**bottom middle**) male gender (%); (**bottom right**) APACHE II score. Data compiled from: Anderson et al. [46], Arlt et al. [33], Biderman et al. [8], Cordell-Smith et al. [75], Michaels et al. [108], Senunas et al. [107], Wu et al. [45, 112].

who are at elevated risk of bleeding is controversial, despite the report finding no substantial elevation in the risk of bleeding among study patients [40].

Another study retrospectively looked at a single-center experience with VV-ECMO over a 10-year period. The authors focused on critically injured trauma patients with mean ISS of nearly 59 and the sequential organ failure assessment (SOFA) scores of 10.5 [111]. Within the sample of 52 patients, 26 received pumpless extracorporeal lung assist (PECLA) and the other 26 underwent VV-ECMO [111]. In this series, mean time to extracorporeal support was 5.2 days, average support duration of was 6.9 days, many patients underwent surgery while on extracorporeal support, and cannula-related complications occurred in 15% of patients (19% PECLA; 12% VV-ECMO) [111]. Overall survival was 79% compared to predicted survival of 59% (estimated from ISS data). The authors additionally noted that patients with elevated risk of hemorrhagic complications or evidence of intracranial bleeding were not started on heparin during the initial 48 h. After securing evidence that bleeding is controlled (e.g., repeat CT scan imaging), heparin was started slowly and target PTT set at approximately 40–50 s [111].

Wu et al. [112] studied 19 patients treated with ECMO for severe lung injury and respiratory failure. The most common mechanism of pulmonary injury was blunt trauma, with median patient age of 38 years, median ISS of 29, median Acute Physiology and Chronic Health Evaluation II (APACHE II) score of 25, and median blood transfusion volume of 5.5 L [112]. The overall survival within this cohort was 68% (13 of 19 patients), with survivors being younger (30 years) than non-survivors (53 years) [112]. There were five patients (26% of total) with traumatic brain hemorrhage, of whom three survived (60% of brain trauma group) [112]. Sixteen out of 19 patients (84%) received heparin during VV-ECMO therapy, with 5 mortalities noted in that group (31%). In addition to demonstrating potential benefits of VV-ECMO in multiply injured patients, the authors also emphasize the value of timely ECMO intervention [112].

Biderman et al. [8] published another important single-center experience using ECMO in trauma. A total of 10 patients (mean age 30 years; mean ISS of 50; 60% male) received ECMO therapy. Within this group, all patients suffered from blunt trauma and severe thoracic injuries, with vascular and abdominal solid organ injuries being the most common. Mean ECMO support time was 9.5 days [8]. Seven patients within the group had traumatic brain injury, with four exhibiting active intracranial hemorrhage. Coagulopathy was prevalent before institution of VV-ECMO in this group. Consistent with other reports outlined in this chapter, the authors point out that complications related to the extracorporeal support therapy were manageable and non-lethal [8]. Reported complications included bleeding from the cannula-tion site, dislodged cannula, and pressure ulcers. Mortalities were attributed to sepsis (two cases) and cardiogenic shock (one case) [8]. Of importance, the authors were able to demonstrate clinical success of high-flow ECMO technique without anticoagulation, especially in patients with coagulopathy or traumatic brain injury. This experience shows that even in patients with acute and active hemorrhage, meaningful benefits can be gained from utilizing ECMO [8].

9. ECMO: weaning and liberation

Because the increasing duration of ECMO support is associated with greater mortality, extracorporeal support weaning should be a constant consideration for patients undergoing this therapy [113]. Thus, as soon as a patient is identified as a candidate for ECMO wean, the process should begin promptly and follow a protocolized course toward the goal of liberation from dependence on extracorporeal oxygenation [113]. In general, weaning for patients on VV-ECMO for severe respiratory failure should be considered based on improvements in pulmonary compliance, chest radiography characteristics, and arterial oxygenation indices [12, 57]. This can be followed by a "weaning trial" where blood flow through the circuit is maintained, but gas transfer is temporarily (up to several hours) stopped [12, 57]. For patients on VA-ECMO for cardiac failure, important considerations prior to weaning therapy should include echocardiographic findings (preferably transesophageal), aortic pulsatility, and a successful "off-ECMO trial" that consists of temporary clamping of the drainage and infusion lines while maintaining a temporary bridge between the arterio-venous conduits [57, 114, 115].

10. The financial impact of ECMO

Due to resource utilization and the overall level of intensive care afforded to affected patients, ECMO is recognized as a labor intensive and costly intervention. In 1993, Schumacher et al. [116] demonstrated that early ECMO in infants was cost-effective when compared to late ECMO or "no ECMO" controls. In 2005, Mahle et al. [117] reported on the cost utility of salvage ECMO following surgery for congenital heart abnormalities. Based on their financial analysis, the authors concluded the calculated cost-utility for salvage extracorporeal membrane oxygenation in this population was $24,386 per quality-adjusted life-year saved, which would be considered within the range of acceptable cost-efficacy. The CESAR trial evaluated cost based on in-hospital expense, as well as the economic burden of services required during follow-up for ECMO patients and their families [72]. The authors reported that mean costs per patient in the group who underwent ECMO were £73,979 (approximately $116,502) over a period of 6 months. Based on cost-benefit analysis, the United Kingdom National Health Service declared ECMO treatment, at a referral center, to be cost-effective even though the mean costs of patients receiving ECMO were higher compared to the control arm. A caveat to this conclusion is that dollar-for-dollar cost in a non-single party payer system (e.g., the USA) may vary considerably [72].

11. Miscellaneous topics

11.1. Analgo-sedation

ECMO applications mandate the ability to control patient activity and ensure adequate analgesia and sedation [118, 119]. It has been noted that VA-ECMO is associated with significantly greater doses of sedation than VV-ECMO [119]. The current understanding of how different ECMO circuits affect pharmacokinetic characteristics of certain drugs (e.g., antibiotics, sedatives, analgesics) is incomplete [118, 120]. Over the past few years, evidence has emerged that periodic sedation and analgesia interruptions, and even allowing patients to remain awake may be beneficial to both short- and long-term ECMO outcomes [118, 121]. In fact, such daily interruptions help facilitate patient mobilization and even ambulation [17, 122, 123]. However, this is not without risks. The importance of adequate analgo-sedation optimization is highlighted by a case of major hemorrhage requiring cardiopulmonary resuscitation following ECMO cannula dislodgement in a conscious, spontaneously breathing patient [124]. The applicability of the "awake ECMO" concept in trauma is probably limited, mainly due to the generally transient requirement for extracorporeal support in this population, as well as the significant analgo-sedation requirement secondary to multiple injuries (e.g., not directly related to ECMO).

11.2. Organ donation

Trauma is one of the leading causes of death, with traumatic brain injury being a major contributor to the overall trauma mortality [39, 125]. Brain death following trauma is numerically one of the major sources of organs donated for transplantation [125]. Balsorano et al. [126] reported on successful use of VA-ECMO as a tool for organ preservation prior to organ procurement. The authors pointed out the myriad of complex physiologic disturbances that occur following brain death, emphasizing potential barriers to organ recovery such as cardiac arrest and refractory cardiopulmonary collapse [126, 127]. The use of ECMO to optimize organs from non-heart-beating donors (e.g., donation after cardiac death) is not a new concept [128]. Gravel et al. [129] describe the use of ECMO to facilitate renal transplantation from organ donors following cardiopulmonary death.

11.3. Multidisciplinary approach to ECMO

The authors of this chapter feel strongly that promotion of a multidisciplinary approach to trauma patients undergoing ECMO therapy is essential. In most of the published literature, patients enrolled in the ECMO arms of the trial were at tertiary referral centers that were replete with expertise in cardiac surgery, perfusion, advanced ventilator strategies, and specialized critical care. Trauma centers embarking on an ECMO program need to ensure that these specialties have reviewed pertinent treatment protocols and safety standards involved in the implementation of extracorporeal support. Also, we recommend involving the ELSO to help with credentialing and performance improvement initiatives for any center considering ECMO as a treatment option. As outlined earlier in this chapter, one of the most significant advantages of modern ECMO circuits is their portability. This facilitates ECMO implementation in a variety of settings, including the emergency department, the operating room, and the ICU [110]. Consequently, multidisciplinary participation in institutional ECMO programs should include representation from all key departments and stakeholders, from cardiovascular surgery to emergency medicine.

12. Conclusions

Improvements in biocompatibility, miniaturization, and portability of modern ECMO circuits have increased the safety profile and clinical utility of this extracorporeal support option. In turn, this has resulted in an expanding range of clinical applications of ECMO, including its increasing use in the trauma patient with refractory circulatory and respiratory failure. Clinical approaches once considered to be futile and controversial are now available as life-saving strategies for patients who otherwise would not be able to survive. Important challenges remain to greater ECMO implementation in the trauma population, including the use of anticoagulation and better optimization of patient selection. Trauma centers contemplating an ECMO program should seek buy-in from the services who will be intimately involved in the care of the patient as well as organizations dedicated to ensuring the quality and efficiency of extracorporeal support program.

Author details

Ronson Hughes, James Cipolla, Peter G. Thomas and Stanislaw P. Stawicki*

*Address all correspondence to: stanislaw.stawicki@sluhn.org

Regional Level I Trauma Center and Department of Surgery, Section of Cardiovascular Surgery, St. Luke's University Health Network, Bethlehem, Pennsylvania, USA

References

[1] Cardona A JM, Valderrama CO, Gaviria UJ, Arboleda VC, Ramirez NG. Clinical and epidemiological characterization of acute respiratory distress syndrome in adult patients with femoral shaft fractures. Rev Colomb Anestesiol. 2014; 42:176–183.

[2] Navarrete-Navarro, P., et al., *Acute respiratory distress syndrome in trauma patients: ICU mortality and prediction factors.* Intensive Care Medicine, 2000. 26(11): p. 1624–1629.

[3] Bone, R.C., et al., *Randomized double-blind, multicenter study of prostaglandin E1 in patients with the adult respiratory distress syndrome. Prostaglandin E1 Study Group.* CHEST Journal, 1989. 96(1): p. 114–119.

[4] Zambon, M. and J.-L. Vincent, *Mortality rates for patients with acute lung injury/ARDS have decreased over time.* CHEST Journal, 2008. 133(5): p. 1120–1127.

[5] Stawicki, S.P., M. Goyal, and B. Sarani, *High-frequency oscillatory ventilation (HFOV) and airway pressure release ventilation (APRV): a practical guide.* Journal of Intensive Care Medicine, 2009. 24(4): p. 215–229.

[6] Dellinger, R.P., et al., *Effects of inhaled nitric oxide in patients with acute respiratory distress syndrome: results of a randomized phase II trial. Inhaled nitric oxide in ARDS study group.* Critical Care Medicine, 1998. 26(1): p. 15–23.

[7] Bein, T., et al., *Transportable extracorporeal lung support for rescue of severe respiratory failure in combat casualties.* The Journal of Trauma and Acute Care Surgery, 2012. 73(6): p. 1450–1456.

[8] Biderman, P., et al., *Extracorporeal life support in patients with multiple injuries and severe respiratory failure: a single-center experience?* The Journal of Trauma and Acute Care Surgery, 2013. 75(5): p. 907–912.

[9] Gatti, G., et al., *Rescue extracorporeal membrane oxygenation in a young man with a stab wound in the chest.* Injury, 2014. 45(9): p. 1509–1511.

[10] Saffarzadeh, A. and P. Bonde, *Options for temporary mechanical circulatory support.* Journal of Thoracic Disease, 2015. 7(12): p. 2102.

[11] Suh, I.-W., et al., *Catastrophic catecholamine-induced cardiomyopathy mimicking acute myocardial infarction, rescued by extracorporeal membrane oxygenation (ECMO) in pheochromocytoma.* Journal of Korean Medical Science, 2008. 23(2): p. 350–354.

[12] Marasco, S.F., et al., *Review of ECMO (extra corporeal membrane oxygenation) support in critically ill adult patients.* Heart, Lung and Circulation, 2008. 17: p. S41–S47.

[13] Stub, D., et al., *Refractory cardiac arrest treated with mechanical CPR, hypothermia, ECMO and early reperfusion (the CHEER trial).* Resuscitation, 2015. 86: p. 88–94.

[14] Skarda, D., J.W. Henricksen, and M. Rollins, *Extracorporeal membrane oxygenation promotes survival in children with trauma related respiratory failure.* Pediatric Surgery International, 2012. 28(7): p. 711–714.

[15] Del Nido, P., et al., *Extracorporeal membrane oxygenator rescue in children during cardiac arrest after cardiac surgery.* Circulation, 1992. 86(5 Suppl): p. II300–II304.

[16] Müller, T., et al., *A new miniaturized system for extracorporeal membrane oxygenation in adult respiratory failure.* Critical Care, 2009. 13(6): p. 1–10.

[17] Tulman, D.B., et al., *Veno-venous ECMO: a synopsis of nine key potential challenges, considerations, and controversies.* BMC Anesthesiol, 2014. 14: p. 65.

[18] Birnbaum, D.E., *Extracorporeal circulation in non-cardiac surgery.* European Journal of Cardio-Thoracic Surgery, 2004. 26(Suppl 1): p. S82–S85.

[19] Midla, G.S., *Extracorporeal circulatory systems and their role in military medicine: a clinical review.* Military Medicine, 2007. 172(5): p. 523–526.

[20] Hintz, S.R., et al., *Decreased use of neonatal extracorporeal membrane oxygenation (ECMO): how new treatment modalities have affected ECMO utilization.* Pediatrics, 2000. 106(6): p. 1339–1343.

[21] Kawahito, K., et al., *Resuscitation and circulatory support using extracorporeal membrane oxygenation for fulminant pulmonary embolism.* Artificial Organs, 2000. 24(6): p. 427–430.

[22] Diaz-Guzman, E., C.W. Hoopes, and J.B. Zwischenberger, *The evolution of extracorporeal life support as a bridge to lung transplantation.* ASAIO Journal, 2013. 59(1): p. 3–10.

[23] Parhar, K. and A. Vuylsteke, *What's new in ECMO: scoring the bad indications.* Intensive care medicine, 2014. 40(11): p. 1734–1737.

[24] Abrams, D. and D. Brodie, *Emerging indications for extracorporeal membrane oxygenation in adults with respiratory failure.* Annals of the American Thoracic Society, 2013. 10(4): p. 371–377.

[25] Stawicki, S.P., et al., *What's new in critical illness and injury science? State of the art in management of ARDS.* International Journal of Critical Illness and Injury Science, 2014. 4(2): p. 95.

[26] Peek, G.J., et al., *Efficacy and economic assessment of conventional ventilatory support versus extracorporeal membrane oxygenation for severe adult respiratory failure (CESAR): a multi-centre randomised controlled trial.* Lancet (London, England), 2009. 374(9698): p. 1351–1363.

[27] Crow, S., A. Fischer, and R. Schears. *Extracorporeal life support: utilization, cost, contro-versy, and ethics of trying to save lives.* Semin Cardiothorac Vasc Anesth. 2009 Sep;13(3): 183–91.

[28] Hsieh, F.T., G.S. Huang, W.J. Ko, and M.F. Lou *Health status and quality of life of survivors of extra corporeal membrane oxygenation: a cross-sectional study.* Journal of Advanced Nursing, 2016 [Epub ahead of print]. DOI: 10.1111/jan.12943.

[29] Dreizin, D., J. Menaker, and T.M. Scalea, *Extracorporeal membranous oxygenation (ECMO) in polytrauma: what the radiologist needs to know.* Emergency Radiology, 2015. 22(5): p. 565–576.

[30] Shaheen, A., et al., *Veno-Venous Extracorporeal Membrane Oxygenation (V V ECMO): indications, preprocedural considerations, and technique.* J Card Surg. 2016 Apr;31(4):248–52.

[31] Makdisi, G. and I.-W. Wang, *Extra Corporeal Membrane Oxygenation (ECMO) review of a lifesaving technology.* Journal of Thoracic Disease, 2015. 7(7): p. E166.

[32] Andrews, A., et al., *Total respiratory support with venovenous (VV) ECMO.* ASAIO Journal, 1982. 28(1): p. 350–353.

[33] Arlt, M., et al., *Extracorporeal membrane oxygenation in severe trauma patients with bleeding shock.* Resuscitation, 2010. 81(7): p. 804–809.

[34] Schmid, C., et al., *Venovenous extracorporeal membrane oxygenation for acute lung failure in adults.* The Journal of Heart and Lung Transplantation, 2012. 31(1): p. 9–15.

[35] Javidfar, J., et al., *Insertion of bicaval dual lumen extracorporeal membrane oxygenation catheter with image guidance.* ASAIO Journal, 2011. 57(3): p. 203–205.

[36] Kohler, K., et al., *ECMO cannula review.* Perfusion, 2013. 28(2): p. 114–124.

[37] Williams, K.E., *Extracorporeal membrane oxygenation for acute respiratory distress syndrome in adults.* AACN Advanced Critical Care, 2013. 24(2): p. 149–168.

[38] Jonathan R. Wisler, Paul R. Beery II, Steven M. Steinberg and Stanislaw P. A. Stawicki (2012). Competing Priorities in the Brain Injured Patient: Dealing with the Unexpected, Brain Injury – Pathogenesis, Monitoring, Recovery and Management, Prof. Amit Agrawal (Ed.), ISBN: 978-953-51-0265-6, InTech, Available from: http://www.intechopen.com/books/brain-injury-pathogenesis-monitoring-recovery-and-management/competing-priorities-in-the-brain-injured-patient-dealing-with-the-unexpected

[39] Bach, J., et al., *Multidisciplinary approach to multi-trauma patient with orthopedic injuries: the right team at the right time.* OPUS 12 Scientist, 2012. 6(1): p. 6–10.

[40] Gothner, M., et al., *The use of double lumen cannula for veno-venous ECMO in trauma patients with ARDS.* Scandinavian Journal of Trauma, Resuscitation and Emergncy Medicine, 2015. 23: p. 30.

[41] Boeckmann, D., et al., *ECMO in trauma patients—should we consider alternative cannulation sites?* Injury Extra, 2006. 37(8): p. 297–298.

[42] Hirose, H., et al., *Right ventricular rupture and tamponade caused by malposition of the Avalon cannula for venovenous extracorporeal membrane oxygenation.* Journal of Cardiothoracic Surgery, 2012. 7(36): p. 1–4.

[43] Riccabona, M., et al., *Venous thrombosis in and after extracorporeal membrane oxygenation: detection and follow-up by color Doppler sonography.* European Radiology, 1997. 7(9): p. 1383–1386.

[44] Stoll, M.C., et al., *Veno-venous extracorporeal membrane oxygenation therapy of a severely injured patient after secondary survey.* The American Journal of Emergency Medicine, 2014. 32(10): p. 1300 e1–1300 e2.

[45] Wu, M.Y., et al., *Venovenous extracorporeal life support for posttraumatic respiratory distress syndrome in adults: the risk of major hemorrhages.* Scandinavian Journal of Trauma, Resuscitation and Emergency Medicine, 2014. 22: p. 56.

[46] Anderson, H.L., et al., *Extracorporeal life support for respiratory failure after multiple trauma.* Journal of Trauma and Acute Care Surgery, 1994. 37(2): p. 266–274.

[47] Minicucci, M.F., et al., *Heart failure after myocardial infarction: clinical implications and treatment.* Clinical Cardiology, 2011. 34(7): p. 410–414.

[48] Kar, B., et al., *Percutaneous circulatory support in cardiogenic shock interventional bridge to recovery.* Circulation, 2012. 125(14): p. 1809–1817.

[49] Mydin, M., et al., *Extracorporeal membrane oxygenation as a bridge to pulmonary endarter-ectomy.* The Annals of Thoracic Surgery, 2011. 92(5): p. e101–e103.

[50] Pagani, F.D., et al., *Extracorporeal life support to left ventricular assist device bridge to heart transplant a strategy to optimize survival and resource utilization.* Circulation, 1999. 100 (suppl 2): p. II-206–II-210.

[51] Kulik, T.J., et al., *Outcome-associated factors in pediatric patients treated with extracorporeal membrane oxygenator after cardiac surgery.* Circulation, 1996. 94(9 Suppl): p. II63–II68.

[52] Rastan, A.J., et al., *Early and late outcomes of 517 consecutive adult patients treated with extracorporeal membrane oxygenation for refractory postcardiotomy cardiogenic shock.* The Journal of Thoracic and Cardiovascular Surgery, 2010. 139(2): p. 302–311. e1.

[53] Friesenecker, B., et al., *Craniotomy during ECMO in a severely traumatized patient.* Acta Neurochirurgica, 2005. 147(9): p. 993–996.

[54] Madershahian, N., et al., *Application of ECMO in multitrauma patients with ARDS as rescue therapy.* Journal of Cardiac Surgery, 2007. 22(3): p. 180–184.

[55] Paden, M.L., et al., *Extracorporeal life support organization registry report 2012.* ASAIO Journal, 2013. 59(3): p. 202–210.

[56] Wydo, S. and R. George, *Extracorporeal membrane oxygenation: a trauma surgeon's perspective.* Mechanical Circulatory Support, 2013. 4:21599.

[57] Haft, J., et al., *Extracorporeal membrane oxygenation (ECMO) in adults.* UpToDate Web site. http://www. uptodate. com/contents/extracorporeal-membrane-oxygenation-ecmo-in-adults, 2012. Accessed May 7, 2016.

[58] Marasco, S.F., et al., *Institution of extracorporeal membrane oxygenation late after lung transplantation – a futile exercise?* Clinical Transplantation, 2012. 26(1): p. E71–E77.

[59] Myat, A., et al., *Percutaneous circulatory assist devices for high-risk coronary intervention.* JACC Cardiovascular Interventions, 2015. 8(2): p. 229–244.

[60] Rupprecht, L., et al., *Pitfalls in percutaneous ECMO cannulation.* Heart, Lung and Vessels, 2015. 7(4): p. 320–326.

[61] Stulak, J.M., et al. *ECMO cannulation controversies and complications.* Semin Cardiothorac Vasc Anesth. 2009 Sep;13(3):176–82.

[62] Field, M., et al., *Open and closed chest extrathoracic cannulation for cardiopulmonary bypass and extracorporeal life support: methods, indications, and outcomes.* Postgraduate Medical Journal, 2006. 82(967): p. 323–331.

[63] Oliver, W.C. *Anticoagulation and coagulation management for ECMO.* Semin Cardiothorac Vasc Anesth. 2009 Sep;13(3):154–75.

[64] Koster, A., et al., *Successful use of bivalirudin as anticoagulant for ECMO in a patient with acute HIT.* The Annals of Thoracic Surgery, 2007. 83(5): p. 1865–1867.

[65] Lappa, A., et al., *Weaning from venovenous extracorporeal membrane oxygenation without anticoagulation: is it possible?* The Annals of Thoracic Surgery, 2012. 94(1): p. e1–e3.

[66] Mejak, B., et al., *Argatroban usage for anticoagulation for ECMO on a post-cardiac patient with heparin-induced thrombocytopenia.* The Journal of Extra-Corporeal Technology, 2004. 36(2): p. 178–181.

[67] Schumacher, R., et al., *Follow-up of infants treated with extracorporeal membrane oxygenation for newborn respiratory failure.* Pediatrics, 1991. 87(4): p. 451–457.

[68] Heiss, K., et al., *Reversal of mortality for congenital diaphragmatic hernia with ECMO.* Annals of Surgery, 1989. 209(2): p. 225.

[69] Ssemakula, N., et al., *Survival of patients with congenital diaphragmatic hernia during the ECMO era: an 11-year experience.* Journal of Pediatric Surgery, 1997. 32(12): p. 1683–1689.

[70] Smedira, N.G., et al., *Clinical experience with 202 adults receiving extracorporeal membrane oxygenation for cardiac failure: survival at five years.* The Journal of Thoracic and Cardiovascular Surgery, 2001. 122(1): p. 92–102.

[71] Nair, P., et al., *Extracorporeal membrane oxygenation for severe ARDS in pregnant and postpartum women during the 2009 H1N1 pandemic.* Intensive Care Medicine, 2011. 37(4): p. 648–654.

[72] Peek, G.J., et al., *Efficacy and economic assessment of conventional ventilatory support versus extracorporeal membrane oxygenation for severe adult respiratory failure (CESAR): a multicentre randomised controlled trial.* Lancet, 2009. 374(9698): p. 1351–1363.

[73] Kao, L.S., et al., *Predictors of morbidity after traumatic pancreatic injury.* Journal of Trauma and Acute Care Surgery, 2003. 55(5): p. 898–905.

[74] Mascia, L., *Acute lung injury in patients with severe brain injury: a double hit model.* Neurocritical Care, 2009. 11(3): p. 417–426.

[75] Cordell-Smith, J., et al., *Traumatic lung injury treated by extracorporeal membrane oxygenation (ECMO).* Injury, 2006. 37(1): p. 29–32.

[76] Hill, J.D., et al., *Clinical prolonged extracorporeal circulation for respiratory insufficiency: hematological effects.* Transactions – American Society for Artificial Internal Organs, 1972. 18(0): p. 546–552, 561.

[77] Ombrellaro, M., et al., *Extracorporeal life support for the treatment of adult respiratory distress syndrome after burn injury.* Surgery, 1994. 115(4): p. 523–526.

[78] Martucci, G., et al., *Veno-venous ECMO in ARDS after post-traumatic pneumonectomy.* Intensive Care Medicine, 2013. 39(12): p. 2235.

[79] Khan, N.U., et al., *Extracorporeal membrane oxygenator as a bridge to successful surgical repair of bronchopleural fistula following bilateral sequential lung transplantation: a case report and review of literature.* Journal of Cardiothoracic Surgery, 2007. 2(1): p. 28.

[80] Goldman, A.P., et al., *Extracorporeal membrane oxygenation as a bridge to definitive tracheal surgery in children.* The Journal of Pediatrics, 1996. 128(3): p. 386–388.

[81] Jacobs, J.V., et al., *The use of extracorporeal membrane oxygenation in blunt thoracic trauma: a study of the Extracorporeal Life Support Organization database.* Journal of Trauma and Acute Care Surgery, 2015. 79(6): p. 1049–1054.

[82] DeBerry, B.B., et al., *Successful management of pediatric cardiac contusion with extracorporeal membrane oxygenation.* Journal of Trauma and Acute Care Surgery, 2007. 63(6): p. 1380–1382.

[83] Giraud, R., et al., *Massive pulmonary embolism leading to cardiac arrest: one pathology, two different ECMO modes to assist patients.* Journal of Clinical Monitoring and Computing, 2015: p. 1–5.

[84] Barreda, E., et al., *Extracorporeal life support in right ventricular rupture secondary to blast injury.* Interactive Cardiovascular and Thoracic Surgery, 2007. 6(1): p. 87–88.

[85] Tisherman, S.A., *Salvage techniques in traumatic cardiac arrest: thoracotomy, extracorporeal life support, and therapeutic hypothermia.* Current Opinion in Critical Care, 2013. 19(6): p. 594–598.

[86] Cohn, S.M., *Pulmonary contusion: review of the clinical entity.* The Journal of Trauma, 1997. 42(5): p. 973–979.

[87] Miller, P.R., et al., *ARDS after pulmonary contusion: accurate measurement of contusion volume identifies high-risk patients.* Journal of Trauma-Injury Infection and Critical Care, 2001. 51(2): p. 223–230.

[88] Maung, A.A. and L.J. Kaplan, *Mechanical ventilation after injury.* Journal of Intensive Care Medicine, 2014. 29(3): p. 128–137.

[89] Muellenbach, R.M., et al., *Prolonged heparin-free extracorporeal membrane oxygenation in multiple injured acute respiratory distress syndrome patients with traumatic brain injury.* The Journal of Trauma and Acute Care Surgery, 2012. 72(5): p. 1444–1447.

[90] Kugai, T. and M. Chibana, *Rupture in a mitral papillary muscle following blunt chest trauma.* The Japanese Journal of Thoracic and Cardiovascular Surgery, 2000. 48(6): p. 394–397.

[91] Brenner, M., J.V. O'Connor, and T.M. Scalea, *Use of ECMO for resection of post-traumatic ruptured lung abscess with empyema.* The Annals of Thoracic Surgery, 2010. 90(6): p. 2039–2041.

[92] Rubin, S., et al., *Traumatic aorto-right atrial fistula and tricuspid valve rupture. Post-operative cardiac and respiratory support with extracorporeal membrane oxygenation.* Interactive Cardiovascular and Thoracic Surgery, 2006. 5(6): p. 735–737.

[93] Brain Trauma, F., et al., *Guidelines for the management of severe traumatic brain injury. I. Blood pressure and oxygenation.* Journal of Neurotrauma, 2007. 24 (Suppl 1): p. S7–S13.

[94] Bermudez, C.A., et al., *Initial experience with single cannulation for venovenous extracorporeal oxygenation in adults.* The Annals of Thoracic Surgery, 2010. 90(3): p. 991–995.

[95] Firstenberg, M.S., et al., *Extracorporeal membrane oxygenation for complex multiorgan system trauma.* Case Reports in Surgery, 2012. 2012: p. 897184.

[96] Zhou, R., et al., *ECMO support for right main bronchial disruption in multiple trauma patient with brain injury—a case report and literature review.* Perfusion, 2015. 30(5): p. 403–406.

[97] Fortenberry, J.D., et al., *Extracorporeal life support for posttraumatic acute respiratory distress syndrome at a children's medical center.* Journal of Pediatric Surgery, 2003. 38(8): p. 1221–1226.

[98] Wen, P.H., et al., *Non-heparinized ECMO serves a rescue method in a multitrauma patient combining pulmonary contusion and nonoperative internal bleeding: a case report and literature review.* World Journal of Emergency Surgery, 2015. 10: p. 15.

[99] Yuan, K.-C., J.-F. Fang, and M.-F. Chen, *Treatment of endobronchial hemorrhage after blunt chest trauma with extracorporeal membrane oxygenation (ECMO).* Journal of Trauma and Acute Care Surgery, 2008. 65(5): p. 1151–1154.

[100] Guest, J. and J. Anderson, *Major airway injury in closed chest trauma.* CHEST Journal, 1977. 72(1): p. 63–66.

[101] Liu, C., et al., *Extracorporeal membrane oxygenation as a support for emergency bronchial reconstruction in a traumatic patient with severe hypoxaemia.* Interactive Cardiovascular Thoracic Surgery, 2014. 19(4): p. 699–701.

[102] Ballouhey, Q., et al., *Benefits of extracorporeal membrane oxygenation for major blunt tracheobronchial trauma in the paediatric age group.* European Journal of Cardiothoracic Surgery, 2013. 43(4): p. 864–865.

[103] Garlick, J., et al., *Differential lung ventilation and venovenous extracorporeal membrane oxygenation for traumatic bronchopleural fistula.* The Annals of Thoracic Surgery, 2013. 96(5): p. 1859–1860.

[104] Tseng, Y.H., et al., *Venoarterial extracorporeal life support in post-traumatic shock and cardiac arrest: lessons learned.* Scandinavian Journal of Trauma, Resuscitation and Emergency Medicine, 2014. 22: p. 12.

[105] Smith, B.P., et al., *Review of abdominal damage control and open abdomens: focus on gastrointestinal complications.* Journal of Gastrointestinal and Liver Diseases, 2010. 19(4): p. 425–435.

[106] Stawicki, S.P., J. Cipolla, and C. Bria, *Comparison of open abdomens in non-trauma and trauma patients: a retrospective study.* OPUS 12 Scientist, 2007. 1(1): p. 1–8.

[107] Senunas, L.E., et al., *Extracorporeal life support for patients with significant orthopaedic trauma.* Clinical Orthopaedics and Related Research, 1997(339): p. 32–40.

[108] Michaels, A.J., et al., *Extracorporeal life support in pulmonary failure after trauma*. The Journal of Trauma, 1999. 46(4): p. 638–645.

[109] Huang, Y.-K., et al., *Extracorporeal life support in post-traumatic respiratory distress patients*. Resuscitation, 2009. 80(5): p. 535–539.

[110] Bonacchi, M., et al., *Extracorporeal life support in patients with severe trauma: An advanced treatment strategy for refractory clinical settings*. The Journal of Thoracic and Cardiovascular Surgery, 2013. 145(6): p. 1617–1626.

[111] Ried, M., et al., *Extracorporeal lung support in trauma patients with severe chest injury and acute lung failure: a 10-year institutional experience*. Critical Care, 2013. 17(3): p. R110.

[112] Wu, S.C., et al., *Use of extracorporeal membrane oxygenation in severe traumatic lung injury with respiratory failure*. American Journal of Emergency Medicine, 2015. 33(5): p. 658–662.

[113] Thiagarjan, R.R. and C.S. Barrett, *ECMO-indications and outcomes. Available from: http://www.sccm.org/Communications/Critical–Connections/Archives/Pages/ECMO——Indications–and–Outcomes.aspx. 2011. Accessed on May 7, 2016.*

[114] Aissaoui, N., et al., *Predictors of successful extracorporeal membrane oxygenation (ECMO) weaning after assistance for refractory cardiogenic shock*. Intensive Care Medicine, 2011. 37(11): p. 1738–1745.

[115] Cavarocchi, N.C., et al., *Weaning of extracorporeal membrane oxygenation using continuous hemodynamic transesophageal echocardiography*. The Journal of Thoracic and Cardiovascular Surgery, 2013. 146(6): p. 1474–1479.

[116] Schumacher, R.E., et al., *Extracorporeal membrane oxygenation in term newborns. A prospective cost-benefit analysis*. ASAIO Journal, 1993. 39(4): p. 873–879.

[117] Mahle, W.T., et al., *Cost-utility analysis of salvage cardiac extracorporeal membrane oxygenation in children*. The Journal of Thoracic and Cardiovascular Surgery, 2005. 129(5): p. 1084–1090.

[118] Wildschut, E., et al., *Determinants of drug absorption in different ECMO circuits*. Intensive Care Medicine, 2010. 36(12): p. 2109–2116.

[119] Shekar, K., et al., *Increased sedation requirements in patients receiving extracorporeal membrane oxygenation for respiratory and cardiorespiratory failure*. Anaesthesia and Intensive Care, 2012. 40(4): p. 648.

[120] Shekar, K., et al., *ASAP ECMO: antibiotic, sedative and analgesic pharmacokinetics during extracorporeal membrane oxygenation: a multi-centre study to optimise drug therapy during ECMO*. BMC Anesthesiology, 2012. 12(1): p. 29.

[121] Fuehner, T., et al., *Extracorporeal membrane oxygenation in awake patients as bridge to lung transplantation*. American Journal of Respiratory and Critical Care Medicine, 2012. 185(7):763–768.

[122] Rehder, K.J., et al., *Active rehabilitation during ECMO as a bridge to lung transplantation.* Respir Care 2013;58(8):1291–1298.

[123] Gulack, B.C., S.A. Hirji, and M.G. Hartwig, *Bridge to lung transplantation and rescue post-transplant: the expanding role of extracorporeal membrane oxygenation.* Journal of Thoracic Disease, 2014. 6(8): p. 1070–1079.

[124] Haneke, F., et al., *Use of extracorporeal membrane oxygenation in an awake patient after a major trauma with an incidental finding of tuberculosis.* Perfusion. 2016 May;31(4):347–8.

[125] Klein, A., et al., *Organ donation and utilization in the United States, 1999–2008.* American Journal of Transplantation, 2010. 10(4p2): p. 973–986.

[126] Balsorano, P., et al., *Extracorporeal life support and multiorgan donation in a severe poly-trauma patient: a case report.* International Journal of Surgery Case Reports, 2015. 9: p. 109–111.

[127] Cipolla, J., S. Stawicki, and D. Spatz, *Hemodynamic monitoring of organ donors: a novel use of the esophageal echo-Doppler probe.* The American Surgeon, 2006. 72(6): p. 500–504.

[128] Ko, W.J., et al., *Extracorporeal membrane oxygenation support of donor abdominal organs in non-heart-beating donors.* Clinical Transplantation, 2000. 14(2): p. 152–156.

[129] Gravel, M., et al., *Kidney transplantation from organ donors following cardiopulmonary death using extracorporeal membrane oxygenation support.* Annals of Transplantation: Quarterly of the Polish Transplantation Society, 2003. 9(1): p. 57–58.

5

Neurologic Issues in Patients Receiving Extracorporeal Membrane Oxygenation Support

Susana M. Bowling, Joao Gomes and
Michael S. Firstenberg

Abstract

Extracorporeal membrane oxygenation (ECMO) is a well-established therapy for patients experiencing acute severe cardiac and/or respiratory failure. Unfortunately, despite noteworthy improvements in patient selection, technology, and multidisciplinary team management, significant complications are still common. The most dramatic and potentially severe complications are neurologic. However, the incidence of neurologic complications (i.e. embolic stroke, intracerebral hemorrhage, seizures, and anoxic injuries) has not been completely defined. Unfortunately, brain death and neurologic injuries are significant causes of morbidity and mortality for patients requiring an ECMO support. Critical to the management of patients requiring ECMO is a broader understanding of neurologic monitoring along with the clinical assessment and management of neurologic events. It is important to evaluate and potentially intervene early in the event of a neurologic problem to minimize its clinical significance. Hopefully, with a better understanding of the pathophysiology, diagnostic and therapeutic tools, and prevention strategies, the true incidence of neurologic complications can be understood and minimized.

Keywords: ECMO, stroke, neurologic, complications, seizures, brain

1. Introduction

Extracorporeal membrane Oxygenation (ECMO) provides cardiopulmonary support to patients with acute severe refractory cardiac and respiratory failure. In veno-veno (VV) support, blood is drained from the venous system, oxygenated, cleared of carbon dioxide, and then pumped back into the central venous system (i.e. into the right atrium or cavoa-trial junction), is typically used for isolated pulmonary failure. For patients with cardiac failure or combined cardiopulmonary failure, venoarterial (VA) support is typically used. Unlike VV support, in VA support, blood is returned back into the arterial system – often as close to the coronary arteries and/or cerebral arterial system as possible. The specifics, including indications, contraindications, techniques, and outcomes are discussed in other chapters of this text. However, as we will discuss in this chapter, the nuances of arterial vs. venous inflow might potentially affect the management, complications, and outcomes, particularly the risks of cerebral complications of these critically ill and high-risk patients.

Since the initial applications in 1960–70, pediatric patients, neonates, and infants with con-genital heart defects or respiratory distress syndrome seem to have been the main recipients of this technique. Better equipment and an exponential increase in the body of knowledge regarding its use have resulted in a dramatic increase in its utilization in the pediatric popu-lation. However, more significantly, there has been a tremendous increase in the adult population for both cardiac and respiratory support [1]. ECMO use in adults covers the spectrum of problems ranging from adults who survive cardiopulmonary resuscitation and post-myocardial infarction-associated cardiogenic and septic shock. ECMO is being commonly used for treatment of acute respiratory failure caused by a variety of problems [2–4]. The role of ECMO during the H1N1 pandemic in 2009 is noteworthy, where the use of ECMO resulted in a survival-to-discharge rate of >50–60%; it has been accepted worldwide as an appropriate rescue therapy for these critically ill patients [5]. There is also a growing experience with the use of ECMO as a bridge to heart and/or lung transplantation in highly selected patients in whom end-organ recovery does not occur or is not expected. Conversely, in the world of acute neurocritical care, ECMO has been thought to be of limited use due to the concomitant need for anticoagulation. However, some case reports have successfully utilized this technique in patients who suffered neurogenic pulmonary edema either In the setting of aneurismal subarachnoid hemorrhage (SAH) preceding surgery or traumatic brain injury (TBI), thereby opening the door to speculation regarding the possible future use in these patient populations [6, 7].

Survival rates for patients undergoing ECMO varies dramatically. Results are often a function of the initial primary pathological insult combined with associated comorbidities. As of 2012, the Extracorporeal Life Support Organization (ELSO)—an international organization dedicat-ed to the study of ECMO (including the voluntary collection/reporting of clinical outcomes) —reported survival rate of 50–60% for adult patients with respiratory failure and 39% for cardiac failure patients [8]. However, survival rates in single-center registries have varied from 15% to 59% [4, 9, 10] with some reporting >80% 30-day survival rates [11]. As we will discuss in this chapter, it is also becoming evident that mortality, morbidity, hospital length of stay, patient care cost, and patient discharge to long-term care (LTAC) facilities appear to be closely related to the development of neurological complications. This is particularly true for those who develop intracerebral hemorrhage (ICH), or ischemic stroke (IS), both of which are considered the most frequent complications and had been found in up to nine of 10 brain studies at autopsy for patients who die after ECMO therapy [1, 9, 11]. The incidence of neurological complications per se vary in the literature and range from 10 to 50% with some investigators speculating as many as 90% of patients treated with ECMO sustain some form of therapy-associated neurologic injury [1, 9, 11]. This huge disparity is a consequence of the lack of structural algorithms for the neurological evaluation of these patients. Most of the outcome data have been obtained from retrospective reviews and are based on clinical exams, imaging, pathology review, or a combination of several diagnostic assessments. Clinically significant events versus imaging or pathological events with no clinical or neurological consequence have also been poorly defined in these case series.

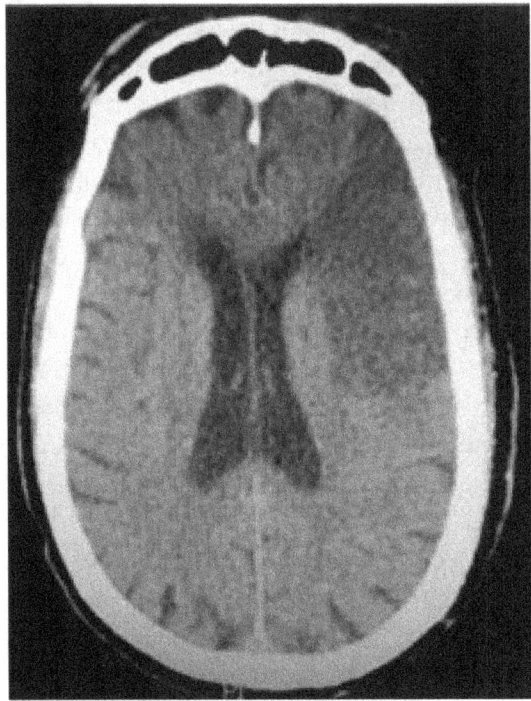

Figure 1. CT scan of a 24-year-old female patient with profound hypoxemia and septic shock. Neurologic evaluation was limited by hemodynamic instability and need for pharmacologic paralysis. Once stabilized on ECMO, imaging demonstrated a large hemispheric stroke of unknown etiology. Despite successful weaning from ECMO and recovery of end-organ function, she remained in coma and family withdrew support.

Regarding the spectrum of neurological complications, embolic ischemic strokes, ischemic watershed infarctions, ICH, SAH, seizures, brain death, and diffuse cerebral edema are the most prevalent, followed by unexplained prolonged coma and hypoxic ischemic encephalopathy. Delirium, severe neuropathy, hearing loss, and vocal cord paralysis are also to be included here; some of these may not be directly related to ECMO, but these are secondary to the need for prolonged intubation, mechanical ventilation, possible tracheostomy, and prolonged ICU stays in these extremely ill and complex patients. Acute disseminated encephalomyelitis has also been reported, but its mechanism remains unclear [9].

Adding to the complexity in the determination of true ECMO-associated complications, patients undergoing ECMO may develop neurological complications prior to the initiation of

ECMO, during, or after decannulation. Patients first receive ECMO in emergent circumstances where neurological examinations are rarely performed. Most patients are paralyzed, sedated, and even undergoing mild to moderate hypothermia during the first 24–72 h giving limited value to the bedside clinical examination [10]. Often critical care teams and neurologists are left with the use of laboratory, electrophysiology, and imaging testing as the only tools for detection of acute complications and determination of outcomes [12]. Unfortunately, sometimes definitive imaging and clinical evaluations cannot be determined until the patient is successfully stabilized (**Figure 1**) or weaned from the ECMO support (**Figure 2**).

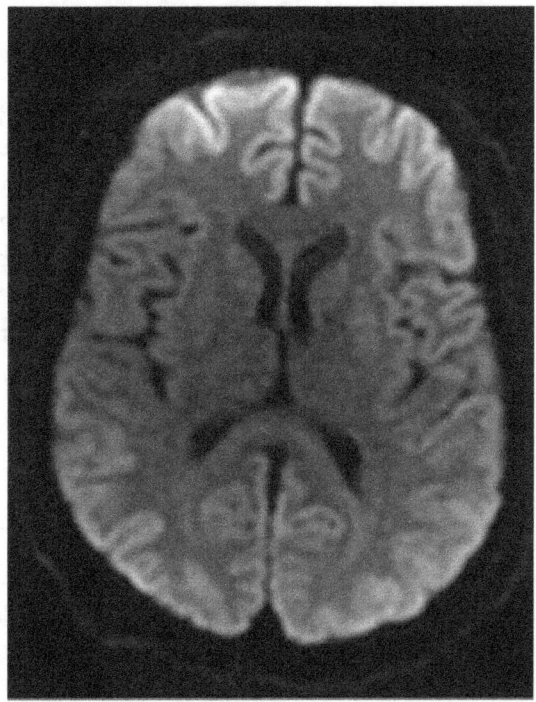

Figure 2. MRI of a 43-year-old patient who sustained an acute respiratory arrest secondary to severe respiratory failure from seasonable influenza. He was transferred immediately to an ECMO center and required 14 days of veno-veno ECMO support. Despite successful weaning from ECMO with good end-organ function, he remained in a coma. Post-ECMO MRI demonstrated an extensive diffusion defect consistent with severe anoxic brain injury/ischemia. Due to these findings and concerns for a poor long-term neurolo The family decided toly withdraw support.

A basic understanding of the physiology of cerebral blood flow (CBF), metabolism, and the management of complications, particularly in the context of long-term extracorporeal support, will be the focus of this chapter as it is critical to understanding the relationships between extracorporeal support and cerebral protection.

2. Principles of cerebral metabolism and blood flow

Under normal conditions, about 15–20% of cardiac output is devoted solely to the brain. This equates to an average perfusion of 50–55 ml/100 g brain tissue/min, with the more metabolically active areas (i.e., gray matter) receiving higher cerebral blood flow (CBF: 75 ml/100 g brain tissue/min), whereas the white matter exhibits a much lower CBF (i.e. 45 ml/100 g brain tissue/min) [13].

Regulation of CBF in the human brain is exceedingly complex, and although not fully understood, three main regulatory paradigms have been identified thus far, namely *cerebral autoregulation, flow-metabolism coupling*, and *neurogenic regulation*. The first mechanism refers to the ability of cerebral arterioles to maintain a constant CBF within a wide range of cerebral perfusion pressures, while a functional hyperemia or coupling between cerebral metabolism in a given area and a matched increase in regional CBF is a well-documented phenomenon. Lastly, the prominent role of *neurovascular units* comprising extensive arborizations of perivascular nerves, endothelial cells, and astrocytes has been increasingly recognized in recent years [14].

Moderate decreases in CBF down to about 30 ml/100 g brain tissue/min are usually well tolerated and do not typically lead to neuronal dysfunction. However, alterations in electrophysiological recordings become apparent once flow drops below 25 ml/100 g brain tissue/min and completely disappear with CBF of ≤12–15 ml/100 g brain tissue/min [15]. The early recognition of hypoperfused but not yet irreversibly injured brain (i.e. penumbra) constitutes one of the main rationales for multimodal brain monitoring of patients undergoing ECMO.

During ECMO support, a number of investigations have shown a significant decrease in cerebral blood flow, with mean flow velocities on transcranial Doppler sonography about half of those predicted for age and gender and a flow pattern characterized by decreased systolic upstroke, lack of dichrotic notch, and continuous diastolic flow [16]. This consistent decrement in CBF with near normalization following decannulation has been ascribed to metabolism-flow coupling secondary to decreased cerebral metabolic rate (i.e. due to the use of sedative agents), cerebral venous congestion secondary to jugular vein ligation (in pediatric and neonatal cases), and left ventricular dysfunction, particularly in patients with venoarterial ECMO [17].

Interestingly, patients who develop intracerebral hemorrhage as a complication of ECMO seem to experience reactive hyperemia with resultant increases in CBF an average of 2–6 days prior to clinical recognition of the acute neurologic injury, likely due to uncoupling of the flow-metabolism regulatory mechanism. In such patients, recent ischemic injury and the use of anticoagulants likely contribute to the elevated risk of cerebral hemorrhage [18].

2.1. Causes of neurological complications during ECMO

As previously mentioned, some of the neurological complications detected during ECMO may be the consequence of the insult that led to the need for ECMO to begin with. The extent of this pre-ECMO injury is impossible to predict prospectively in most cases. These patients are either hypoxic or hypotensive before ECMO and represent a wide range of circumstances, from cardiac arrest to severe respiratory failure and sepsis, thereby making it impossible to identify common denominators as predictors of outcome in the front end. Data suggest that pre-ECMO lactic acidosis levels >10 mmol/L are associated with poor outcomes as well as the presence of hyperpyrexia, hyperglycemia, and metabolic acidosis. Other potential contributors to the overall injury to the central nervous system prior and during ECMO that may be considered as independent predictors of poor outcome include high ventilatory pressures, disseminated septic embolism, and air embolism.

In children, the ECMO cannulation approach represents a significant risk by altering blood flow after ligation of the internal jugular vein and common carotid arteries. In adults with extensive aortic atherosclerotic disease, arterial cannulation might result in retrograde disruption of debris from the high pressure and flow and result in diffuse microvascular embolic events. Cases of retrograde aortic (and carotid) dissection have also been discussed as the potential causes of acute catastrophic injuries during cannulation and therapy. Other similar procedures that require vascular access complications may includ currently reported causes of embolic neurologic system to oxygenate, development of pump head thrombus, and intracardiac thrombus are among the currently reported causes of embolic neurologic [18, 19].

All patients undergoing ECMO should be systemically anticoagulated. Exposure of blood to non-biological surfaces leads to a chain of biological reactions, increased inflammatory response, and increase in acute-phase reactants. This results in hypercoagulability and potential thrombotic events. This may occur acutely within 24–48 h after initiation of the circuit and can lead to ischemic complications including stroke. Embolic areas that become ischemic are subsequently prone to associated hemorrhagic transformation and intra-cranial bleeding complication. Similarly, these biological reactions, which can increase the bleeding risk via thrombocytopenia, impaired platelet function, and consumption of clotting factors as well as fibrinolysis associated with the therapeutic anticoagulation, increase dramatically the risk for hemorrhagic complications, among which ICH is the most feared [20].

Different considerations for neurologic risk are based upon VA versus VV cannulation. This is particularly true in neonates where VV ECMO has a significantly lower risk for neurologic complications when comparing with VA ECMO [11]. However, the same findings have not been consistently replicated in adult population. It is important to recognize that neurologic complications increase the risk of a poor outcome, but such events are not inherently futile [21]. In the absence of a specific diagnosis of brain death, clinically significant neurologic events are often used for justification to withdraw support on patients requiring ECMO. In one study of 87 patients treated with ECMO (for all indications), 65 experienced a neurologic event. Of these 66, 25 survived to discharge, 25 had support withdrawn, and 16 died. The distinction between the 16 patients who were listed as having "died" versus the 25 who had "support withdrawn" and presumed to have died remained unclear [11]. Given the potential implications and link between neurologic events and clinical outcomes, without a doubt, a better understanding, definitions, and management protocols are necessary.

3. Specific complications

3.1. Intracranial hemorrhage (ICH)

ICH is most frequently reported in neonates due to easy detection using transcranial Doppler (TCD), with the incidence varying between 26% and 52% and also the cerebellum being the most common location at this age. Independent of the use of ECMO, the overall mortality from ICH is 60–70% [2, 22, 23]. This contrasts dramatically with lower incidence reported in adult population, with 2–19% patients developing ICH. The range in incidence varies depending on the variability in the use of computed tomography (CT) scanning for diagnosis or postmortem pathology data [10, 11, 20]. Conversely, the most common location in adult patients is supratentorial [11]. The existence of proven independent risk factors for ICH is limited at this time. While the duration of ECMO support and site of cannulation did not seem to affect the rates of ICH in adults, a correlation has been noted between female gender, thrombocytopenia, acute renal failure (Cr > 2.6 or the need for dialysis). Being female with thrombocytopenia (<50.000) is the most important predictor. In the case of infants, prematurity, venous cannulation, carotid artery ligation, sepsis, and acidosis carried an increased risk [20]. In adults, outcomes after ICH while on ECMO are felt to be catastrophic with mortality as high as 92.3% [24], but successful outcomes are not uncommon [25] (**Figure 3**).

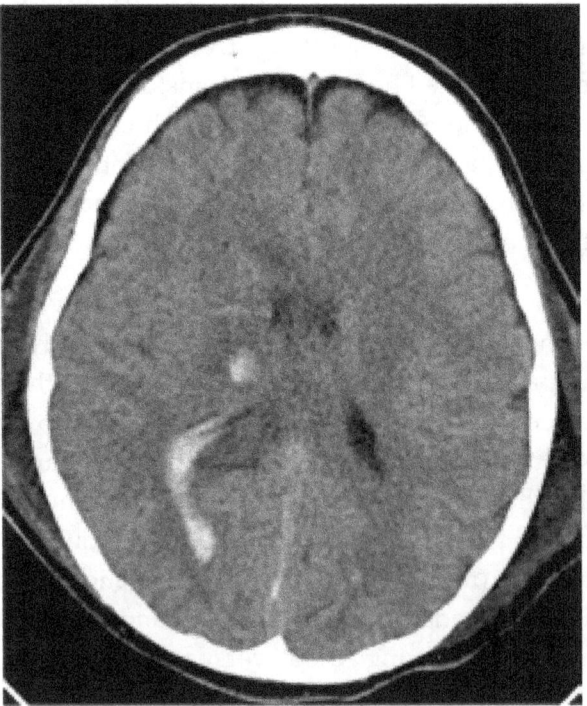

Figure 3. CT scan of a 25-year-old male patient who sustained a motor vehicle accident. He presented with hypothermia and refractory hypoxemia from severe pulmonary contusions. Despite intraventricular hemorrhage, he was supported on veno-veno ECMO for 4 days, 2 days without the use of systemic heparin. He was successfully weaned from ECMO, extubated, and discharged to a rehabilitation facility 21 days postinjury (see text for reference).

3.2. Stroke

Ischemic strokes are among the most common complications in patients on ECMO; however, the true incidence is not known. Data currently available do not differentiate among the mechanism of stroke, characteristics of the infarctions (for example, large vessel occlusions versus microembolization) or the timing of the infarction with regard to outcomes. Events caused by hypoperfusion that may have occurred during CPR leading to watershed infarctions are thought to have completely different presentations, mechanisms, and outcomes as cardioembolic events in patients with CHF, septic embolization, thrombosis caused by hypercoagulability; however, these are lump together at the time of discussing incidence and outcomes. It is therefore impossible to generalize the prediction of the prognosis of ischemic strokes in patients with ECMO, which should be considered in a case-to-case bases, rather than assuming that the presence of ischemic stroke equals poor prognosis.

Limited information exists regarding the true incidence of stroke as mentioned before. The work by Omar HR et al. [26] is worth mentioning, wherein a retrospective review of all ECMO patients at the Tampa General Hospital from 2004 to 2014 has been reviewed for detection of incidence of radiologically proven ischemic stroke. Detecting a 5.8 % of incidence, however in the report, they recognize the limitation of the study based on the lack of systematic studies with the possibility of a falsely low incidence due to underreported events. In this report, the presence of high lactic acid of >10 mmol/L prior to ECMO appeared related to an increased incidence of stroke. Literature review has associated stroke with an increased morbidity of up to 14% [11]. However, unfortunately, most of the adult studies tend to combine mortality for both ischemic and hemorrhagic cases. No stroke correlation has been proven with the duration of ECMO treatment; however, the association with high levels of lactic acid suggests that systemic post-anoxic events is more common than ischemic strokes caused by cardiac embolization. While cannula embolization or air or atherothrombotic embolisms as mechanism are far more common with venoarterial therapies in which abnormal or high pressure (and often retrograde) flows in the arterial system might predispose to this complication. Unless air is iatrogenically introduced into the system, post-oxygenator, the intrinsic filtering of modern oxygenators has virtually eliminated the risk of ECMO circuit-induced embolic complication [27]. Nevertheless, there is clearly much to learn in this specific area of neurologic complications [21].

3.3. Seizures

Post-anoxic encephalopathy, stroke, and ICH are all associated with an increased risk for development of seizures. Therefore, it is not surprising that ECMO patients also have an increased risk. Fever, metabolic changes, and medications all contribute to this risk. Their presentation may vary from post-anoxic myoclonus, focal, generalized seizures to subclinical seizures. Any indication of abnormal motor function, especially while under heavy sedation, or concern should prompt a formal evaluation. Unrecognized seizure activity, if left untreated, can result in catastrophic neuronal ischemia/anoxic injury. Formal recommendations for the systematic use of electroencephalography in this patients do not exist, thereby resulting in a potentially under reported incidence and therefore poor understanding of the role that this entity plays in the overall outcome. Continuous EEG recording could assist with the detection of not only seizure activity but also focal suppression of the background that could indirectly herald the presence of a structural abnormality.

4. General brain edema/brain death

The presence of generalized brain edema is clinically heralded by either persistent coma or physical examination findings suggestive of brain death. Systemic conditions resulting in severe hypoxia or hypotension will result in a global decrease in cerebral blood flow or cerebral oxygenation, which if sustained and above what the cerebral autoregulation or metabolic coupling can compensate for, the result can be general brain edema neuronal cell death Many of these patients are diagnosed with general brain edema within 3 days of cannulation for ECMO [11]. This would suggest that is the brain insult suffered during the condition that led to the need for ECMO what cause the injury and subsequent edema. Brain death occurred in 7–21% of the ECMO patients treated in academic centers [28–30].

In one recent series, 295 adult patients treated with ECMO, 21% of patients where given a diagnosis of brain death [24]. Unfortunately, given the retrospective nature of this voluntary registry data, no specific criteria were given to validate the method for making the diagnosis.

Brain death is a formal diagnosis for which there can be little margin of error in assessment. Once these diagnostic criteria are met, the diagnosis is established, which thereby provides both medical and legal grounds for terminating any and all care. Prolongation of therapies after the establishment of brain death is unethical and potentially illegal with grounds for litigation. Because many of the physiologic criteria and responses to bedside testing used for the assessment of cerebral and brainstem function can be influenced by the physiologic benefits of ECMO, the diagnosis of brain death while on ECMO can be challenging. In addition, while several authors have advocated criteria for determining brain death in a patient supported by ECMO, formal guidelines to assist in the making of such a critical, life-ending, diagnosis are lacking. This topic will be further discussed below.

4.1. Neurological monitoring during ECMO

The role of the ongoing neurological assessment while patients are on ECMO support is of particular importance in this patient population due to the high incidence of neurological complications [1, 11, 31, 32]. Findings from neurological monitoring either physical exam, laboratory, electrophysiological, or neuroimaging data have a high probability to result in a change in care plan or goals of care that may definitely lead to change in outcomes and potentially prevent further deterioration. There is no consensus regarding minimal recommended neurological assessment ether prior, during, or after ECMO. Nevertheless, to the extent possible, all patients on ECMO – even when heavily sedated and pharmacologically paralyzed – require very close and frequent neurologic assessment consistent with routine ICU clinical monitoring. Given the high risk and incidence for adverse neurologic complications, as discussed, any and all neurologic changes in patients undergoing ECMO therapy require early and aggressive evaluation and management. Limited data exist regarding the predictive value of the different monitoring modalities and in particular physical examination prior and during treatment on ECMO outcomes.

4.2. Physical exam

As itor response to noxious stimulation. Most of this could be continued during ECMO support, limited only by sedation and paralysis, in which case, only pupillary studies may be followed. The latest can be done using an automatic computerized measure to avoid examiner variability (**Figure 4**). As with any critical care patient, we suggest the establishment of sedation vacation protocols that would facilitate clinical examination whenever possible. Identification of changes in physical exam findings has been followed traditionally by a need in cranial imaging.

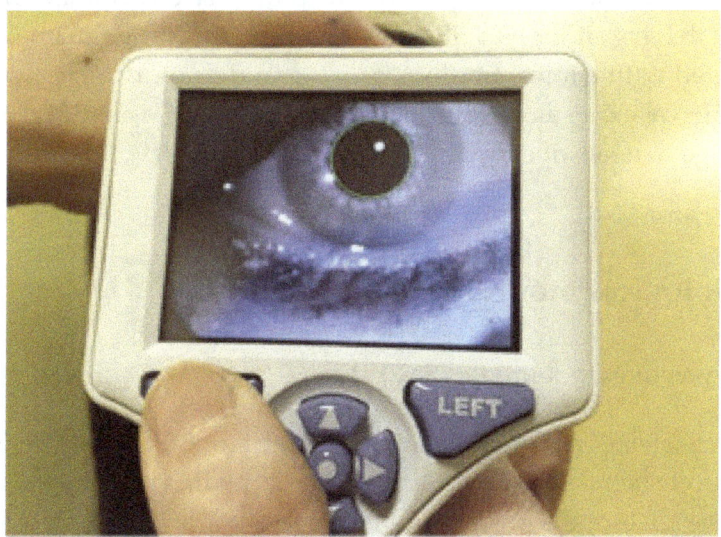

Figure 4. The NPi-200 Pupillometer (Neuroptics Inc, Irvine CA, USA, http://www.neuroptics.com) uses quantitative infrared technology that objectively and accurately measures and trends the pupillary size and reactivity in critically ill patients. Eliminating inaccuracies caused by interpreter reliability. Measurement of NPi, (Neurologic pupillary index), maximal diameter at rest and maximal constriction as well as calculating % change and latency time between initiation of stimulation and onset of constriction. MCV, (maximum constriction velocities, mm/sec) is also calculated in each eye.

4.3. Imaging

Choices for imaging techniques are also limited during ECMO. While in infants, transcranial Doppler (TCD) provides extraordinary bedside imaging data prior to the closure of the fontanels; in adults, cranial computed tomography (CT) is preferred and TCD is limited to assessment of cerebral blood flow dynamics, detection of increase in ICP, and detection of microembolism [33]. Due to the ferrous properties of the ECMO pump and circuit, magnetic resonance imaging while on ECMO is obviously contraindicated.

4.4. Cranial computed tomography (CT)

Transportation of these patients outside of the ICU is not only technically and physically difficult but also potentially dangerous [34]. For the most part, presumably, only a few patients undergo CT during actual ECMO and most are tested after decannulation. Up to 95 % of the complications found in infants and 85 % in pediatric and adult patients are found in the first 3–4 days on ECMO support, undelaying the need of imaging technique protocols during ECMO [9, 18]. The availability of portable CT scans is of particular use in the ECMO centers. With wider availability of portable CT scanning or easier transport of patient due to more compact ECMO circuit design, the hope is that closer monitoring or more frequent imaging might improve the overall understanding of ECMO therapies on clinical neurologic events and outcomes. Clearly, more comprehensive, and potentially prospective data and studies, are required in this area.

In a study by Marika K et al., 37% of patients who underwent cranial CT scanning during ECMO were found to have either ICH, IS, or generalized brain edema. Imaging findings were not always associated with clinical findings proving underreporting of neurological complications based on clinical exam alone, but the results of CT had a significant impact in clinical management, change in goals of care, and surgical indications [9, 11].

5. Electrophysiological monitoring

5.1. Somatosensory-evoked potentials (SSEPs)

Evoked potentials are electrical signals generated by the nervous system in response to sensory stimuli. In SSEPs, an electrical stimulus is applied to the median nerve at the wrist, the common peroneal nerve at the knee, or the posterior tibial nerve at the ankle, while electrodes are placed along the neuraxis measure latency and amplitude. The median nerve is the most commonly stimulated site and scalp electrodes overlying the contralateral somatosensory cortex record the so-called N20 component of the evoked potential.

The cortical generators of the N20 component are located in the territory of the middle cerebral artery and various studies have correlated decreased N20 amplitude (by >50%) with cerebral hypoperfusion in this vascular distribution [35, 36]. Furthermore, the absence of SSEPs in the setting of cardiac arrest and global cerebral ischemia strongly correlates with poor neurologic outcome, while its presence is not sensitive enough to predict a favorable one [37].

In patients undergoing ECMO, SSEP responses can be asymmetric between right and left hemispheres in up to 15% of cases [38]. Abnormalities (or absence) of the N20 component following median nerve stimulation seem to have a prognostic value for poor neurologic outcome, similar to other instances of global cerebral ischemia [39]. Future studies are warranted to further refine its role in ECMO patients.

5.2. Electroencephalography (EEG)

In major medical centers, frequent or even continuous EEG monitoring of patients with devastating neurologic injuries is becoming commonplace, and patients undergoing ECMO support should not be an exception to this rule. Akin to cardiac telemetry, this form of monitoring ("neurotelemetry") can assist in the identification and early treatment of reversible conditions, which could then lead to improved neurologic outcomes in this patient population. With this in mind, EEG monitoring can serve three main purposes: early identification of cerebral ischemia, recognition of seizure activity, and assisting with prognostication. While a review of the complexities of EEG testing and interpretation are beyond the scope of this chapter, an understanding of the basics – particularly as applied to ECMO patients – is important to clinical management (**Figure 5a** and **b**).

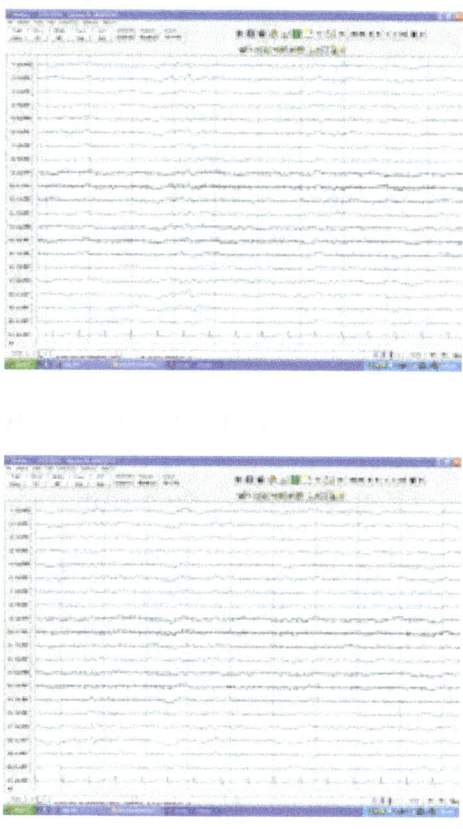

Figure 5. (a) Initial EEG in a 40-year-old, status post cardiopulmonary arrest and initiation of ECMO therapy for acute respiratory failure. CPR had been conducted on and off for over 60 min, at home, during transport to hospital and then during salvage cardiac catheterization. A 16-channel digital EEG recording 1 h after arrival to the ICU demonstrating low amplitude and severe suppression of the background rhythms with superimposed drug effect. No evidence of asymmetry or paroxysmal discharges. (b) Follow-up EEG (approximately 1 week later). A 16-channel digital EEG recording of the same patient with clinical examination concerning persistent coma off sedation and after discontinuation of ECMO. EEG demonstrates generalized suppression, which however has improved in amplitudes. No paroxysmal or asymmetric patterns were detected, despite concern for an asymmetric tone of limbs in the clinical exam. Patient recovered consciousness 48 h, following this EEG and was discharged 2 weeks later with no neurological deficits.

Following decreased CBF and ensuing cerebral ischemia, EEG changes progress from the loss of faster frequencies (i.e. beta and alpha) to slowing, first with excess theta and, as ischemia worsens, with excess delta waves. Finally, suppression of all frequencies usually indicates neuronal cell death and infarction. Periodic lateralized epileptiform discharges (PLEDs), stimulus-induced periodic rhythmic or ictal discharges (SIRPIDs), unilateral attenuations, and asymmetric triphasic waves can all be seen in patients with cerebral ischemia and aid in early recognition and prevention of irreversible injury [40].

The relatively high risk of both ischemic and hemorrhagic stroke during ECMO support leading to irreversible brain injury can in turn elevate the risk of clinical as well as non-convulsive seizures (as mentioned above). The incidence of clinical seizures during ECMO ranges from 2 to 10%, with somewhat higher rates in younger children [41]. However, the rates of subclinical seizures have been reported to be as high as 17%, including 11% with non-convulsive status epilepticus [42]. Furthermore, the occurrence of seizures seems to be associated with neurodevelopmental disorders in neonates as well as an increased risk of death and worse functional outcomes [43]. Continuous EEG monitoring can help with early identification of ictal patterns and guidance of pharmacologic treatment.

While more studies are still required, the presence of EEG background abnormalities and certain electrographic patterns can aid in the prediction of neurologic outcome after ECMO support. In one study, the presence of an unexplained burst suppression pattern was associated with an increased risk of death or severe disability [44], while low voltage or isoelectric EEG patterns are usually correlated with poor outcomes after global cerebral ischemia [45].

6. Laboratory studies as predictors of neuronal injury and clinical outcome

6.1. Biomarkers as predictors of neuronal injury and clinical outcome

Given that neuromonitoring modalities during ECMO vary widely among institutions and their reported use is limited to small studies, the introduction of plasma biomarkers has emerged as a monitoring tool to aid in outcome prediction for patients on ECMO. An ideal biomarker would have high sensitivity for detection of both ischemic and hemorrhagic injury, provide real-time information, and allow detection of injury at the cellular level that precedes cellular death. While such an ideal marker is not available yet, a number of plasma proteins have been studied to date.

In general, these biomarkers can be divided into three groups, those that reflect glial injury (glial fibrillary acidic protein [GFAP] and S100b), those indicative of neuronal injury (neuron-specific enolase [NSE], intercellular adhesion molecule-5 [ICAM-5], and brain-derived neurotrophic factor [BDNF]), and those suggestive of increased neuroinflammation (ICAM-5 and monocyte chemoattractant protein 1/chemokine (C-C motif) ligand 2 [MCP-1/CCL-2]) [43]. For instance, elevated plasma levels of GFAP in patients with ECMO were associated with a higher risk of brain injury and death (odds ratio of 11.5 and 13.6, respectively) [44]. Similarly, S100B may serve as an early indicator of cerebral complications, in particular intracerebral hemorrhage [46].

In a more recent investigation, a combination of six different biomarkers measured daily for the duration of ECMO demonstrated that GFAP, MCP-1/CCL-2, NSE, and S100b were all significantly higher in patients with unfavorable outcomes and that peak concentrations of GFAP, NSE, S100b, and MCP-1/CCL-2 were higher in non-survivors [47]. Even after adjusting for potentially confounding variables, GFAP and NSE remained significantly associated with unfavorable outcome and NSE associated with increased mortality. Lastly, elevated concentrations of GFAP and ICAM-5 predicted abnormal neuroimaging in this cohort. Taken together, while validation in larger studies is still required, these results suggest that the biomarkers mentioned above could serve as indicators for obtaining further investigations (i.e. neuroimaging) and for initiation of neuroprotective therapies.

7. Brain death examination

The America Academy of Neurology (AAN) has outlined criteria for the determination of brain death [48]. Given the high reported mortality rates—and in particular, brain death—in patients treated with ECMO, a thorough understanding of the definition and determinations of brain death is critical. Despite the importance of the assessment of brain death, objective protocols for patients on ECMO are clearly lacking.

A key component to the determination of brain death in the ECMO patient is the bedside clinical exam—ideally performed by a neurologist or clinician specifically skilled, or credentialed, in the assessment of brain function in ICU patients. The first step is to evaluate for coma. Coma is defined by the lack of all responsiveness, including eye opening or movement (spontaneous or provoked) and motor function in response to painful stimuli (not including spinal reflexes). The potentially reversible causes of coma must be excluded (**Table 1**):

Acid-base abnormalities
Electrolyte abnormalities
Endocrine complications
Presence of central nervous system depressants (neuromuscular blockade, suppressive drugs/medications
Hypothermia
Hypotension
Hypovolemia

Table 1. Potentially reversible causes of coma.

Other components to the clinical exam must include assessment of brainstem reflects and cranial nerve testing. Any evidence of brainstem function, or an incomplete assessment, is, by definition, inconsistent with a diagnosis of brain death (**Table 2**).

Continuous electroencephalographic (EEG) testing can be helpful when positive, but external electromagnetic energy sources, including the pump and ECMO circuitry, can make conclusive interpretation of results difficult. Cerebral angiography or nuclear scanning may document the absence of cerebral blow flow, but such testing in patients on ECMO can be difficult as transporting the patient and all of the mechanical equipment (ventilator, ECMO system, etc.) to remote areas of the hospital for testing can be dangerous and sometimes logistically impossible (i.e. will all of the equipment, the patient, and necessary clinical staff fit in a transport elevator?).

Prerequisites
Exclude the presence of central nervous system depressant drugs, neuromuscular blocking agents.
Rule out severe electrolyte, acid-base, or endocrine disturbance
Achieve normal core temperature
Achieve normal blood pressure (systolic blood pressure >100 mmHg)
Clinical evaluation of a coma
Absence of eye opening or movement to noxious stimuli
Absence of motor response other than spinally mediated reflexes to noxious stimuli
Absence of brainstem reflexes
Absence of pupillary response to a bright light in both eyes
Absence of ocular movement using oculocephalic and oculovestibular testing
Absence of corneal testing
Absence of facial muscle movement to noxious stimuli
Absence of pharyngeal and tracheal reflexes
Apnea test absence of breathing drive to carbon dioxide challenge
Ancillary tests
Electroencephalography, cerebral angiography, nuclear scan, transcranial Doppler, cerebral tomography angiography, and magnetic resonance imaging/angiogram

Table 2. Brain death criteria.

Formal apnea testing is the key procedure used in the establishment of brain death. The principle behind the test is that the absence of an appropriate respiratory drive, as manifested by an increased in $PaCO_2$ following a CO_2 challenge, is indicative of a potentially irreversible brain-stem injury and, therefore, when positive, supportive of the diagnosis of brain death. Specific criteria must be met prior to attempting an apnea test. In the absence of a history of comorbidities that might predispose to abnormalities in, or blunted responses to, CO_2 retention (e.g. COPD, sleep apnea, and/or morbid obesity), such testing can be diagnostic. Proper conduct of the test involves insuring an adequate blood pressure, preoxygenation with 100% oxygen for at least 10 min with a goal $PaO_2 > 200$ mmHg, normo-capnia with a ventilatory rate of 10 breaths/min, and a reduction of positive end-expiratory pressure to ~ 5 mmHg. If the patient remains hemodynamically stable and blood saturation remains >95%, then a baseline, pretest, arterial blood gas is obtained. The patient is then disconnected from the ventilator, but given a source of oxygen. A continuous source of oxygen, such as a T-piece or cannula placed directly into the trachea, is mandatory to prevent acute hypoxemia and therefore in validating the test. Continuous monitoring of the patient, looking for any evidence of respiratory function, gasping, or chest rise is required. Any signs of initiating a breath during the test should prompt discontinuation of the test and rule out a diagnosis of "brain death". Hypotension or desaturation mandate test termination. After 8 min of observation, a repeat blood gas is obtained. If the PCO_2 level is >60 mmHg or 20 mmHg above the baseline, then the test is considered positive and diagnostic of brain death. Longer periods of apnea (10–15 min), provided the patient remains hemodynamically stable, can be used when the initial blood gas results or clinical findings are inconclusive. Unfortunately, patients who require ECMO support often have physiologic conditions that might further challenge apnea testing. For patients being support-ed on veno-arterial ECMO, pulsatile flow and blood pressures might be too low as mandated by the AAN prior to attempting an apnea test. As discussed above, a systolic blood pressure >100 mmHg is a prerequisite for apnea testing – a threshold that might be very difficult to accomplish in patients on VA-ECMO with non-pulsatile flow in the absence of significant doses of vasoactive agents. In such circumstances, some experts have advocated using mean arterial pressure of 75-80 mmHg as an appropriate surrogate [49].

To compensate for the confounding influence of the inherent ability of the ECMO circuit to not only provide hemodynamic stability, but more importantly, to maintain adequate oxygenation and normal PCO2 levels, some investigators have proposed modifications of ECMO flows and gas exchange during apnea testing. However, such experiences are limited to a small series of patients. For example, Reddy and colleagues from the Mayo Clinic advocating preoxygenation with 100% oxygen using the ECMO circuit. An initial blood gas is obtained and the ECMO sweep flow was then reduced to 0.5 liters/min to minimize CO_2 removal while providing some degree of continuous oxygen support. It has been advocated that at minimal sweep levels, supplemental oxygen (i.e. given directly to the trachea or airways) is not necessary. With an adequate flow (75–80% of cardiac output) and oxygen through the ECMO, significant decreases in PO_2 and hypoxemia should not occur [47]. Patients were disconnected from the ventilator and after 8 min of observation (for clinical evidence of a respiratory drive), a repeat blood gas was obtained. In two patients, a rise in $PaCO_2$ over 60 mmHg or greater than 20 mmHg above baseline was reported, which confirmed brain death [50]. This group of investigators also reported a series of three critically ill patients on ECMO support, each of who experienced catastrophic neurologic complications consistent clinically with brain death. However, in each of these patients, apnea testing could not be safely performed due to the absence of a defined protocol and hemodynamic instability. Neverthe-less, they advocated the use of apnea testing using the protocol they described in their initial patients to assist in the timely diagnosis of brain death in appropriate patients. The benefits of a timely and definitive diagnosis include increased potential for organ donation, decreased resource utilization in futile cases, and most importantly definitive information for the family [51]. Such testing can be difficult because decreasing the sweep gas too much may theoretically result in a significant hypoxemia – and mandate cessation of the test – before a significant increase in $PaCO_2$ can occur to yield a definitive result [52].

Because apnea testing is dependent on intrinsic brainstem response to initiate a breath in the setting of increasing levels of carbon dioxide, it has been suggested that in patients treated with ECMO the addition of exogenous CO2 could safely and more efficiently facilitate this test. A significant concern for apnea testing is the ability to safely provide an oxygen source during testing. Oxygen depravation, particularly in an already compromised and potentially brain injured patient, may worsen an anoxic injury. While ECMO is used to eliminate CO_2 (while supplementing oxygen), in theory, ECMO can be used to increase $PaCO_2$ levels. Pirat and colleagues describe the addition of a CO_2 source to the ECMO circuit gas blender and the flow was initiated at 0.5 liters/min and titrated to an end titer of CO_2 of 60 mmHg. The PaO_2 level was then confirmed with blood gas after a period of clinical observation. They suggested that the addition of carbon dioxide was safer by minimizing hypoxemia and hemodynamic instability that might come with the removal of ventilatory (or gas sweep/flow) support [53]. Clearly, while such an approach sounds intriguing and physiologically possible, confirmatory studies are necessary prior to wider use.

8. Conclusions

Without a doubt, ECMO has proven to be a valuable therapy for patients with severe acute respiratory and/or cardiac failure. Early initiation of the therapy, prior to the development of irreversible end-organ function, has been shown to improve outcomes in critically ill patients. Unfortunately, despite improved technologies, earlier and more aggressive therapy and a better understanding of the complex pathophysiology and human-extracorporeal circuit interface, complications are still common. Neurologic complications, either as a function of preECMO comorbidities, presenting illnesses, or as a consequence of the intricacies of either veno-veno or veno-arterial support are unfortunately not uncommon. Such complications can manifest in a variety of anoxic, embolic, hemorrhagic, metabolic, or functional ways and are often a source of significant morbidity and mortality. Early and aggressive monitoring, diagnostic testing, optimization of cerebral perfusion, and oxygenation might not prevent complications, but might limit their impact by allowing for optimization of neuroprotective interventions. In addition, earlier testing might also provide better prognostic implications of therapy and allow for optimal resource utilization, including patient selection for ECMO. As many patients experience neurologic complications, even in the absence of definitive and comprehensive testing, a more thorough understanding of the problem will allow for better management tools and therapies. Hopefully, this review not only illustrates the complex scope of this problem but provides the foundation for further explorations into how to better protect the brain while on extracorporeal membrane oxygenation support.

Author details

Susana M. Bowling[1], Joao Gomes[1] and Michael S. Firstenberg[2*]

*Address all correspondence to: msfirst@gmail.com

1 Department of Neurology, Division of Internal Medicine, Summa Health Care System – Akron City Hospital, Akron, OH, USA

2 Department of Surgery – Cardiothoracic, Summa Health Care System – Akron City Hospital, Akron, OH, USA

References

[1] Nasr DM, Rabinstein AA. Neurologic complications of extracorporeal membrane oxygenation. J Clin Neurol. 2015;11(4):383–9.

[2] Bulas DI, Taylor GA, O'Donnell RM, Short BL, Fitz CR, Vezina G. Intracranial abnormalities in infants treated with extracorporeal membrane oxygenation: update on sonographic and CT findings. Am J Neuroradiol. 1996;17(2):287–294.

[3] Fowler RA, Lapinsky SE, Domınguez-Cherit G. Extracorporeal membrane oxygenation for ARDS due to 2009 influenza A (H1N1). JAMA. 2009;302(17):1888–95.

[4] Cheng A, Sun HY, Lee CW, Ko WJ, Tsai PR, Chuang YC, Hu FC, Chang SC, Chen YC. Survival of septic adults compared with nonseptic adults receiving extracorporeal membrane oxygenation for cardiopulmonary failure: a propensity-matched analysis. J Crit Care. 2013;28(4):532–e1.

[5] Paden ML, Conrad SA, Rycus PT, Thiagarajan RR. Extracorporeal life support organization registry report 2012. ASAIO J. 2013;59(3):202–210.

[6] Biscotti M, Gannon WD, Abrams D, Agerstrand C, et al. Extracorporeal membrane oxygenation use in patients with traumatic brain injury. Perfusion. 2015 Jul 1;30(5):407–9.

[7] Beurtheret S, Mordant P, et al. Emergency circulatory support in refractory cardiogenic shock patients in remote institutions: a pilot study (The cardiac – RESCUE program). European heart journal. 2012 Apr 17:ehs081.

[8] Firstenberg MS, Galloway J, Abel E, Mast D, Tripathi RS. Extra-corporeal circulatory support: a resurgence of a life saving therapy in the digital information age. Surgery: Current Research. 2012 Mar 24;2011.

[9] Marika K, Lidegran M, Mosskin M, et al. Cranial CT diagnosis of intracranial complications in adult and pediatric patients during ECMO: clinical benefits in diagnosis and treatment. Acad Radiol 2007;14:62–71.

[10] Extracorporeal Life Support Organization. ECLS Registry Report. Ann Arbor, MI: Extracorporeal Life Support Organization, 2006. Int J Acad Med. 2016;2(1):22–26.

[11] Mateen FJ, Muralidharan R. Neurologic injury in adults treated with extracorporeal membrane oxygenation. Arch Neurol. 2011;68(12):1543–1549. Published online August 8, 2011. doi: 10.1001/archneurol.2011.209

[12] Firstenberg MS, Blais D, Abel E, Louis LB, Sun B, Mangino JE. Fulminant Neisseria meningitidis: role for extracorporeal membrane oxygenation. Heart Surg Forum. 2010;13(6):E376–E378.

[13] Lassen NA, Christensen MS. Physiology of cerebral blood flow. Br J Anaesth. 1976;48:719–734.

[14] Peterson EC, Wang Z, Britz G. Regulation of cerebral blood flow. Int J Vasc Med. 2011;2011:823525. doi: 10.1155/2011/823525. Epub 2011 Jul 25.

[15] Prior PF. EEG monitoring and evoked potentials in brain ischemia. Br J Anaesth. 1985;57:63–81.

[16] Raju TN, Kim SY, Meller JL, et al. Circle of Willis blood velocity and flow direction after common carotid artery ligation for neonatal extra-corporeal membrane oxygenation. Pediatrics. 1989;83:343–347. PubMed: 2645565.

[17] O'Brien NF, Hall MW. Extracorporeal membrane oxygenation and cerebral blood flow velocity in children. Pediatr Crit Care Med. 2013;14(3):e126–134. doi: 10.1097/PCC. 0b013e3182712d62

[18] Kasirajan V, Smedira NG, et al. Risk factors for intracranial hemorrhage in adults on extracorporeal membrane oxygenation. Eur J Cardiothoracic Surg. 1999;15:508–514.

[19] Mendoza JC, Shearer LL, Cook LM. Lateralization of brain lesions following extracorporeal membrane oxygenation. Pediatrics. 1991;88:1004–1009.

[20] Oliver WC. Anticoagulation and coagulation management for ECMO. Semin Cardiothorac Vasc Anesth. 2009;13(3):154–175.

[21] Hill S, Hejal R, Bowling SM, Firstenberg MS. Neurologic complications in patients receiving extracorporeal membrane oxygenation for influenza H1H1: morbid but not futile. Int J Acad Med. In press.

[22] Dalton HJ, Day SE. Neurologic outcome following ECLS in pediatric patients with respiratory or cardiac failure. In Van Meurs K, Lally KP, Peek G, et al., eds. ECMO Extracorporeal Cardiopulmonary Support in Critical Care. 3rd ed. Ann Arbor, MI: Extracorporeal Life Support Organization, 2005; pp. 383–392.

[23] Biehl DA, Stewart DL, et al. Timing of intracranial hemorrhage during extracorporeal life support. ASAIO J 1996;42:938–941.

[24] Thiagarajan RR, et al. Extracorporeal membrane oxygenation to support cardiopulmonary resuscitation in adults. Ann Thorac Surg. 2009;87(3):778–785.

[25] Firstenberg MS, Nelson K, Abel E, McGregor J, Eiferman D. Extracorporeal membrane oxygenation for complex multiorgan system trauma. Case reports in surgery. 2012 Mar 29;2012.

[26] Omar HR, Mirsaeidi M, Shumac J, Enten G, Mangar D, Camporesi EM. Incidence and predictors of ischemic cerebrovascular stroke among patients on extracorporeal membrane oxygenation support. J Crit Care. 2016 April (32):48–51.

[27] Pokersnik JA, Buda T, Bashour CA, Gonzalez-Stawinski GV. Have changes in ECMO technology impacted outcomes in adult patients developing postcardiotomy cardiogenic shock? J Cardiac Surg. 2012;27(2):246–252.

[28] Lan C, Tsai PR, Chen YS, Ko WJ. Prognostic factor for adult patients receiving extracorporeal membrane oxygenation as mechanical circulatory support: a 14-year experience at a medical center. Atif Organs. 2010;34(2):E59–E64.

[29] Ko WJ, Lin CY, et al. Extracorporeal membrane oxygenation support for adult postcardiotomy cardiogenic shock. Ann Thorac Surg. 2002;73(2):538–545.

[30] Risnes I, Wagner K, Nome T, et al. Cerebral outcome in adult patients treated with extracorporeal membrane oxygenation. Ann Thorac Surg. 2006;81(4):1401–1406.

[31] Mehta A, Ibsen LM. Meurologic complications and neurodevelopmental outcome with extracorporeal life support. World J Crit Care Med. 2013;2(4):40–47.

[32] Auvil B, Mattiola R, et al. Outcomes of patients on extracorporeal membrane oxygenation (ECMO) for periods of time without anticoagulation at LVHN in the past 3 years. Poster presented at the LVHN Research Scholar Program Poster session, Lehigh Valley Health Network, Allentown, PA.

[33] Taylor G, Fitz CR, Miller MK, et al. Intracranial abnormalities in infants treated with extracorporeal membrane oxygenation: imaging with US and CT. Radiology. 1987;165:675–678.

[34] Lidegram M, Palmer K, Joruf H, et al. CT in the evacuation of patients on ECMO due to acute respiratory failure. Pediatr Radiol. 2002;32:567–574.

[35] Horsch S, De Vleeschauwer P, Ktenidis K. Intraoperative assessment of cerebral ischemia during carotid surgery. J Cardiovasc Surg. 1990;31:599–602.

[36] Guerit JM, Witdoeckt C, de Tourtchaninoff M, et al. Somatosensory evoked potential monitoring in carotid surgery. I. Relationships between qualitative sep alterations and intraoperative events. Electroencephalogr Clin Neurophysiol. 1997;104:459–469.

[37] Koenig MA. Brain resuscitation and prognosis after cardiac arrest. Critical care clinics, 30(4), pp.765–783.

[38] Carter BG, Butt WW. Median nerve somatosensory evoked potentials in children receiving ECMO. Pediatr Neurol. 1995;12(1):42–46.

[39] Amigoni A, Pettenazzo A, Biban P, et al. Neurologic outcome in children after extracorporeal membrane oxygenation: prognostic value of diagnostic tests. Pediatr Neurol. 2005;32(3):173–179.

[40] Hirsch LJ, Brenner RP. EEG in cerebrovascular disease. In Atlas of EEG in Critical Care. Oxford UK: Wiley-Blackwell, 2010.

[41] Abend NS, Dlugos DJ, Clancy RR. A review of long-term EEG monitoring in critically ill children with hypoxic-ischemic encephalopathy, congenital heart disease, ECMO, and stroke. J Clin Neurophysiol. 2013;30(2):134–142. doi: 10.1097/WNP. 0b013e3182872af9

[42] Hahn JS, Vaucher Y, Bejar R, Coen RW. Electroencephalographic and neuroimaging findings in neonates undergoing extracorporeal membrane oxygenation. Neuropediatrics. 1993;24:19–24. PubMed: 8474607.

[43] Bembea MM, Rizkall N, Freedy, J et al. Plasma biomarkers of brain injury as diagnostic tools and outcome predictors after extracorporeal membrane oxygenation. Crit Care Med. 2015;43(10):2202–2211.

[44] Bembea MM, Savage W, Strouse JJ, et al. Glial fibrillary acidic protein as a brain injury biomarker in children undergoing extracorporeal membrane oxygenation. Pediatr Crit Care Med. 2011;12(5):572–579. doi: 10.1097/PCC.0b013e3181fe3ec7

[45] Cloostermans MC, van Meulen FB, Eertman CJ, Hom HW, van Putten MJ. Continuous electroencephalography monitoring for early prediction of neurological outcome in postanoxic patients after cardiac arrest: a prospective cohort study. Crit Care Med. 2012;40(10):2867–2875.

[46] Gazzolo D, Masetti P, Meli M, et al. Elevated S100B protein as an early indicator of intracranial haemorrhage in infants subjected to extracorporeal membrane oxygenation. Acta Paediatr. 2002;91:218–221.

[47] Hoskote SS, Fugate JE, Wijdicks EFM. Performance of an apnea test for brain death determination in a patient receiving venoarterial extracorporeal membrane oxygenation. J Cardiothoracic Vasc Anesth. 2014;28(4):1027–1029.

[48] Wijdicks EF, Varelas PN, Gronseth GS, et al. American academy of neurology: evidence-based guideline update: determining brain death in adults: report of the Quality Standards Subcommittee of the American Academy of Neurology. Neurology. 2010;74:1911–1918.

[49] Shah V, Lazaridis C. Apnea testing on extracorporeal membrane oxygenation: case report and literature review. J Crit Care. 2015;30(4):784–786.

[50] Reddy DR, Hoskote S, Guru P, Fugate J, Crow S, Wijdicks EFM. Brain death confirmation on extracorporeal membrane oxygenation (ECMO): a novel technique. Crit Care Med. 2014;42(12):523.

[51] Muralidharan RN, Mateen FJ, Shonohara RT, Schears GJ, Wijdicks EFM. The challenges with brain death determination in adult patients on extracorporeal membrane oxygenation. Neurocrit Care. 2011;14:4239–4426.

[52] Goswami S, Evans A, Das B, Prager K, Sladen RN, Wagener G. Determination of brain death by apnea test adapted to extracorporeal cardiopulmonary resuscitation. J Cardiothoracic Vasc Anesth. 2013;27(2):312–314.

[53] Pirat A, Kömürcü Ö, Yener G, Arslan G. Apnea testing for diagnosing brain death during extracorporeal membrane oxygenation. J Cardiothoracic Vasc Anesth. 2014;28(1):e8–e9. doi: 10.1053/j.jvca.2013.09.013

6

Sedation, Analgesia Delirium in the ECMO Patient

SV Satyapriya, ML Lyaker, AJ Rozycki and Papadimos

Abstract

The goal of this chapter is to identify medications frequently utilized for sedation and analgesia in Extracorporeal Membrane Oxygenation (ECMO) patients. In addition to describing basic pharmacologic principles of these medications, we discuss their benefits and disadvantages and explain the effects the ECMO circuitry will have on pharmacokinetics of each drug. We also discuss need for various depths of sedation and the utility of neuromuscular blocking agents. Emerging techniques for achieving appropriate sedation will be identified. An explosion of literature in recent years has led to Intensive Care Unit (ICU) delirium increasingly being recognized as an indicator of poor outcomes in the general ICU population. We discuss strategies to manage this complex and multifactorial issues, and how they can be applied to our particular subpopulation of ECMO patients.

Keywords: sedation, analgesia, agitation, delirium, neuromuscular blocking agents, ECMO sequestration

1. Introduction

The basic principles of initiation and titration of sedatives and analgesics in the critically ill apply to those on Extracorporeal Membrane Oxygenation (ECMO). There are, however, some unique characteristics that pertain to the patient as well as the ECMO device itself that may help guide the intensivist in this particular subset. We will describe the basic pharmacologic principles of commonly used medications for providing sedation and analgesia and nonpharmacologic interventions. Emerging techniques for achieving appropriate sedation will be identified that include ECMO in the awake patient.

The ECMO circuitry has its own unique effects on the pharmacokinetics of each drug. We will also discuss the need for various depths of sedation and the utility of neuromuscular blocking agents. This chapter also includes a discussion of monitoring and identifying the emerging techniques for management of sedation, analgesia, and delirium that include ECMO in the awake patients.

The reader should be able to identify the most commonly used analgosedation practices in ECMO patients after reading this chapter as well as the emerging techniques. They should understand the effect of the ECMO circuitry on pharmacokinetics of each drug described. We also hope to increase the understanding of the complex issue of Intensive Care Unit (ICU) delirium. The authors hope the readers will use the information to develop a systematic approach for delivering and titrating targeted analgosedation as well as for identifying and managing delirium in the critically ill ECMO patient.

2. Sedation and analgesia

The American College of Critical Care Medicine task force recently revised its clinical practice guidelines for the management of pain, agitation, and delirium in critically ill adult patients [1]. These guidelines recognize that pain is common in Intensive Care Unit (ICU) patients and may lead to both acute and long-term sequelae. In the acute setting, pain increases the proinflammatory balance of cytokines and may contribute to tissue hypoperfusion due to arteriolar vasoconstriction [2,3]. Opiates decrease this stress response and decrease tissue metabolic oxygen consumption [2]. Later, acute pain may lead to PTSD and Chronic Pain in patients who survive their critical illness [4,5]. Sedatives such as benzodiazepines may be used to decrease the stress response; however, they may have negative consequences that could worsen outcomes in ICU patients [1]. The 2013 guidelines thus advocate for pain assessment in ICU patients and an "analgesia-first" approach to sedation [1]. For patients undergoing ECMO, many considerations are similar to those encountered in other critically ill populations; however, certain factors will require additional consideration in this vulnerable group. Ultimately, the choice of medication for sedation and analgesia in a patient on ECMO will rely on multiple pharmacokinetic and pharmacodynamics considerations, clinical circumstances, patient's variables, and the goals of the team managing the patient [6].

Although intravenous opioids have been a mainstay of ICU analgesia for many years, much of the pharmacokinetic data comes from single-dose studies in healthy volunteers [7,8]. ECMO further complicates the situation by altering the pharmacokinetics of analgesics and sedatives [9,10]. The depth and duration of sedation as well as the titratability of the medication(s) selected must be considered. Often the level of sedation tolerated will depend on the patient's stability and sedation goals may vary considerably over time. This is especially true during the initial period after initiation of ECMO. At this stage, greater levels of sedation and sometimes chemical paralysis may be required. At the same time, the patient is frequently still in a state of hemodynamic or metabolic shock. Patients with an open chest due to central cannulation and those who require multiple painful procedures will require a greater degree of sedation to decrease movement and the consequent risk of cannula dislodgement. Medication interactions with the ECMO circuit itself must also be taken into account. Circuit sequestration of highly lipophilic medications will decrease their bioavailability. This issue will be discussed in more detail in a later part of this chapter. Renal and hepatic functions are often impaired in patients requiring ECMO [11]; thus, the half-life of many medications can be prolonged; metabolites and compounding agents such as propylene glycol may accumulate leading to unwanted side-effects.

Route of administration is another concern with critically ill patients on ECMO. Enteral administration is cheaper and decreases reliance on parenteral access but may result in erratic and unpredictable absorption [6]. Submucosal and IM administration is generally unreliable in patients suffering from shock [8]. The 2013 Clinical Practice Guidelines from the Society of Critical Care Medicine consequently recommend intravenous opioids as the first-line drug class of choice to treat nonneuropathic pain in critically ill patients [1]. Intravenous administration provides faster onset, higher bioavailability, and rapid titratability [8]. This proves advantageous when administering medication prior to an invasive procedure or when following a sedation protocol. As the patient progresses in their course, lesser levels of sedation and analgesia may be required and minimal analgesia and sedation may be necessary [12]. At this point, continuous infusions may be discontinued and intermittent dosing of analgesics may prove sufficient.

All the available IV opioids can be titrated to achieve equally effective levels of analgesia [1]; thus the main difference between opiates comes down to cost, pharmacokinetic properties, and pharmacodynamic distinctions [6]. Opioids with agonist-antagonist properties should be avoided in critically ill patients in general due to decreased analgesic efficacy and the potential for triggering withdrawal in opiate dependent patients [6]. Meperidine is an undesirable choice because of potential drug interactions with serotonergic and dopaminergic agents, vagolytic side effects and the buildup of normeperidine, a metabolite which lowers the seizure threshold [8]. Fentanyl, a synthetic opioid with a rapid onset and short distribution half-life, is one of the most commonly used opioids in the ICU [13]; however, because fentanyl and its derivatives, sufentanil, alfentanil, and remifentanil, are highly lipophilic, they are extensively consumed by the ECMO circuit [10]. It has been demonstrated that within hours of administration, nearly the entire dose of fentanyl is lost in an ex vivo ECMO circuit primed with blood [14,15]. With such rapid absorption rates, exceedingly high doses of fentanyl would be required to maintain the desired level of analgesia. Furthermore, a patient previously exposed to high doses of opiates may experience withdrawal if placed on ECMO while already receiving fentanyl analgesia. Fentanyl may thus best play the role of a rapid onset analgesic used for brief but painful procedures.

From a pharmacokinetic standpoint morphine may be the preferred analgesic during ECMO. Because it is hydrophilic, it shows little absorption into the ECMO circuit [14,15]. Morphine was in fact considered the "preferred analgesic agent for critically ill patients" by the older 1995 guidelines for analgesia and sedation published by the Society of Critical Care Medicine [16]. Some of morphine's attributes however make it less desirable for use in the critically ill population. Histamine release from morphine may contribute to bronchospasm and hypotension [6]. In renal failure, accumulation of the active metabolite morphine-6-glucuronide may lead to prolonged sedation. Hydromorphone, a semisynthetic opiate, may thus prove a more suitable option for IV analgesia in patients on ECMO. Although there is no specific study of hydromorphone's pharmacokinetics in an ECMO circuit, the drug's hydrophilic nature should keep sequestration at acceptable levels. There is no histamine release associated with large doses of hydromorphone, and although the parent drug may accumulate in renal and hepatic impairment, there are no active metabolites. The half-life of hydromorphone is 2–3 h, allowing for either intermittent bolus dosing or a continuous infusion to maintain the desired level of analgesia. Oxycodone, another semisynthetic opioid, may be given enterally for patients who are expected to have adequate absorption from their gastrointestinal tract. It is metabolized by the cytochrome P450 system, thus the dose should be reduced in hepatic dysfunction. Peak effect is reached after approximately 30 minutes to an hour and the duration of its effect is approximately 3–6 h. Oxycodone is relatively hydrophilic and so should not significantly bind to the ECMO circuit.

Analgesic adjuncts such as intravenous (IV) acetaminophen, gabapentin, ketamine, and dexmedetomidine may be used to decrease reliance on opioid analgesics and minimize their side effects. Unfortunately, many of these medications have only been studied on a limited basis in the ICU population, and data for patients receiving ECMO is remarkably limited. IV acetaminophen has been approved by the US Food and Drug Administration (FDA) for use along with opioids for pain management after major and cardiac surgery [17,18]. However, it has not been studied for extended periods of time or in a population with a high incidence of organ failure such as ECMO patients [19]. Additionally, the benefits of acetaminophen may not be as apparent or relevant in a population that requires long-term ICU level care. Neuropathic pain in settings such as burns, neuralgia, and neuropathy tends to be poorly treated by opioids [1]; however, it may respond to medications such as gabapentin and pregabalin that target calcium channels in the central nervous system [6,20]. If patients have been started on these medications due to pre-existing conditions, continuation of the therapy is prudent to avoid withdrawal. Unfortunately, pharmacokinetics can be complicated by unpredictable absorption from the GI tract, renal dysfunction, renal replacement therapy, and uncertain interactions with the ECMO circuit.

Since ECMO is frequently complicated by hemodynamic instability and rapidly escalating requirements for sedation and analgesia [9], ketamine infusions have been used to optimize patient comfort without increasing the depth of sedation or contributing to hypotension. Ketamine is an NMDA antagonist that has been shown to augment opiate analgesia without decreasing sympathetic tone [21]. Limited data exists on long-term ketamine use in critically ill patients; however, some trials have shown decreased opiate usage, improved gastrointestinal motility, and decreased vasopressor requirements in patients treated with ketamine [22]. Similarly, a retrospective review of ketamine in 26 ECMO patients treated at a single center demonstrated a decrease in vasopressor requirements and a decrease in sedation requirements while maintaining the same level of sedation [23]. The doses of ketamine used in the ECMO trial (50–150 mg/H) were substantially higher than those described for analgesia in other studies. Since ketamine is lipophilic, this may be attributable to circuit sequestration of ketamine. A possible concern with ketamine analgesia in patients, who have cardiogenic shock, is that the increase in blood pressure may come at the expense of a decrease in cardiac output and an increase in systemic and pulmonary vascular resistance [24].

When an analgesia-based regimen is insufficient to provide adequate patient comfort, or a greater depth of sedation is required due to clinical circumstances, a sedative may be initiated. Just as opiates have been the mainstay of analgesia in the ICU, benzodiazepines have traditionally been used for sedation in critically ill patients. Benzodiazepines activate -aminobutyric acid A receptors in the central nervous system leading to anxiolysis, amnesia, sedation, and an increase in the seizure threshold [8]. Recent evidence however has identified these agents as a leading, modifiable cause of delirium in hospitalized patients and implicated them in prolonging the duration of mechanical ventilation and ICU stays [25–27]. Other agents such as propofol and dexmedetomidine have shown superiority in comparison to benzodiazepines by reducing ICU stays and duration of delirium [26–28].

Of the benzodiazepines, midazolam is frequently used as an infusion for short to intermediate duration sedation of ICU patients [8]. It is water soluble, has a rapid onset of action, and a relatively shorter half-life of 2–5 h. However, with prolonged infusion, midazolam and its active metabolite 1-hydroxymidazolam glucuronide may accumulate, contributing to prolonged sedation and respiratory depression. Liver and renal failure may both prolong this effect. Lorazepam is metabolized by glucuronidation in the liver to an inactive metabolite and is thus less affected by renal and hepatic dysfunction. Since it has a longer half-life of 10–20 h, it may be given as an infusion or bolused on an as needed basis. Midazolam is highly lipophilic and is to a large extent absorbed by the ECMO circuit. In one study 50% of midazolam remained available after 30 min of in vitro ECMO circulation, and only 13% was detected after 24 h [29]. On the other hand, another study evaluated lorazepam and showed that 70% of lorazepam remained at 24 h [61]. Since lorazepam is somewhat less lipophilic, a lesser degree of sequestration would be anticipated.

Of the nonbenzodiazepine sedatives, propofol is extensively absorbed by the ECMO circuit [30]. This property and its tendency to cause hypotension would make propofol a less desirable agent for the sedation of patients on ECMO. Dexmedetomidine, a selective alpha-2 receptor agonist, with sedative and analgesic properties, has demonstrated substantial advantages over benzodiazepines in the care of critically ill patients. Patients sedated with dexmedetomidine are more easily aroused, have a reduced incidence of delirium, decreased sympathetic tone, and less respiratory depression [1,28]. A recent study showed that addition of dexmedetomidine to standard care of agitated, mechanically ventilated patients resulted in more rapid resolution of delirium and more ventilator free days [31]. Dexmedetomidine may not be appropriate in patients requiring a deep level of sedation or those with hypotension or bradycardia [6]. Dosage adjustments will likely be required for patients on ECMO due to significant interactions with the PVC tubing of the circuit [32].

Monitoring levels of sedation and analgesia is crucial in decreasing the likelihood of undesired outcomes [1]. Chanques et al. demonstrated that a protocol for systematically assessing and treating pain and agitation in critically ill patients not only decreased pain and agitation but also decreased the duration of mechanical ventilation and the incidence of nosocomial infections in a mixed medical-surgical population [33]. Although a patient's self-assessment of pain is considered the "gold standard" for pain assessment, this is frequently difficult to obtain in the ICU setting. Hemodynamic indicators of pain are not validated or reliable [1]. Behavioral scales have been developed as an objective tool for measuring pain in patients unable to communicate. Two scales in particular, the Behavioral Pain Scale and the Critical Care Pain Observation Tool have been found to be both reliable and valid in patients who are unable to report pain but have intact motor function [34]. Although further validation and study is warranted, implementation of these scales has been shown to be feasible and to lead to improved pain management and clinical outcomes [33,35,36]. Whether such protocols of pain assessment and titration would improve outcomes in ECMO patients remains to be seen.

With regard to sedation, the Richmond Agitation-Sedation Scale (RASS) and the Sedation-Agitation Scale (SAS) are considered the most valid and reliable sedation assessment tools for measuring depth of sedation. They demonstrate high inter-rater reliability as well as convergent and discriminant validation in a relatively high number of subjects [1]. The RASS additionally provides a goal for the titration of sedation. In patients who are chemically paralyzed, as ECMO patients may be immediately after cannulation, one of several objective sedation monitors, such as the bispectral index (BIS), Narcotrend Index, Patients State Index or state entropy, should be used [1]. Electroencephalogram monitoring should be used in patients suspected of having nonconvulsive seizures.

3. Neuromuscular blockade and ECMO/ARDS

Neuromuscular blocking agents (NMBAs) have been controversial with regard to their efficacy in treating acute respiratory distress syndrome (ARDS) (we will not discuss the use of NMBAs for the initial intubation of the patient). Due to lack of evidence on a large scale, no clear recommendations exist regarding the use of NMBAs in ARDS. Early work suggested that anesthesia and paralysis cause a ventilation/perfusion mismatch and impair gas exchange [37]. The traditional view on NMBA use in the critical care setting is largely negative, with a number of potential complications associated with this therapeutic modality [38,39]. However, other work over the past 12 years has indicated that use of NMBAs in acute respiratory distress syndrome (ARDS) has been shown to improve oxygenation and decrease mortality in most hypoxemic patients [40]. What is applicable in ARDS is also applicable in ECMO because ECMO is just a further device extension beyond ventilators and high-frequency oscillators [41,42].

Gannier et al. asserted that the hypoxemia in ARDS reaches its worst levels in the first 48 h. In a study of 56 patients with ARDS, improved oxygenation was seen in patients randomized to NMBAs in the first 48 h while receiving volume assist control with a tidal volume of 6–8 ml/kg [43]. Another similar study reported that early NMBA use may contribute to modulation of the pro-inflammatory response [44]. Additionally, a third study of 340 patients where cis-atracurium was administered in the first 48 h of development of ARDS found that the NMBAs improved the adjusted 90-day survival and increased time off of the ventilator without increasing muscle weakness [45].

Two recent meta-analyses based on randomized control trials analyzed the use of NMBAs in ARDS. Neto et al. performed a systematic review of the literature and meta-analysis of studies conducted between 1966 and 2012, and the three abovementioned studies were the only acceptable, high-quality trials performed [46]. The authors concluded, based on these three studies, that that the use of NMBAs in the early stages of ARDS leads to an improved outcome. Alhazzani et al., in a second meta-analysis, demonstrated a decreased mortality rate at 28 days among those receiving NMBAs in early ARDS [47]. They stated that nine patients need to be treated to save one life. They also found that there was a reduced risk of barotrauma and an increased number of days without mechanical ventilation during the first four weeks in those receiving NMBAs. Furthermore, they showed that the PaO2:FiO2 ratio was improved at one, two, and three days.

Physicians must be aware of the potentially important pathophysiological events that can occur with the use of NMBAs in hypoxemic patients [40]. These include increases in thoraco-pulmonary compliance, functional residual capacity, perfusion of ventilated spaces, and recruitment of portions of the lung that have little compliance. There can be decreases in pulmonary shunt, muscular O_2 consumption, overdistention of high-compliance areas, derecruitment, end-expiratory collapse, asynchronous patient-ventilator dynamics, barotrauma, volutrauma, biotrauma, and atelectrauma. The debate continues as to the best ventilation practices/strategy in ARDS. The problem with NMBAs is that they seem to eliminate the opportunity for the use of spontaneous modes [40].

Additionally, every practicing intensivist must be aware of ICU-acquired weakness (ICUAW), a polyneuropathy and/or myopathy, that occur in 34–60% of the patients with ARDS [48–50]. It was associated with independent risk factors such as organ dysfunction, female gender, length of time on a ventilator, and corticosteroid administration [51], and there is some evidence it is related to hypothermia, hyperglycemia, ICU length of stay, low albumin, and vasopressors [52–54]. While NMBAs have historically been associated with ICUAW, recent evidence contradicts this view, at least with nonsteroidal NMBAs [40].

It is of great importance to use a nerve stimulator for the monitoring of neuromuscular blockade [55]. If the dose of NMBAs is limited, there may be a decrease in the subsequent risks of ICUAW and complications from residual neuromuscular blockade [56]. Peripheral nerve stimulator use is mandatory in order to facilitate appropriate titration of NMBAs. Train of four (TOF) monitoring is the primary method for assessment of NMBA and generally involves the use of supramaximal electrical impulses every 0.5 s applied to the ulnar, facial, or posterial tibial nerve with a resultant identifiable pattern or response [55]. Instruction in TOF monitoring is beyond the scope of this chapter.

Hraiech et al. make the observation that based on the available evidence provided by random-ized control trials, NMBAs can be integrated safely into the concept of protective ventilation [40]. The use of NMBAs should be confined to the acute phase of ARDS. Spontaneous breathing must be encouraged when the severe phase has passed and in those with mild and moderate ARDS from the outset. Finally, never forget to sedate a patient in which a NMBA is used. In some countries, such as the USA, this can be a cause of legal action or discipline [57]. While the above suppositions related to NMBAs were not directly related to ECMO, the difficulty in oxygenating an ECMO patient should at least lead to the consideration of pharmacologic paralysis.

4. Drug sequestration in ECMO

Drug therapy while a patient is on ECMO may be affected by multiple pharmacokinetic alterations, including volume of distribution and protein binding. One of the reasons a patient's volume of distribution may be increased is due to sequestration of drug within the ECMO circuit. Sequestration of drugs into the ECMO circuit is a well-known phenomenon with certain drug properties predicting which medications may bind to the ECMO circuit [15]. Medications that are considered lipophilic, such as propofol, will have a high octanol/water partition coefficient (log P) and will be soluble in organic materials such as PVC tubing [15]. Conversely, medications that are considered hydrophilic may be unaffected by the ECMO circuit. In an ex vivo study performed by Lemaitre and colleagues, the concentration of propofol decreased to 11% of expected values after 24 h in a closed ECMO circuit [30], while concentrations of vancomycin, a relatively hydrophilic drug, remained unchanged.

In addition to lipophilicity, the degree of a drug's protein binding may affect sequestration in the ECMO circuit. Shekar and colleagues performed an ex vivo study and determined that drugs with significantly reduced concentrations at 24 h were either highly protein bound (>80%), highly lipophilic (log P > 2.3), or both [60]. For medications with the similar lipophilicity, the degree of drug recovery was based on protein binding. Both ciprofloxacin and thiopentone have similar lipophilicity (log P 2.3; however, greater reductions were seen in the drug with higher protein binding, thiopentone (88%), compared with ciprofloxacin (4%). This held true when comparing two hydrophilic drugs vancomycin and ceftriaxone. Circuit drug recovery at 24 h was higher for vancomycin (91%) compared with ceftriaxone (80%), which is more highly protein bound. It is unclear of why highly protein bound drugs bind to the ECMO circuit. It is postulated that proteins in the priming solution or in the patient's blood bind to the circuit and then the drug in turn binds to the protein sequestered in the circuit. Drugs that are both lipophilic and highly protein bound may be more prone to sequestration in the circuit. As an example, fentanyl a highly protein bound and lipophilic drug has been studied in ECMO with extreme reductions in concentrations (97%) at 24 h [14]. However, it is still unclear if the presence of both properties results in additive binding within the circuit.

In addition to considering drug properties to predict sequestration, it is imperative to evaluate the ECMO circuit components and their materials. Wildschut and colleagues showed significant differences in drug recovery for both fentanyl and midazolam in neonatal centrifugal pumps compared to neonatal roller pumps [15]. The neonatal centrifugal pumps had nearly one hundred fold increases in drug recovery for fentanyl and midazolam compared with the roller pumps, which may be due to the fact that roller pumps require more PVC tubing, potentially increasing the amount of drug-binding sites. The PVC tubing and membrane oxygenators used in ECMO have both been shown to sequester drug within the ECMO circuit; however, the PVC tubing is presumed to be responsible for the removal of a vast majority of the drugs [61,62]. It is unclear if saturation of drug-binding sites on the PVC tubing occurs, as studies comparing drug recovery in new and used ECMO circuits show variable results [15,32,61]. The limitation of all of these studies is the short duration (<48 h) of drug exposure to the ECMO circuit. As ECMO has been used clinically for much longer periods of time, it is unclear if or when saturation of the ECMO circuit occurs and how this may impact drug therapy.

Once a patient is placed on the ECMO, drug sequestration is just one of the factors that can cause pharmacokinetic changes. Data for sequestration of drugs in the ECMO circuits are limited, and it is important to understand the majority of the data is derived from ex vivo experiments. When caring for a patient on the ECMO, it is imperative to consider the drug properties, type, and duration of ECMO, and patient's factors that influence drug dosing in order to prevent harm and/or therapeutic failure.

5. Delirium

Often used interchangeably with the term "acute brain dysfunction," delirium has consistently been shown to be an independent predictor of poor short-term outcomes in the critically ill. This includes increased mortality in mechanically ventilated patients as well as prolonged hospital and ICU stays [63,64]. There is now increasing evidence of delirium's ill effects in the long term as well. Long-term cognitive impairment has been linked to the development and duration of delirium in the ICU setting [65].

Delirium is defined as a disturbance in attention and awareness which is an acute change from baseline. Typically, it develops over a short period of time (over hours to days) and fluctuates throughout the course of the day. Patients often present with additional disturbances in cognition (e.g., memory deficit, disorientation, language, visuospatial ability, or perception) [66,67].

There are three subtypes of delirium that are based on the patient's level of alertness: "hyper-active," "hypoactive," and "mixed." Often hypoactive delirium goes unrecognized and has been linked to poorer outcomes [68].

Patients on the ECMO are particularly vulnerable to the development of delirium given their severity of illness and comorbidities. Four independent risk factors for transition to delirium have been identified: pre-existing dementia, history of hypertension, and/or alcoholism, and a high severity of illness at admission [6]. However, there are many other factors that have been associated with this form of acute brain dysfunction—these can be further stratified based on (1) illness (2) patient's factors, and (3) environmental or iatrogenic factors [69] **(Table 1)**.

Care of the delirious patient in the ICU should focus on a three-step approach of monitoring, preventing, and treating delirium. At this time, there is limited data on delirium in the ECMO patients. Further research is essential in determining an evidence-based algorithm in the ECMO patient as there are many unique patient- and equipment-related factors specific to these patients that need to be investigated. The Confusion Assessment Method for the

Intensive Care Unit (CAM-ICU) is the most frequently applied screening and monitoring tool in the ICU setting (**Figure 1**) [70]. Proper assessment will guide further interventions.

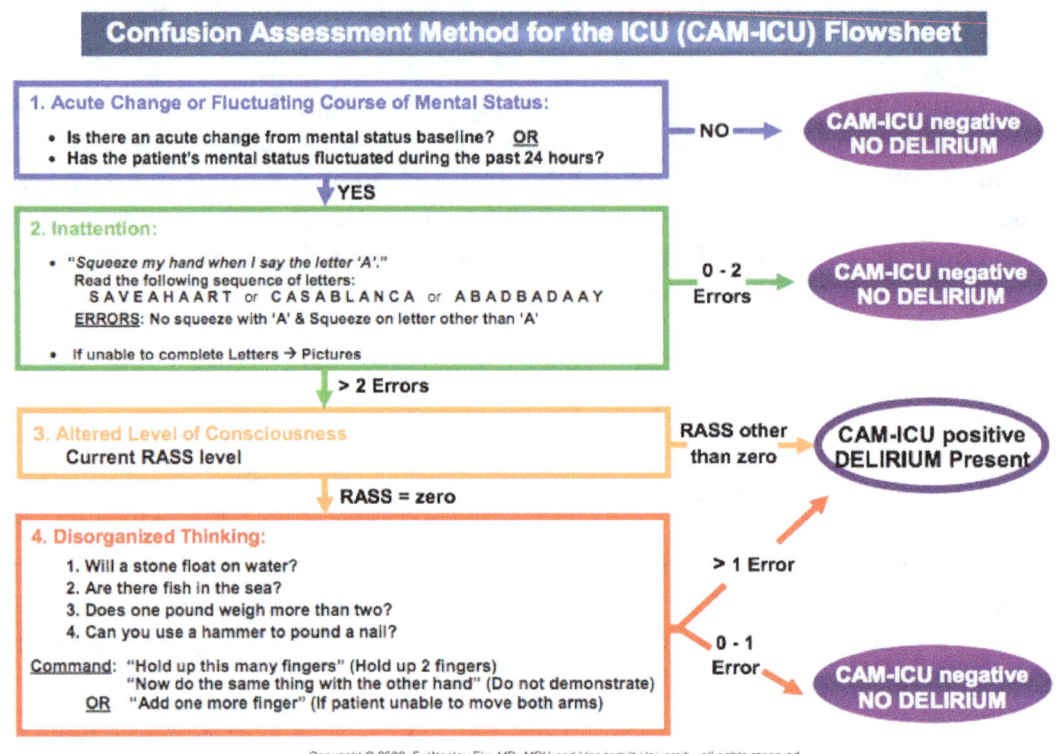

Figure 1. Confusion assessment method for the ICU (CAM-ICU) Flow sheet.

Illness	Patient's factors	Environmental/iatrogenic factors
Cardiovascular instability	Cognitive impairment, pre-existing dementia, and depression	Diagnostic procedures and therapeutic interventions
Acid base disorders	Age > 65	Use of restraints
Electrolyte abnormalities		Sensory deprivation: need for hearing aids and glasses
Sepsis		Sleep deprivation
Respiratory distress		
Acute CNS abnormalities		
http://www.mc.vanderbilt.edu/icudelirium/ terminology.html		

Table 1. Factors that have been associated with delirium.

Primary prevention should focus on decreasing the risk factors and minimizing iatrogenic causes known to increase the likelihood of transition to delirium. Management for both prevention and treatment can be further subcategorized into nonpharmacologic and pharmacologic interventions. These include minimizing loud noises and interruptions, a nonpharmacologic sleep protocol, stimulation during the day, and frequent reorientation to person, place, and time. Pharmacologic prevention of delirium has not been shown to decrease the likelihood of its occurrence [6]. The authors believe this practice may actually lead to over sedation and increase the likelihood of transition to delirium and do not recommend this approach based on existing evidence at this time. Daily assessment of analgesia and sedation requirements and deliberate choices in agents are an important part of the management (**Figure 2**).

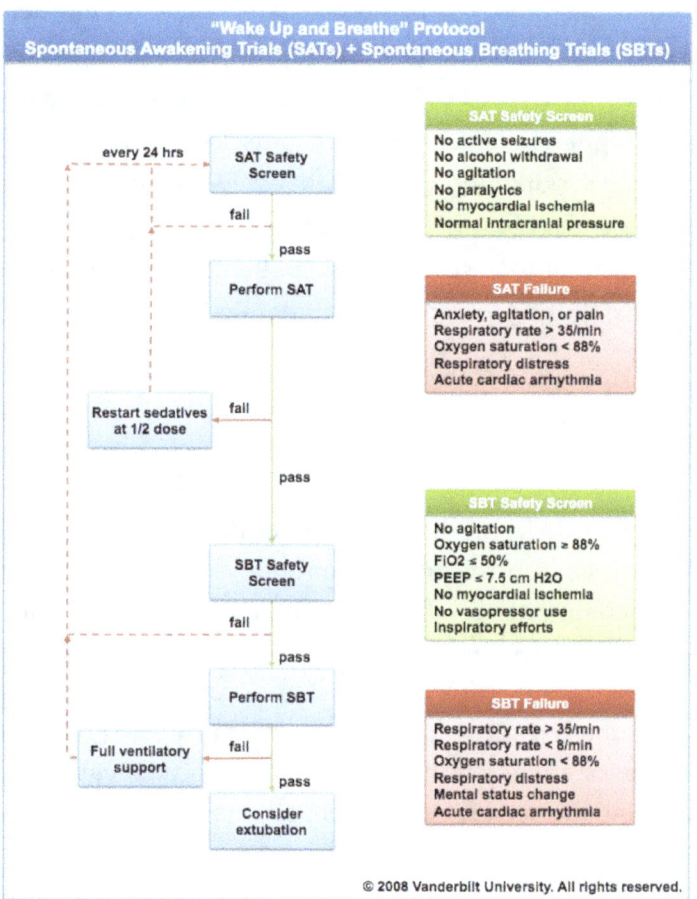

Figure 2. 'Wake up and breathe' protocol.

Benzodiazepines have been proven in multiple ICU settings to increase the likelihood of transition to delirium [71, 72]. Traditionally, they have been used for deep sedation in the ECMO patients because of their relative preservation of hemodynamic stability and unique pharmacologic property of lorazepam that would ensure adequate plasma concentrations in patients on the ECMO. In the future, the use of deep sedation with medications that remain in the system long after titrating off may lead to this practice being called into question. Deep sedation may be provided with multiple other sedatives that were discussed in the section regarding sedation and analgesia.

As further evidence emerges, prevention and treatment of delirium in the ECMO patient will become more standardized. Early mobilization and liberation from mechanical ventilation should be included in goals for prevention and management of delirium in the ECMO patient. There is compelling evidence that protocol-based treatment with these goals in mind can improve clinical outcomes in the general ICU population [73].

In keeping with the goal of early liberation of mechanical ventilation, many centers are exploring strategies for the use of ECMO in the awake patient. This may decrease the morbidity and mortality associated with mechanical ventilation, deep sedation, and immobility that have traditionally accompanied the use of ECMO. Additionally, it is possible for patients to breathe spontaneously, which might prevent respiratory muscle atrophy. While this has been best documented in the pediatric population and adult VV-ECMO patients being bridged to lung transplantation, this could also be utilized in the VA-ECMO patient. In such a case, close monitoring would be essential to ensure that the patient's breathing pattern and neurologic status are not compromising the patient's hemodynamics and respiratory status [74–76].

6. Conclusion

Increasingly, complications related to sedation, analgesia, and delirium are being recognized as factors that may play a role in morbidity of the critically patient. The decision to initiate medications for sedation, pain control, or agitation should be made by a clinician with intimate knowledge of the most commonly used agents. The use of deep sedation, light sedation, or minimal sedation should be decided upon based on the clinical picture specific to each individual patient on VA or VV ECMO. Pain must be accurately assessed in patients who may or may not be able to verbally express pain scores and titrated to response. The initiation of medications for agitation or anxiety must be decided upon with careful consideration in this critically ill population and the need for these medications should be reviewed on a daily basis.

Author details

SV Satyapriya*, ML Lyaker, AJ Rozycki and Papadimos

*Address all correspondence to: sree.satyapriya@osumc.edu

Department of Anesthesiology, Ohio State University Wexner Medical Center, Columbus, OH, United States of America

References

[1] Barr J, Fraser G, Puntillo K, Clinical practice guidelines for the management of pain, agitation and delirium in adult patients in the intensive care unit, Critical Care Medicine 2013; 41:263–306.

[2] Molina P, Opioids and opiates: analgesia with cardiovascular, haemodynamic and immune implications in critical illness, Journal of Internal Medicine 2006; 259(2):138–154.

[3] Akça O, Melischek M, Hellwagner K, Postoperative pain and subcutaneous oxygen tension, Lancet 1999; 354(9172)41–42.

[4] Wade D, Hardy R, Howell D, Identifying clinical and acute psychological risk factors for PTSD after critical care: a systematic review, Minerva Anestesiologica 2013; 79(8): 944–963.

[5] Schelling G, Stoll C, Haller M, Health-related quality of life and posttraumatic stress disorder in survivors of the acute respiratory distress syndrome, Critical Care Medicine 1998; 26(4):651–659.

[6] Erstad B, Puntillo K, Gilbert H, Pain management principles in the critically ill, Chest 2009; 135(4):1075–1086.

[7] Lindenbaum L, Milia D, Pain management in the ICU, Surgical Clini North America 2012; 92(6):1621–1636.

[8] Devlin J, Roberts R, Pharmacology of commonly used analgesics and sedatives in the ICU: benzodiazepines, propofol, and opioids, Anesthesiology Clinics 2011; 29(4):567–585.

[9] Shekar K, Roberts J, Mullany D, Increased sedation requirements in patients receiving extracorporeal membrane oxygenation for respiratory and cardiorespiratory failure, Anaesthesia and Intensive Care 2012; 40(4):648–655.

[10] Shekar K, Frasier J, Smith M, Pharmacokinetic changes in patients receiving extracorporeal membrane oxygenation, Journal of Critical Care 2012; 27(6) 741.e9–e18.

[11] Makdisi G, Wang I, Extra Corporeal Membrane Oxygenation (ECMO) review of a lifesaving technology, Journal of Thoracic Disease 2015; 7(7): E166–E176.

[12] ELSO Guidelines for cardiopulmonary extracorporeal life support, Extracorporeal Life Support Organization, Version 1.3 November 2013; Ann Arbor, MI, USA.

[13] Payen J, Chanques G, Mantz J, Current practices in sedation and analgesia for mechanically ventilated critically ill patients: a prospective multicenter patient-based study, Anesthesiology 2007; 106(4):687–695.

[14] Shekar K, Roberts JA, Mcdonald CL, et al. Sequestration of drugs in the circuit may lead to therapeutic failure during extracorporeal membrane oxygenation, Critical Care 2012; 16(5): R194.

[15] Wildschut E, Ahsman M, Allegaert K, Determinants of drug absorption in different ECMO circuits, Intensive Care Medicine 2010; 36(12):2109–2116.

[16] Shapiro B, Warren J, Egol A, Practice parameters for intravenous analgesia and sedation for adult patients in the intensive care unit: an executive summary. Society of Critical Care Medicine, Critical Care Medicine 1995; 23(9):1596–1600.

[17] Memis D, Inal M, Kavalci G, Intravenous paracetamol reduced the use of opioids, extubation time, and opioid-related adverse effects after major surgery in intensive care unit, Journal of Critical Care 2010; 25(3):458–462.

[18] Pettersson P, Jakobsson J, Owall A, Intravenous acetaminophen reduced the use of opioids compared with oral acetaminophen after coronary artery bypass grafting, Journal of Cardiothoracic and Vascular Anesthesia 2005; 19(3):306–309.

[19] Candiotti K, Bergese S, Viscusi E, Safety of multiple-dose intravenous acetaminophen in adult patients, Pain Medicine 2010; 11(12):1841–1848.

[20] Retrouvey H, Shahrokhi S, Pain and the thermally injured patient-a review of current therapies, Journal of Burn Care &Research 2015; 36(2):315–323.

[21] Subramaniam K, Subramaniam B, Steinbrook R, Ketamine as adjuvant analgesic to opioids: a quantitative and qualitative systematic review, Anesthesia and Analgesia 2004; 99(2): 482–495.

[22] Patanwala A, Martin J, Erstad B, Ketamine for analgosedation in the intensive care unit: a systematic review, Journal of Intensive Care Medicine 2015; Dec 8 (Epub)

[23] Tellor B, Shin N, Graetz T, Ketamine infusion for patients receiving extracorporeal membrane oxygenation support: a case series, F1000 Research 2015; 4:16.

[24] Christ G, Mundigler G, Merhaut C, Adverse cardiovascular effects of ketamine infusion in patients with catecholamine-dependent heart failure, Anaesthesia and Intensive Care 1997; 25(3):255–259.

[25] Carson S, Rodgers J, Vinayak A, A randomized trial of intermittent lorazepam versus Propofol with daily interruption in mechanically ventilated patients, Critical Care Medicine 2006; 34(5):1326–1332.

[26] Hall R, Sandham D, Cardinal P, Propofol vs midazolam for ICU sedation: a Canadian multicenter randomized trial, Chest 2001; 119(4):1151–1159.

[27] Pandharipande P, Sanders R, Girard T, Effect of dexmedetomidine versus lorazepam on outcome in patients with sepsis: an a priori-designed analysis of the MEDDS randomized controlled trial, Critical Care 2010; 14(2):R38.

[28] Riker R, Shehabi Y, Bokesch P, Dexmedetomidine vs midazolam for sedation of critically ill patients:a randomized trial, Journal of the American Medical Association 2009; 301(5):489–499.

[29] Shekar K, Roberts J, Welch S, ASAP ECMO: antibiotic, sedative and analgesic pharmacokinetics during extracorporeal membrane oxygenation: a multi-centre study to optimize drug therapy during ECMO, BMC Anesthesiology 2012; 12:29.

[30] Lemaitre F, Hasini N, Leprince P, Propofol, midazolam, vancomycin and cyclosporine therapeutic drug monitoring in extracorporeal membrane circuits primed with whole blood, Critical Care 2015; 19:40.

[31] Reade M, Eastwood G, Bellomo R, Effect of dexmedetomidine added to standard care on ventilator-free time in patients with agitated delirium: a randomized clinical trial, JAMA 2016; 315(14):1460–1468.

[32] Wagner D, Pasko D, Phillips K, et al. In vitro clearance of dexmedetomidine in extracorporeal membrane oxygenation, Perfusion 2013; 28(1):40–46.

[33] Chanques G, Jaber S, Barbotte E, Impact of systematic evaluation of pain and agitation in an intensive care unit, Critical Care Medicine 2006, 34(6):1691–1699.

[34] Li D, Puntillo K, Miaskowski C, A review of objective pain measures for use with critical care adult patients unable to self-report, Journal of Pain 2008; 9(1):2–10.

[35] Gelinas C, Arbour C, Michaud C, Implementation of the critical-care pain observation tool on pain assessment/management nursing practices in an intensive care unit with nonverbal critically ill adults: a before and after study, International Journal of Nursing Studies 2011; 48(12):1495–1504.

[36] Payen, J, Bosson J, Chanques G, Pain assessment is associated with decreased duration of mechanical ventilation in the intensive care unit: a post hoc analysis of the DOLOREA study, Anesthesiology 2009; 111(6):1308–1316.

[37] Rehder K, Sessler AD, Rodarte JR. Regional Intrapulmonary gas distribution in awake an anesthestized-paralyzed man. Journal of Applied Physiology: Respiratory, Environmental and Exercise Physiology 1977;42:391–401.

[38] Ohsone J, Yamakage M, Murouchi T. Reversal of neuromuscular blockade and complications of remaining blocking effect. Mansui 2008;57:838–844.

[39] Casale LM, Seigel RE. Neruomuscular blockade in the ICU. Chest 1993;104:1639–1641.

[40] Hraiech s, Dizier S, Papazian L. The use of paralytics in patients with acute respiratory distress syndrome. Clinics in Chest Medicine 2014;35:753–763.

[41] Tulman D, Stawicki SPA, Whitson BA, Gupta SC, Tripathi RS, Firstenberg MS, Hayes Jr. D, Xu X, Papadimos TJ. Veno-venous ECMO: a synopsis of nine key potential challenges, considerations, and controversies. BMC Anesthesiology 2014;14:65.

[42] Burry LD, Seto K, Rose L, Lapinsky sC, Mehta S. Use of sedations and neuromuscular blockers in critically ill adult receiving high-frequency oscillatory ventilation. Annals of Pharmacotherapy 2013;47:1122–1129.

[43] Gannier M, Roch A, FOrel JM, Thirion X, Amal JM, Donati S, Papazian L. Effect of neuromuscular blocking agents on gas exchange I patients presenting with acute respiratory distress syndrome. Critical Care Medicine 2004;32:113–119.

[44] Forel JM, Roch Am Marin V, Michelet P, Demory D, Blache JL, Perrin G, Gannier M, Bongrand P, Papazian L. Neuromuscular blocking agents decrease inflammatory response in patients presenting with acute respiratory distress syndrome. Critical Care Medicine 2006;34:2749–2757.

[45] Papazian L,Forel JM, Gacouin A, Penot-Ragon c, Perrin G, Loundou A, Jaber S, Arnal JM, Perez D, Seghboyan JM, Constantin JM, Courant P, Lefrant JY, Guerin C, part G, Morange S, Roch A. Neuromuscular blocking agents in patients with acute respiratory distress syndrome. New England Journal of Medicine 2010;363:1107–1116.

[46] Neto AS, Pereira VG, Esposito DC, Damasceno MC, Schultz MG. Neuromuscular blocking agents in patients with acute respiratory distress syndrome: a summary of the current evidence from three randomized control trials. Annals of Intensive Care 2013;2:33.

[47] Alhazzani W, Alshahrani M, Jaeschke R, Forel JM, Papazian L, Sevransky J, Meade MO. Neuromuscular blocking agents in acute respiratory distress syndrome: a systematic review and meta-analysis of randomized control trials. Critical Care 2013;17:R43.

[48] Dalton RE, Tripathi RS, Abel EE, Kothari DS, Firstenberg MS, Stawicki SP, Papadimos TJ. Polyneuropathy and myopathy in the elderly. HSR Proceedings in Intensive Care and Cardiovascular Anesthesia 2013;4:15–19.

[49] Latronico M, Bolton CF. Critical illness polyneuropathy and myopathy: a major cause of muscle weakness and paralysis. Lancet Neurology 2011;10:931–941.

[50] Bolton CF. The discovery of critical illness polyneuropathy: a memoir. Canadian Journal of Neurological Sciences 2010;37:431–438.

[51] De JB, Sharshar T, Lefaucheur JP, Authier FJ, Durand-Zaleski I, Boussarsar M, Cerf C, Renaud E, Mesrati F, Carlet J, Raphael JC, Outin H, Bastuji-Garin S: Groupe de Reflexion d'Etude des Neuromyopathies en Reanimation. Paresis acquired in the intensive care unit: a prospective multicenter study. JAMA 2002;288:2857–2867.

[52] Witt NJ, Zochodne DW, Bolton CF, Grand'Maison F, Wells G, Young GB, Sibbald WJ. Peripheral nerve function in sepsis and multi organ failure. Chest 1991;99:176–184.

[53] Latronico N, Peli E, Botteri M. Critical Illness myopathy and neuropathy. Current Opinion in Critical Care 2005;11:126–132.

[54] Van den Berghe G, Schoonheydt K, Becx P, Bruyninckx F, Wouters PJ. Insulin therapy protects the central and peripheral nervous system of intensive care patients. Neurology 2005;64:1348–1353.

[55] Greenberg SB, Vender J. The use of neuromuscular blocking agents in the ICU: Where are we now? Critical Care Medicine 2013;41:1332–1334.

[56] Vender JS, Szokol J, Murphy GS. Sedation, analgesia, neuromuscular blockade in sepsis: An evidence based review. Critical Care Medicine 2004;32:S554–S561.

[57] Kent CD, Domino KB. Awarenes:, practice, standards, and the law. Best Practice & Research: Clinical Anaesthesiology 2007;21:369–383.

[58] Wildschut ED, Ahsman MJ, Allegaert K, et al. Determinats of Drug Absorption in Different ECMO circuits. Intensive Care Medicine 2010;36:2109–2166

[59] Lemaitre F, Hasni N, Leprince P, et al. Propofol, midazolam, vancomycin and cyclosporine Therapeutic Drug Monitoring in Extracorporeal Membrane Oxygenation Circuits Primed with Whole Human Blood. Critical Care 2015;40:1–6.

[60] Shekar K, Roberts JA, Mcdonald CI, et al. Protein bound drugs are prone to sequestration in the extracorporeal membrane oxygenation circuit: results from an ex vivo study. Critical Care 2015;49:164.

[61] Bhatt-Mehta V, Annich G. Sedative clearance during extracorporeal membrane oxygenation. Perfusion 2005;20:309–315.

[62] Preston TJ, Hodge AB, Riley JB, et al. In vitro drug adsorption and plasma free hemoglobin levels associated with hollow fiber oxygenators in the extracorporeal life support circuit. Journal of Extracorporeal Life Support 2007;39:234–237.

[63] Ely, E. Wesley, et al. Delirium as a predictor of mortality in mechanically ventilated patients in the intensive care unit. Journal of the American Medical Association 291.14 (2004): 1753–1762.

[64] Ouimet, Sébastien, et al. Incidence, risk factors and consequences of ICU delirium. Intensive Care Medicine 33.1 (2007): 66–73.

[65] Pandharipande, Pratik P., et al. Long-term cognitive impairment after critical illness. New England Journal of Medicine 369.14 (2013): 1306–1316.

[66] DSM-IV, Diagnostic and Statistical Manual of Mental Disorders, fourth edition.

[67] DSM-5, Diagnostic and Statistical Manual of Mental Disorders, fifth edition.

[68] Pandharipande, Pratik, et al. Motoric subtypes of delirium in mechanically ventilated surgical and trauma intensive care unit patients. Intensive Care Medicine 33.10 (2007): 1726–1731.

[69] Hipp, Dustin M., and E. Wesley Ely. Pharmacological and nonpharmacological management of delirium in critically ill patients. Neurotherapeutics 9.1 (2012): 158–175.

[70] Ely EW, Inouye SK, Bernard GR, et al. Delirium in mechanically ventilated patients: validity and reliability of the confusion assessment method for the intensive care unit (CAM-ICU). Journal of the American Medical Association. 2001;28621:2703–2710.

[71] Pandharipande P, Shintani A, Peterson J, et al. Lorazepam is an independent risk factor for transitioning to delirium in intensive care unit patients. Anesthesiology. 2006;1041:21–26

[72] Pandharipande P, Cotton BA, Shintani A, et al. Prevalence and risk factors for development of delirium in surgical and trauma intensive care unit patients. Journal of Trauma. 2008;651:34–41

[73] Morandi, Alessandro, Nathan E. Brummel, and E. Wesley Ely. Sedation, delirium and mechanical ventilation: the 'ABCDE' approach. Current Opinion in Critical Care 17.1 (2011): 43–49.

[74] Sommer, Wiebke, et al. Cardiac Awake Extracorporeal Life Support—Bridge to Decision? Artificial Organs 39.5 (2015): 400–408.

[75] Mohite, Prashant N., et al. Extracorporeal life support in "awake" patients as a bridge to lung transplant. Thoracic and Cardiovascular Surgery (2015): 1–7.

[76] Hoeper, Marius M., et al. Extracorporeal membrane oxygenation instead of invasive mechanical ventilation in patients with acute respiratory distress syndrome. Intensive Care Medicine 39.11 (2013): 2056–2057.

Extracorporeal Membrane Oxygenation During Lung Transplantation

Young-Jae Cho

Abstract

Lung transplantation is increasing as a widely accepted surgical treatment for certain type of end-stage lung disease. Recent technical improvements in extracorporeal membrane oxygenation (ECMO) have been able to expand the role of ECMO during lung transplantation. The evolution of oxygenators, introduction of the new-type pump and tube, and improvement of percutaneous cannulation including dual lumen single catheter resulted in the technical renaissance of ECMO for lung transplantation. Now, beyond the traditional support for patients with severe primary graft dysfunction, ECMO can be established as essential perioperative roles for patients undergoing lung transplantation, such as preoperative lung protective support as a bridge to transplantation, replacement cardiopulmonary bypass during intraoperative support, and rescue of various life-threatening situations after post-transplant. After all, ECMO will be a fundamental, life-saving modality for patients during lung transplantation.

Keywords: Perioperative procedures, lung transplantation, Perioperative procedures, Ventilator-induced lung injury, Intensive care unit

1. Introduction

Recent expanded role of extracorporeal membrane oxygenation (ECMO) is switching the paradigm of organ transplantation, especially in the lung. Traditionally, the role of ECMO in the area of lung transplantation was focused in supporting patients with severe primary graft dysfunction (PGD) after post-transplant; however, as the technical ECMO environments such as new type of pump, oxygenator, catheter and tubing are improving, ECMO is now applied to the whole process of lung transplantation, from "bridge-to-transplant" to "rescue post-transplant" [1, 2].

The prevalence of lung transplantation has also increased over several decades especially in the specific end-stage lung diseases, such as cystic fibrosis, interstitial lung disease, and chronic obstructive lung disease. Contrary to successful early survival rate, the long-term survival rate of lung transplantation has still seen modest improvement. In addition, the mortality of patients on the waiting list is also concerning, consequently the interest in looking for alternative strategies for patients with end-stage lung disease who wait lung transplantation has risen considerably.

Mechanical ventilation has been applied to support the failing lung in peritransplant patients; however, per se can aggravate respiratory failure and hemodynamic instability by increasing the risk of ventilator-associated pneumonia and ventilator-induced lung injury [3]. Traditionally, mechanically ventilated pretransplant patients have been reported to have higher post-transplant mortality rates than nonventilated patients [4].

At this point, ECMO can be considered an alternative bridging strategy in lung transplantation, and now despite the complexity and side effects, the use of ECMO during lung transplantation has risen by 150% in the recent last 2 years compared to the previous decades (1970–2010; **Figure 1**). Besides the increase of amount, the characteristics of using ECMO are also evolving (**Table 1**) [5].

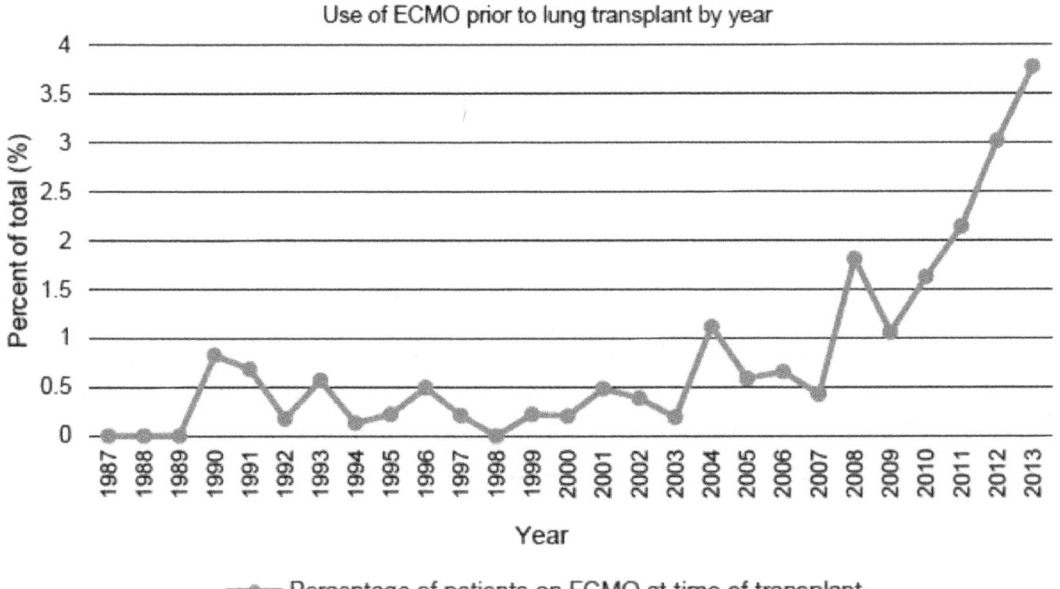

Figure 1. Percentage of patients on ECMO at the time of transplant by year. Data obtained from the United Network for Organ Sharing (UNOS) database 1987–2013. Published un-der AME Publishing Company. Promotional and commercial use of the mate-rial in print, digital or mobile device format is prohibited without the permission from the publisher AME Publishing Company.

	1970s	1980s	1990–2000	2000–2010	2010–June 2011
Patients listed for lung transplantation on ECMO	1	1	22	104	58
Modes of ECLS used	VA	VA	VA	VV, VA, iLA™	VV, VA, iLA™, hybrid
Pump configuration	CPB	Roller pump	Roller pump	Centrifugal	Centrifugal
Oxygenator membrane	Silicone membrane	Polypropylene and silicone	Polypropylene	PMP	PMP
Cannulation approach innovation	Central	Central	Central	Peripheral Novalung®	Peripheral Avalon™

CPB, cardiopulmonary bypass; ECLS, extracorporeal life support; ECMO, extracorporeal membrane oxygenation; ILA™, interventional lung assist; PMP, polymethylpentene; VA, venoarterial; and VV, venovenous.

Table 1. Evolution of ECMO as a bridge to lung transplant by decade. Promotional and commercial use of the material in print, digital or mobile device format is prohibited without the permission from the publisher Wolters Kluwer Health.

2. Extracorporeal membrane oxygenation as a bridge to lung transplantation

The first report of the use of ECMO as a bridge-to-transplant was published in the 1970s [6]. The patient was successfully transplanted and wean from ECMO, he died at 10 days of post-transplant. Successful cases were reported in 1993 [7]; however, still controversies of using ECMO as a bridge-to-transplant were noted at that time because of poor clinical outcomes, for example, the estimated 1-year survival for the transplant of ECMO was only 40%. In addition, the resources have been considerable for a successful transplant through ECMO bridge, such as prolong intensive care and hospital stays, need of tracheostomy, substantial blood requirement, and consequent neuromuscular complications that also required prolonged periods of postoperative rehabilitation.

The lung allocation scoring (LAS) system, begun in 2005, can be attributable to increase the use of ECMO as a bridge-to-transplant. Contrary to it patients before 2005 would receive lungs only based on the length of time on the waiting list, both medical urgency and net benefit from transplantation were incorporated to create a standardized scoring system. Since the adoption of LAS system, patients receiving continuous mechanical ventilation get higher scores, more likely to receive a transplant. Simultaneously, issues were arisen that ventilator-dependent patient before transplantation may be too sick for transplantation, which may affect the post-transplant outcomes. Direct or indirect risk factors could be considered in these patients: one is the increased risk of "ventilator-induced lung injury (VILI)" or "ventilator-associated pneumonia" during waiting period, and the other is "ICU-acquired weakness."

ECMO has been associated with avoidance of mechanical ventilation and it facilitates perioperative rehabilitation. As far as minimizing VILI when using ECMO as a bridge-to-transplant,
ECMO may be beneficial for the patients waiting lung transplantation who have refractory
hypercapnic respiratory failure, which was followed by most patients with end-stage lung
disease combined with hypoxic respiratory failure. Extracorporeal CO_2 removal (ECCO2R),
more commonly called as this concept instead of ECMO, reduces mechanical ventilation
requirements, enabling the use of low tidal volume and high PEEP at relatively lower respiratory rates. Recently, technological improvements, such as interventional lung-assisted
device pumpless venovenous ECMO (NovalungGmbH, Germany), a low-resistance oxygenator that offers good decarboxylation, and the CardioHelp venovenous ECCO2R device
(Maquet, Germany), have led to remove CO_2 selectively including partial or full oxygenation
support [8].

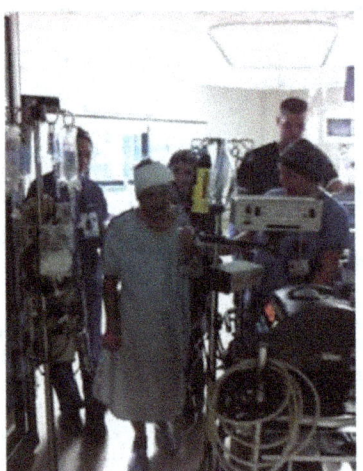

a.

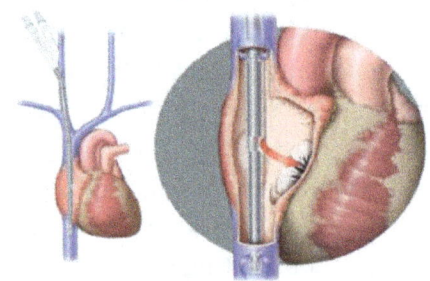

b.

Figure 2. (a) Patient ambulating on venovenous-ECMO, (b) Avalon Elite Double lumen catheter and catheter placement. Promotional and commercial use of the material in print, digital or mobile device for-mat is prohibited without
the permission from the publisher Wolters Kluwer Health.

Compared to the conventional mechanical ventilation strategy, patients who received "awake"
ECMO as a bridge-to-transplant can be liberated from bed and participate in a preoperative
"active" rehabilitation program, which consequently mitigated ICU-acquired weakness

(**Figure 2a**). For this purpose, new-type single catheters, configured by double lumen, such as "Avalon" (**Figure 2b**) or "Novatwin" cannula, can be preferable, which facilitate easier patient mobilization to prevent decline in skeletal muscle dysfunction in postoperative period. Although a direct causal relationship between preoperative rehabilitation enhanced by a bridge-to-transplant using ECMO and postoperative exercise tolerance with ultimate clinical outcomes has not been established, it is generally considered a standard of care to enlist all patients into an active pulmonary rehabilitation program before transplantation or a "destination therapy" like that seen with left ventricular-assisted devices in the area of heart transplantation. There appears to be a benefit even in a common selected group of extremely sick conditions before transplant despite the scarcity of data currently [9].

Until now, there are no randomized controlled trials showing the beneficial effect of ECMO as bridge to lung transplant, several retrospective studies reported acceptable survival and its feasibility. Because most of these analyses were composed of many heterogeneous patients' feature, whether ECMO as an alternative, rather than an adjunction, to invasive mechanical ventilation is a better bridging strategy during lung transplantation still remains an unresolved issue. A meta-analysis of 14 retrospective studies [10–23] reported from 50 to 90% of the post-transplant 1-year survival rate, which was significantly better in spontaneously breathing patients or when the ECMO bridge duration was shorter than 14 days.(**Tables 2** and **3**) [4].

Author, year	Patients, number	Age (years)	Sex male, n (%)	Diagnosis	Ventilation strategy	Bridge time (days)	Severity score prebridge
Mason, 2010 [19]	51	39±22	25 (49%)	PF 27%; COPD 1996; CF 12%; PH 9.8%; sarcoidosis 2%; other 20%	na	na	LAS 54±21
Bermudez, 2011 [11]	17	40±14	7 (41%)	PF 35%; Re-LTx 35%; CF 23%; COPD 6%	MV	3.2 (0–49)	na
Hammainen, 2011 [15]	16	41±8[a]	7 (58%)	PF 37%[a]; PH 15%[a]; CF 8%[a]; ARDS 8%[a]; IP 8%[a]; PVOD 8%[a]; BOS 8%[a]; PGD 8%[a]	na	12 (1–59)	na
Shafii, 2012 [21]	19	44 (23–60)	10 (53%)	IP 68%; CF 16%; PH 16%	MV 13	6±5	LAS 87 (64–95)
Nosotti, 2012 [20]	11	34±13	5 (45%)	na	Awake 7 MV 4	12.1±14.7	SOFA 4.9±1.4
Javidfar, 2012 [17]	18	34 (22–50)	8 (45%)	CF 44%; PF 33%; PH 11%; Other 11%	Awake 6	11.5 (6–18)	LAS 93(90–94)
George, 2012 [14]	122	48±16	74 (60%)	PF 29.5%; CF 11.5%; COPD 10.7%; PH 2.5%; other 45.8%	na	na	LAS 73.9±21.4
Fuehner, 2012 [13]	26	44 (23–62)	21 (81%)	PF 35%; PH 27%; CF 19%; BOS 12%; sarcoidosis 4%	Awake 19 MV 7	9 (1–45)	SOFA 7 (6–12)

Author, year	Patients, number	Age (years)	Sex male, n (%)	Diagnosis	Ventilation strategy	Bridge time (days)	Severity score prebridge
Hoopes, 2013 [16]	31	45±15	21 (67%)	PF 29%; CF 23%; ILD 13%; ARDS 10%; PVOD 10%; PH 6%; BOS 3%; IP 3%; CWP 3%	Ambulatory 18 13 VM	11 (2–53)	LAS > 50
Anile, 2013 [10]	12	na	na	CF 92%; histiocytosis 8%	Awake 2 MV 10	6±2.1	na
Toyoda, 2013 [22]	31	46±15[a]	10 (43%)[a]	Pf 33%[a]; CF 21%[a]; Re-LTx 13%[a]; scleroderma 13%[a]; bronchiectasis 8%[a]; COPD 4%[a]; sarcoidosis 4%[a]; PH 4%[a]	MV[a]	7.1±10	Las 87±9 [a]
Weig, 2013 [23]	26	36 (30–51)[a]	14 (54%)	PF 62%; CF 23%; COPD 4%; Re-LTx 4%; lung cancer 4%; sarcoidosis 4%	na	16 (88–25)[a]	SOFA 9 (8.5–10.5)[a]
Crotti, 2013 [12]	25	41±12	na	PF 52%; CF 16%; PH 16%; Re-LTx 12%; ARDS 4%	Awake 10 MV 15	5.8±4.5 versus 29.8±11.5[a]	SOFA 5.6±1.9
Lafarge, 2013 [18]	36	31 (22–48)	19 (53%)	CF 56%; PF 30%; other 14%	MV	3.5 (2–7)	na

Data presented in this table refer to patients underwent ECMO support with the intention to bridge to lung transplantation.

[a]Transplanted patients (when data for all enrolled patients are not available; Hemmainen et al., all data; Toyoda, all data; Weig et al., ECMO bridge time and SOFA; Anile, diagnosis). ECMO bridge time (days) and the prebridge severity score are expressed as mean± standard deviation or median and range. When no descriptive cumulative data for the overall population are provided, they are calculated from raw data presented in the original papers.
[b]Data refer to patients divided according to waiting time on ECMO: up to 14 days or longer.
Pts, patients; ECMO, extracorporeal membrane oxygenation; PF, pulmonary fibrosis; COPD, chronic obstructive pulmonary disease; CF, cystic fibrosis; PH, pulmonary hypertersion; Re-LTx, Re-lung transplantation; ARDS, acute respiratory distress syndrome; IP, interstitial pneumonia; PVOD, pulmonary veno-occlusive disease, bronchiolitis obliterans syndrome; PGD, primary graft dysfunctions ILD, interstitial lung disease; CWP, coal workers, pneumoconiosis; MV, mechanical vertilation; LAS, lung allocation score; SOFA, sequential organ failure assessment; and na, not available.

Table 2. Characteristics of patients who underwent ECMO bridge to lung transplant.

Author, year	Ltx/total patients, n	Died before Ltx, n (%)	Type of bypass	Survival at 1 year post-LTx (%)	Length of stay post-LTx (days)	MV (days post-LTx)
Mason, 2010 [19]	51/51	na	na	50%	24 (9–55) H	na
Bermudez, 2011 [11]	14/17	3 (17%): neurologic dysfunction, thrombosis	W, VA	74%	16 (3–40) ICU	12 (2–20)

Author, year	Ltx/total patients, n	Died before Ltx, n (%)	Type of bypass	Survival at 1 year post-LTx (%)	Length of stay post-LTx (days)	MV (days post-LTx)
Hammainen, 2011 [15]	13/16	3 (19%): septic MOF	W, VA	92%	22 (3–63) ICU	na
Shafii, 2012 [21]	14/19	5 (26%): septic MOF 2, DC 2, and anoxic brain injury 1	W, VA	75%	42 (19–175) H	22 (5–125)
Nosotti, 2012 [20]	11/11	na	W	87% and 50%[b]	47.6±21.9 H 30±20.4 ICU	27.1±20.7
Javidfar, 2012 [17]	10/18[a]	8 (44%): pneumonia 1, MOF 6, and CA 1	W, VA	60%	22 (18–33) H 47 (41–52) ICU	na
George, 2012 [10]	122/122	na	na	57.6%	32 (16.5–60) H	na
Fuehner, 2012 [13]	20/26	6 (23%): CA 2, septic MOF 4	W, VA	6 months 80%	38 (20–87) H 18 (1–69) ICU	14 (0–64)
Hoopes, 2013 [16]	31/31	na	VA, W	93%	31 (12–86)[e]H	na
Anile, 2013 [10]	7/12	5 (41%)	W, VA	85.7%	29 (15–59) H	<5
Toyoda, 2013 [22]	24/31	7(22%)	W, VA	74%	46 median H	na
Weig, 2013 [23]	13/26	13 (50%): acute liver failure 7, thoracic bleeding 3, cerebral hemorrhage 1, and PE 2	W, VA	54%	na	na
Crotti, 2013 [12]	17/25	8 (32%): MOF 3, septic shock 2, cardiogenic shock 2, and intestinal ischemia 1	W, VA	82% and 29%[c]	na	12.2±11.9[d]
Lafarge, 2013 [18]	30/36	6 (17%): GI bleeding 1, DIC 1, cerebral hemorrhage 1, CA 1, septic shock 1, and therapeutic limitation 1	W, VA,CPB	66.5%	na	na

Data are expressed as mean±standard deviation or median and range. Mason et al., Nosotti et al., and George et al. enrolled transplanted patients.

[a]Three of the eight patients who died had transiently recovered their baseline function and were weaned from ECMO support; they subsequently died before LTx.

[b]ECMO group: 87% awake (7 pts); mechanical ventilation ECMO group: 50% (4 pts);

[c]82% patients on ECMO bridge <14 days (early); 29% patients on ECMO bridge >14 days (late);

[d]12.2±11.9 days (early group) −45.3±33.5 (late group).

[e]LTx, lung transplant; CA, cardiac arrest; MOF, multiorgan failure; DIC, disseminated intravascular coagulation; GI, gastrointestinal; VV, venovenous; VA, venoarterial; CPB, cardiopulmonary bypass; MV, mechanical ventilation; LOS, length of stay; H, hospital; and na, not available.

Table 3. Summary of outcomes.

3. Extracorporeal membrane oxygenation during lung transplantation

There is little evidence or protocol about how to manage ECMO during intraoperative situation; however, the intraoperative use of ECMO may be necessary at any stage of developing hypoxia, hypercapnia, and/or hemodynamic instability. In bilateral lung transplantation, ECMO can stabilize hemodynamic variables and prevent "first lung syndrome," the hyperperfusion of the first implanted lung during implantation of the second lung. In addition, it can also be used at every phase during lung transplantation to enhance a protective ventilation strategy and avoid 100% oxygen so as to mitigate the reperfusion syndrome especially during one-lung ventilation or to support when there was a lung size mismatch, auto-PEEP, and dynamic hyperinflation [8].

Because of many advantages mentioned earlier, ECMO has replaced CPB as the first option for intraoperative support during lung transplantation in many transplant centers. A recent published study from Germany showed 5-year experience with intraoperative ECMO in lung transplantation since April 2010 [10]. Compared with patients who underwent lung transplantation without ECMO, overall survival at 1 and 4 years was not inferior in patients in whom the indication for ECMO support and the intraoperative use of ECMO did not emerge as a risk factor for mortality. Though small numbers were included, many studies showed overall clinical beneficiary of ECMO over CPB during lung transplantation, such as lesser intraoperative blood transfusion requirement, lesser mechanical ventilation requirement, shorter ICU stay, and higher postoperative complications.

Bermudez et al. [11] compared 49 VA-ECMOs with 222 CPBs using intraoperative lung transplantation. In this study, there was a higher requirement for reintubation, tracheostomy, and dialysis in the CPB group; however, the lack of significant differences in perioperative blood transfusion requirement and hospital length of stay may have been caused by the ECMO group including a sicker population, such as the higher LAS (73.3 vs. 52.9) and higher pretransplantation ECMO requirement (42.8% vs. 7.2%). Though most of these studies did not show any difference in the survival curve between two groups, one study [12] revealed the hospital mortality gain of CPB over ECMO (39% vs. 13%); however, it should be considered that there were more planned ECMOs than CPBs (61% vs. 28%) in this study, which may not be ignored showing the different mortality between two groups.

4. Extracorporeal membrane oxygenation as a rescue postlung transplant

In the postopertative setting of lung transplantation, early primary graft dysfunction (PGD), which is a syndrome consisting of lung injury during the first 72 hours following lung transplant defined as a physiologically decreased oxygenation and radiologically diffuse infiltrates, continues to be a major situation of morbidity and mortality. There is no doubt that ECMO has been applied as a pivotal management strategy to support severe PGD because none of interventions to ameliorate the effects of PGD on transplanted lung have been successful, including inhaled nitric oxide and prostaglandins. Although about 5% of lung transplantation requires ECMO support for PGD, this remains the most common indication for ECMO use as a rescue strategy and consequently it is reasonable that the concept of "bridge-to-transplant" has been arisen from the intermittent successes of a bridge to redo transplant in selected patients [1].

The goal of ECMO for severe PGD after lung transplant, same as mentioned in bridging-to-transplant, should be to minimize ventilator-induced lung injury such as elevated airway pressures or high inspired oxygen concentration by mechanical ventilation with positive pressure. While about this no uniform guidelines exist, one recommendation how to use ECMO to support PGD after lung transplant consists of initiating it when peak inspiratory pressure reaches up to 35 cm H_2O or 60% FiO_2 [13]. In addition, if possible, it could not be delayed greater than 48 hours to initiate ECMO after transplantation because of alleged worse outcomes. Hartwig et al. [14] reported surprising survival result in this group patients supported with VV-ECMO. Of the recipients from VV-ECMO following transplant, 96% weaned successfully with a 1-year survival of 64%.

Promisingly, *ex vivo* lung perfusion (EVLP), a novel technique used to evaluate and recondition marginal or rejected grafts, is also adapted during lung transplantation. The retrieved donor lung can be perfused in an *ex vivo* circuit, providing an opportunity to reassess its function before transplantation for the purpose of increasing successful transplantation with high-risk donor lungs. Cypel et al. [15] showed physiologically stable donor lung during 4 hours of *ex vivo* perfusion and its feasibility regarding less PGD event. Although the result was statistically not significant, this was the first report that demonstrates the possibility of *ex vivo* using ECMO for lung transplantation, remained and cited as the reference protocol. Recently, Boffini et al. [16] also revealed that the use of initially rejected grafts treated with EVLP did not increase severity of PGD after lung transplantation, suggesting a protective role of EVLP against PGD.

5. Conclusions

Recently, Biscotti et al. suggested the decision algorithm of how to use ECMO during entire lung transplantation (**Figure 3**) [2]. Though the details are not described in this chapter, the interhospital transport of lung transplantation candidate during ECMO is also feasible and this is opening a kind of new future episode [17].

Modern experience with ECMO and reported institutional experience on survival challenge historical assumptions about the treatment of end-stage lung disease and suggest that "bridging" to transplant with ECMO is both technically feasible and logistically viable. It is clear at this point that continued advances in the technologies and further research will help determine how best to include ECMO as a bridging strategy for lung transplantation.

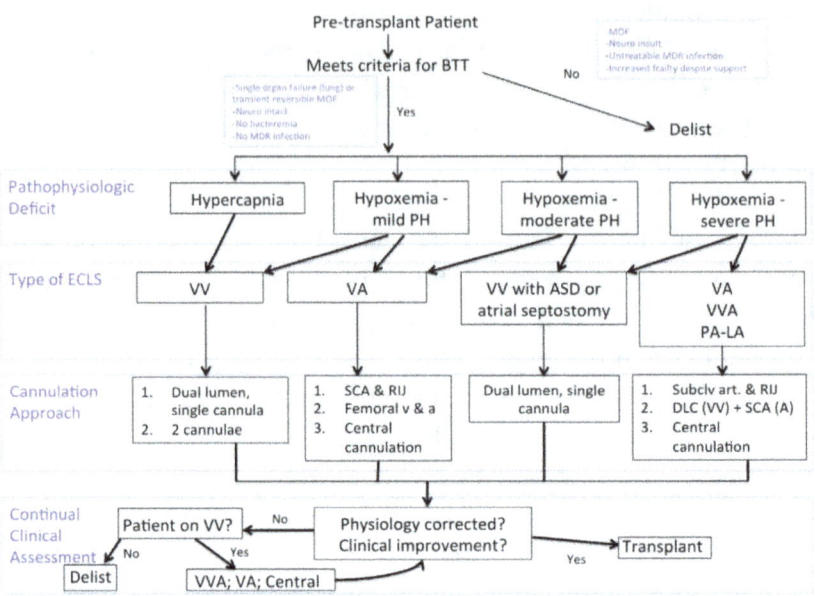

Figure 3. Decision algorithm of ECMO for lung transplantation. DLC, double lumen cannula; MDR, multidrug resistant; MOF, multiorgan failure; PALA, pulmonary artery to left atrium; PH, pulmonary hypertension; RIJ, right internal jugular vein; and SCA, subclavian artery. Promotional and commercial use of the material in print, digital or mobile device format is prohibited without the permission from the publisher Elsevier.

Author details

Young-Jae Cho

Address all correspondence to: lungdrcho@snubh.org

Division of Pulmonary and Critical Care Medicine, Department of Internal Medicine, Seoul National University Bundang Hospital, Seongnam-Si, South Korea

References

[1] Gulack, B.C., S.A. Hirji, and M.G. Hartwig, *Bridge to lung transplantation and rescue posttransplant: the expanding role of extracorporeal membrane oxygenation.* J Thorac Dis, 2014. 6(8): p. 1070–9.

[2] Biscotti, M., J. Sonett, and M. Bacchetta, *ECMO as bridge to lung transplant.* Thorac Surg Clin, 2015. 25(1): p. 17–25.

[3] Slutsky, A.S. and V.M. Ranieri, *Ventilator-induced lung injury.* N Engl J Med, 2013. 369(22): p. 2126–36.

[4] Chiumello, D., et al., *Extracorporeal life support as bridge to lung transplantation: a systematic review.* Crit Care, 2015. 19: p. 19.

[5] Diaz-Guzman, E., C.W. Hoopes, and J.B. Zwischenberger, *The evolution of extracorporeal life support as a bridge to lung transplantation.* ASAIO J, 2013. 59(1): p. 3–10.

[6] Nelems, J.M., et al., *Extracorporeal membrane oxygenator support for human lung transplantation.* J Thorac Cardiovasc Surg, 1978. 76(1): p. 28–32.

[7] Barankay, A., et al., *[Successful resuscitation using extracorporeal perfusion].* Orv Hetil, 1975. 116(49): p. 2898–9.

[8] Soluri-Martins, A., et al., *How to minimise ventilator-induced lung injury in transplanted lungs: The role of protective ventilation and other strategies.* Eur J Anaesthesiol, 2015. 32(12): p. 828–36.

[9] Abrams, D. and D. Brodie, *Novel Uses of Extracorporeal Membrane Oxygenation in Adults.* Clin Chest Med, 2015. 36(3): p. 373–84.

[10] Anile, M., et al., *Extracorporeal membrane oxygenation as bridge to lung transplantation.* Transplant Proc, 2013. 45.

[11] Bermudez, C.A., et al., *Extracorporeal membrane oxygenation as a bridge to lung transplant: midterm outcomes.* Ann Thorac Surg, 2011. 92.

[12] Crotti, S., et al., *Organ allocation waiting time during extracorporeal bridge to lung transplant affects outcomes.* Chest, 2013. 144.

[13] Fuehner, T., et al., *Extracorporeal membrane oxygenation in awake patients as bridge to lung transplantation.* Am J Respir Crit Care Med, 2012. 185.

[14] George, T.J., et al., *Outcomes and temporal trends among high-risk patients after lung transplantation in the United States.* J Heart Lung Transplant, 2012. 31.

[15] Hammainen, P., et al., *Usefulness of extracorporeal membrane oxygenation as a bridge to lung transplantation: a descriptive study.* J Heart Lung Transplant, 2011. 30.

[16] Hoopes, C.W., et al., *Extracorporeal membrane oxygenation as a bridge to pulmonary transplantation.* J Thorac Cardiovasc Surg, 2013. 145.

[17] Javidfar, J., et al., *Extracorporeal membrane oxygenation as a bridge to lung transplantation and recovery.* J Thorac Cardiovasc Surg, 2012. 144.

[18] Lafarge, M., et al., *Experience of extracorporeal membrane oxygenation as a bridge to lung transplantation in France.* J Heart Lung Transplant, 2013. 32.

[19] Mason, D.P., et al., *Should lung transplantation be performed for patients on mechanical respiratory support? The US experience.* J Thorac Cardiovasc Surg, 2010. 139.

[20] Nosotti, M., et al., *Extracorporeal membrane oxygenation with spontaneous breathing as a bridge to lung transplantation.* Interact Cardiovasc Thorac Surg, 2013. 16.

[21] Shafii, A.E., et al., *Growing experience with extracorporeal membrane oxygenation as a bridge to lung transplantation.* ASAIO J, 2012. 58.

[22] Toyoda, Y., et al., *Efficacy of extracorporeal membrane oxygenation as a bridge to lung transplantation.* J Thorac Cardiovasc Surg, 2013. 145.

[23] Weig, T., et al., *Parameters associated with short- and midterm survival in bridging to lung transplantation with extracorporeal membrane oxygenation.* Clin Transplant, 2013. 27.

[24] Ius, F., et al., *Five-year experience with intraoperative extracorporeal membrane oxygenation in lung transplantation: Indications and midterm results.* J Heart Lung Transplant, 2016. 35(1): p. 49–58.

[25] Bermudez, C.A., et al., *Outcomes of intraoperative venoarterial extracorporeal membrane oxygenation versus cardiopulmonary bypass during lung transplantation.* Ann Thorac Surg, 2014. 98(6): p. 1936–42; discussion 1942–3.

[26] Ius, F., et al., *Lung transplantation on cardiopulmonary support: venoarterial extracorporeal membrane oxygenation outperformed cardiopulmonary bypass.* J Thorac Cardiovasc Surg, 2012. 144(6): p. 1510–6.

[27] Diaz-Guzman, E., et al., *Lung function and ECMO after lung transplantation.* Ann Thorac Surg, 2012. 94(2): p. 686–7; author reply 687.

[28] Hartwig, M.G., et al., *Improved survival but marginal allograft function in patients treated with extracorporeal membrane oxygenation after lung transplantation.* Ann Thorac Surg, 2012. 93(2): p. 366–71.

[29] Cypel, M., et al., *Normothermic ex vivo lung perfusion in clinical lung transplantation.* N Engl J Med, 2011. 364(15): p. 1431–40.

[30] Boffini, M., et al., *Incidence and severity of primary graft dysfunction after lung transplantation using rejected grafts reconditioned with ex vivo lung perfusion.* Eur J Cardiothorac Surg, 2014. 46(5): p. 789–93.

[31] Lee, S.G., et al., *The feasibility of extracorporeal membrane oxygenation support for inter-hospital transport and as a bridge to lung transplantation.* Ann Thorac Cardiovasc Surg, 2014. 20(1): p. 26–31.

Management of Mechanical Ventilation During Extracorporeal Membrane Oxygenation

David Stahl MD and Victor Davila MD

Abstract

This chapter explores the best practices of mechanical ventilation during extracorporeal membrane oxygenation (ECMO) through a detailed discussion of the physiologic theory and clinical evidence. Future areas of study and unanswered questions about mechanical ventilation during ECMO are also delineated.

Keywords: mechanical ventilation, venovenous extracorporeal membrane oxygenation, venoarterial extracorporeal membrane oxygenation, ECMO, lung protective ventilation, positive end expiratory pressure

1. Introduction

Extracorporeal membrane oxygenation (ECMO) has been used as rescue therapy for hypoxemic, hypercarbic, and cardiogenic respiratory failure for decades, despite high complication rates [1, 2]. Venovenous (VV) ECMO was implemented internationally to great success during the recent H1N1 pandemic, and continues to be used as a last hope in refractory hypoxemia [3, 4]. Venoarterial (VA) ECMO is often employed when respiratory failure is secondary following hemodynamic collapse (most commonly cardiogenic in origin).

In a global effort to improve both the application and outcomes of VV and VA ECMO, all aspects of ECMO patients' care have been called into question. In this chapter, we explore both the theory and data behind specific mechanical ventilation (MV) strategies used in patients receiving ECMO to better understand current practice and propose areas of future study.

2. Ventilator associated lung injury

The landmark studies of lung protective ventilation in acute respiratory distress syndrome (ARDS) were published nearly 20 years ago, but the goal of lung protective ventilation remains to avoid ventilator associated lung injury (VALI) while permitting healing from the initial pathologic state [5, 6]. VALI is commonly described as a series of related injurious phenomena.

Barotrauma was the first, distinct aspect of VALI to be described. It can be defined as alveolar injury resulting from elevated transpulmonary pressures [7, 8]. Volutrauma is a related process where overdistension of alveolar volume results in lung injury [7, 8]. Barotrauma and volutrauma are both clinical explanations to approximate the physiologic principles of lung stress and strain using commonly measured variables including tidal volume, plateau pressure and positive end expiratory pressure (PEEP) [9]. MV strategies commonly aim to prevent barotrauma or volutrauma by limiting plateau airway pressures to ≤30 cm H_2O or tidal volumes to ≤6 ml/kg predicted body weight (PBW) [5].

Atelectrauma, conversely, occurs when low (or negative) end-expiratory transpulmonary pressures result in cyclic opening and closing of alveoli, generating disruptive forces on the basement membrane, resulting in lung injury [7, 10]. PEEP is commonly used to prevent atelectrauma by minimizing alveolar closure at the end of exhalation. Mechanical activation of the lung creates a biological reaction (e.g., neutrophil recruitment, cytokine release) known as biotrauma [8, 10–12]. Evidence of biotrauma may serve as a surrogate marker of the response to mechanical ventilation, and is often employed as an outcome measure when comparing MV strategies.

3. Mechanical ventilation strategies during venovenous extracorporeal membrane oxygenation

Guidelines for MV during ECMO are sparse. The Extracorporeal Life Support Organization 25 (ELSO) has published guidelines that include pressure assist-control ventilation (PCV) with low inflation 26 pressures (10 cm H2O), higher PEEP (15 cm H2O), low respiratory rate (5 bpm), and FiO2 of 0.5 27 or less [13]. The European Network of Mechanical Ventilation had similar guidelines in a 2009 response to the H1N1 pandemic recommending tidal volumes to obtain a plateau pressure of 20–25 cm H_2O, PEEP above 10 cm H_2O and with a respiratory rate of 6–20 cycles per minute and an FiO_2 between 0.3 and 0.5 [14]. However, in practice, there is significant variation in the mode of mechanical ventilation used in patients receiving ECMO [15, 16].

In the past 20 years, significant progress has been made in identifying the specific mechanical ventilation strategies that benefit patients with ARDS and acute respiratory failure [5, 17–20]. However, during this time, little progress has been made on the optimal method of mechanical ventilation in ECMO patients [14]. While volume assist-control ventilation (VCV) remains the most common mode of MV in ARDS, an observational study of current practice demonstrated pressure controlled modes of ventilation to be the most common mode of MV during ECMO [16, 21]. In many circumstances, ECMO may even facilitate ultraprotective MV, loosely defined as ventilation with tidal volumes below 4 ml/kg PBW. Although surrogate outcomes such as inflammatory markers may be improved by using this strategy, clinical benefit has not been demonstrated [22–24].

Experts continue to advocate for particular variations of VCV, PCV, or airway pressure release ventilation (APRV) predominantly based on physiologic 7 rationale and surrogate outcome studies demonstrating the avoidance of VALI [13]. However, there is a growing body of clinical evidence to guide the use of MV during ECMO [25, 26].

3.1. Lung rest: prevention of barotrauma or volutrauma

In a 2014 survey of ELSO centers, the majority (77%) reported "lung rest" to be the primary goal of mechanical ventilation during ECMO [15]. Although the definition of lung rest was not prespecified, one can assume that an intended goal was to limit both tidal volume and inspiratory airway pressures in that 81% of participants used tidal volumes ≤ 6 ml/kg PBW, including 34% who used ultraprotective tidal volumes ≤ 4 ml/kg PBW [15].

Initial studies of very low tidal volume ventilation in lung-injured rats demonstrated that tidal volumes of 3 ml/kg decreased pulmonary edema formation and improved pulmonary epithelial fluid clearance even when compared to 6 ml/kg [27]. Decreased levels of pulmonary inflammatory markers have also been found in humans ventilated with very low tidal volumes [22, 28]. These findings parallel a *post hoc* analysis of five large ARDS trials, which demonstrated a continuous mortality benefit to very low tidal volumes even when plateau pressures were less than 30 cm H_2O [29]. Case reports of tidal volumes as low as 1.9 ml/kg PBW have also shown positive outcomes [30]. However, prospective studies have failed to show a mortality benefit to ultralow tidal volume ventilation [24]. The Xtravent study compared very low tidal volume ventilation (~ 3 ml/kg PBW) plus $ECCO_2R$, to conventional low tidal volume ventilation (~ 6 ml/kg PBW) without $ECCO_2R$ in 79 patients with ARDS and did not find a difference in ventilator-free days or mortality at 60 days [24]. There was, however, an improvement in ventilator-free days in the more hypoxemic subgroup ($PaO_2/FiO_2 \leq 150$) [24].

Although it is generally accepted that limiting tidal volumes and plateau pressures with controlled ventilation modes should minimize VALI in the population requiring VV ECMO, preferences for volume control vs. pressure control ventilation vary significantly [4, 16, 25]. Advocates of volume control ventilation cite the ease of setting and studying a pre-specified tidal volume, as well as the added benefit of preventing large tidal volumes as lung compliance improves. However, VCV requires manually checking plateau pressures to analyze the compliance of the respiratory system. PCV has the benefit prespecifying a maximal inspiratory pressure and of being able to visually observe improving lung compliance by noting the change in tidal volume for a given driving pressure.

The most likely reason for the abundant use of PCV during ECMO is its use during the CESAR trial, the largest and most widely accepted comparison of ECMO to conventional ventilation in patients with potentially reversible respiratory failure [25]. In the CESAR trial, PCV settings included a peak inspiratory pressure of 20–25 cm H_2O, PEEP of 10–15 cm H_2O, respiratory rate of 10 bpm, and FiO_2 of 0.3. Similar settings were used in 54% of ECMO patients in a recent observational study in three major centers [16]. Only 10% of patients received a volume controlled mode of ventilation again suggesting the widespread acceptance of the CESAR trial and the ESLO guidelines [16]. However, it remains unclear how these potential risks and benefits of VCV versus PCV translate into clinical outcomes.

The disadvantage to lung protective ventilation is primarily hypercarbia (and subsequent effects of increase $PaCO_2$) that can often be mitigated by ECMO or $ECCO_2R$. Right ventricular (RV) heart function must be considered in this setting as pulmonary vascular resistance and right ventricular stroke work index is likely to increase significantly even with relatively small (10 mm Hg) increases in $PaCO_2$ [31]. Lung recruitment may result in decreased hypoxemic pulmonary vasoconstriction and increased available pulmonary vasculature which may offset some of the increase in pulmonary vascular resistance seen with hypercarbia [32]. Alternative therapies for refractory hypoxemia including aerosolized prostacyclin may also mitigate hypercarbia-induced pulmonary hypertension, but prospective studies have failed to demonstrate a mortality benefit [33].

Finally at the extremes of ultralow tidal volume ventilation (nearing or below physiologic dead space), high levels of PEEP are required to maintain convective ventilation and prevent small airway closure and progressive atelectasis as seen during apneic oxygenation [34, 35].

3.2. Lung recruitment: prevention of atelectrauma

Lung recruitment does not exist in a vacuum, isolated from lung protection. Some strategies designed to maximize lung rest may exacerbate atelectrauma, other strategies selected to prevent atelectrauma may worsen alveolar overdistension. Ideally, these strategies can be combined to balance lung rest with lung recruitment. For example, most studies of ultralow tidal volume ventilation use relatively high amounts of PEEP to prevent atelectasis and ventilation/perfusion mismatch [7, 22, 24].

The goal of lung recruitment is to prevent atelectrauma by maintaining open all available lung units. The primary strategy to accomplish this is through the use of PEEP. The optimal PEEP for acute respiratory failure remains unknown [17–20, 36]. Even less data exists about the optimal PEEP for patients receiving ECMO. One retrospective observational study demonstrated an increase in mortality for lower PEEP during the first 7 days of ECMO [16]. It is notable that "lower PEEP" in this study was <12 cm H_2O which would include all patients at the ELSO guideline-recommended PEEP of 10 cm H_2O [16]. The SOLVE ARDS study is currently enrolling to compare PEEP set for optimal lung compliance versus zero PEEP (ZEEP), in patients receiving ECMO [37].

One alternative strategy to maintain an open lung is the regular use of recruitment maneuvers [18, 38]. Recruitment maneuvers have not been systematically studied in the ECMO population. Data on their use in acute respiratory failure is conflicting. When incorporated into a multifaceted open lung strategy, recruitment maneuvers failed to show mortality benefit when compared to conventional low tidal volume ventilation [18]. The lack of benefit of recruitment maneuvers is often attributed to the bundling of many lung protective strategies in one intervention or to studies being underpowered to detect significant differences in outcomes [39]. Neither a systematic review nor the Cochrane meta-analysis demonstrated a mortality benefit to recruitment maneuvers [39, 40].

One downside of recruitment maneuvers relates to the heterogeneity of the lung in the setting of ARDS that may result in simultaneous alveolar overdistension and atelectasis during lung recruitment, particularly if PEEP is not adjusted or re-optimized following recruitment [41]. Alveolar overdistension may also be caused by excess use of PEEP with manifold negative consequences including decrease in venous return, decrease in cardiac index and increase in RV afterload [42].

Some centers have advocated the use of airway pressure release ventilation (APRV) during ECMO to augment lung recruitment. APRV is a "time-triggered, time-cycled, bi-level, pressure-regulated ventilation mode that allows a patient's spontaneous breathing pattern to be superimposed upon the mechanical ventilation pattern" [43]. Functionally, the patient is held at an inspiratory pressure level ($PEEP_{High}$) and with short "releases" to $PEEP_{Low}$ (typically less than 1.5 s) while able to breathe spontaneously throughout. Oxygenation is typically improved by increasing airway pressure (both $PEEP_{High}$ and $PEEP_{Low}$) or FiO_2, while ventilation is achieved through the number and duration of "releases" as well as by spontaneous ventilation. When the mode is adjusted so that the time spent at $PEEP_{High}$ is equal to, or less than $PEEP_{Low}$ the mode is often referred to as bilevel, bipap, or biphasic positive airway pressure.

Advocates of APRV assert that higher mean airway pressures improve both lung recruitment (decreasing microstrain) and functional residual capacity (FRC) (improving lung compliance) [43, 44]. They also add that facilitating spontaneous ventilation improves V/Q matching by increasing ventilation near the diaphragm in well-perfused areas, and may enhance venous return and cardiac output [43–46]. Alternatively, these benefits may simply reflect improved lung recruitment due to higher mean airway pressures, as similar beneficial effects are seen during lung protective ventilation with higher PEEP [44]. Furthermore, permissive hypercarbia during APRV either results in an increased work of breathing for the patient, or undesirably high release volumes, which likely offsets the benefits of lung recruitment by increasing tidal strain [43]. Given the lack of large trials comparing the use of APRV to conventional lung protective ventilation, the benefit of using APRV during ECMO remains theoretical at best. The in-progress EOLIA trial does permit APRV and subgroup analyses may delineate the role of APRV in the future management of MV during ECMO [26].

3.3. Additional concerns

In adults with acute respiratory failure undergoing MV, high plateau pressures due to decreased respiratory system compliance often trigger clinicians to limit tidal volumes (or driving pressures) and PEEP. In a subset of patients, however, the decrease in respiratory system compliance reflects a decrease in chest wall compliance rather than lung compliance. In these patients attempts to measure surrogates of pleural pressure such as esophageal manometry may facilitate further optimization of MV [47, 48]. Future studies, including the currently enrolling EPVent2 may help elucidate the benefits of esophageal pressure monitoring in the management of MV in patients with acute respiratory failure [49]. Specifically, esophageal manometry may help select patients who can avoid VV ECMO, and those in whom atypical MV settings should be considered even during ECMO.

A high fraction of inspired oxygen increases shunt by increasing absorption atelectasis [50, 51]. In most settings, ECMO facilitates weaning of ventilator FiO_2 to ≤0.5. However, during ECMO weaning, ventilator FiO_2 is often increased. Given that ECMO weaning is a priority for 84% of ELSO centers surveyed, future studies should examine the optimal timing of ECMO weaning, including the necessary changes to MV to facilitate ECMO weaning and the negative effects of premature weaning [15].

4. Mechanical ventilation strategies during venoarterial extracorporeal membrane oxygenation

The lung protective principles described are generally applicable to all patients on ECMO. For VA ECMO patients, however, the cardiovascular effects of mechanical ventilation can be especially relevant. RV dysfunction is a predictor of poor outcomes and increased mortality for patients with left ventricular assist devices (LVADs) [52]. These devices are often the bridge/destination therapy for patients requiring VA ECMO [52]. Also, because VA ECMO may limit blood flow through the lungs, the optimal amount of alveolar ventilation may be different compared with patients requiring VV ECMO [53].

4.1. Lung volume and right ventricular afterload

The primary measurement of RV afterload is pulmonary vascular resistance (PVR) [54]. PVR is comprised of the resistance imparted by (1) alveolar vessels and (2) parenchymal vessels. PVR is altered significantly by increasing lung volumes and is minimized when the lung is at functional residual capacity (FRC). As lung volumes increase and alveoli become distended, alveolar pressure exceeds pulmonary arteriolar pressure, leading to vascular compression, and increased PVR. However, that same increase in lung volume also increases the radial traction on parenchymal lung vessels and improves their geometry; decreasing the contribution of parenchymal vessels to PVR [54]. Thus, generally, as lung volume increases, the contribution of alveolar vasculature to total PVR increases, while the contribution of parenchymal vasculature decreases. The net effect is a balance between these two phenomena in which PVR is relatively stable at normal lung volumes [54].

In normal individuals, PVR is optimized (at its lowest point) when the lung is at FRC [54]. It is important to note that lung volumes slightly below FRC may be more deleterious to PVR than lung volumes slightly above FRC. As alveolar units collapse, decreased oxygenation leads to hypoxic vasoconstriction, which further increases PVR above the expected increase from parenchymal lung vessels. Thus, one approach to decreasing RV afterload using MV would be ventilation with relatively low tidal volumes at or slightly above FRC. This would optimize pulmonary mechanics to decrease PVR while also minimizing volutrauma to the susceptible segments of the lung.

4.2. PEEP and venoarterial extracorporeal membrane oxygenation

In the ideal physiologic scenario during VA ECMO, PEEP would be optimized to maintain FRC thus optimizing PVR, and minimizing the negative effects on RV preload (unless clinically desired). However, little is known clinically about the optimal PEEP in the setting of VA ECMO.

The use of PEEP to maintain FRC is clinically challenging. Helium dilution and other traditional methods of determining FRC are highly impractical in the clinical setting. While techniques involving nitrogen washout or partial CO_2 rebreathing have been proposed, and may be automated on some ventilators, they have not been widely adopted [55, 56]. Thus, "optimal" PEEP is often determined by the PEEP that maximizes oxygenation, improves lung compliance, or decreases lung stress [57]. Optimal PEEP has rarely been studied in the presence of ECMO, and is often extrapolated from studies of ARDS. For example, in animal studies of ARDS, optimal PEEP is often cited as the point at which thoracopulmonary dynamic and static compliance is maximized, which correlates with the PEEP value immediately above that at which FRC begins to decrease [58, 59]. In these studies, PEEP was incrementally decreased to determine the point at which respiratory system compliance decreased—thereby approximating the minimal amount of "open lung" PEEP required to maintain FRC. There is mixed evidence on whether optimal PEEP should be determined using this methodology [60, 61]. Others argue that incremental PEEP combined with dynamic compliance monitoring allows for the simultaneous evaluation of recruitment and compliance [61]. More recent studies using computed tomography-guided optimal PEEP have reported that lung recruitability and the amount of PEEP required to maintain alveolar recruitment are independent and therefore the optimal PEEP may not be related to lung recruitability [62].

PEEP, when it contributes to total intrathoracic pressure, affects venous return to the heart [63]. As PEEP increases above resting pleural pressure, intrathoracic pressure increases; decreasing venous return to the right heart and therefore decreasing RV preload [64]. These effects are often seen as negative, but in the correct setting may be beneficial [64, 65]. For example, patients with afterload-dependent left ventricular (LV) heart failure, including many patients on VA ECMO, may benefit from the decreased RV preload associated with the addition of PEEP, particularly if PEEP is helping to minimize PVR [64, 66]. Conversely, patients with a preload dependent cardiac output (CO) could potentially benefit from lower levels of positive pressure ventilation and PEEP. In this patient population, if PEEP is required, careful attention should be paid to minimizing the effects on cardiac preload.

Many argue that in the ARDS patient, true optimal PEEP does not exist, maintaining that it is not clinically realistic to expect all of the beneficial effects of PEEP to converge on a particular value for a given patient [67]. A similar argument could be extended to patients on ECMO. As such, given a lack of direct evidence, it remains in the hands of the clinician to determine which parameters are most important to optimize for their individual patients.

4.3. Inhaled pulmonary vasodilators and right ventricular function

RV dysfunction is common in patients receiving both VV and VA ECMO. In patients with moderate-to-severe ARDS (likely candidates for VV ECMO), the prevalence of RV dysfunction is approximately 20%. RV dysfunction is more common in patients with pneumonia, those with high driving pressures ($\geq$18 cm H_2O), low PaO_2/F_iO_2 ratio (<150 mmHg), and high $PaCO_2$ ($\geq$48 mmHg); patients who would also be more likely to meet criteria for VV ECMO [68]. Similarly, in LVAD patients (a cohort related to VA ECMO patients), RV dysfunction may be seen in up to 40% of cases [69].

While inhaled pulmonary vasodilators have long served as adjuvant therapies for patients with increased PVR receiving LVADs [69], the data supporting their use in ARDS and VV ECMO is less clear [70]. Inhaled nitric oxide (iNO) is commonly used in pediatric patients with persistent pulmonary hypertension [71], and adults with LVADs [69]. It may temporarily improve oxygenation in patients with acute respiratory failure [72, 73], but has not been shown to improve mortality [70], comes with substantial cost (**Table 1**) and at doses above 20 ppm has an escalating side effect profile [72, 74]. Inhaled aerosolized prostacyclin (iAP) has also been used in the treatment of pulmonary hypertension [75], as well as refractory hypoxemia [72]. Similar to iNO, no mortality benefit has been demonstrated for its noncardiac use [33], and drug delivery depends on delivery setup [74]. However, the cost savings compared with iNO may be as large as 17-fold [76]. Controlled studies on the use of inhaled vasodilators specifically on ECMO patients are currently lacking.

Medication	Administration methods	Dosing	Cost per day
Inhaled aerosolized prostacyclin	Nebulization	5–50 ng/kg/min (can be fixed or weight-based and delivered drug will vary according to setup)	$100–900
Inhaled nitric oxide	Direct gas delivery (diluted with nitrogen and oxygen)	5–20 ppm (range 1–80 ppm)	$2000–5000

Table 1. Inhaled vasodilators dosing and cost [75, 76].

Although inhaled nitric oxide and prostacyclins are well-established therapies for patients with RV dysfunction, associated with increased transpulmonary gradients, there are other agents that may be beneficial. Milrinone, a type III phosphodiesterase inhibitor, typically used intravenously as an inotrope with systemic vasodilatory effects, has been used successfully as inhaled pulmonary vasodilator [77, 78]. The use of inhaled sodium nitroprusside has also been reported [79]. Despite a lack of firm scientific evidence, these agents are often used as adjuvants in patients with RV dysfunction on ECMO (given a plausible physiologic benefit and lack of evidence of harm) and may be considered in patients with elevated transpulmonary gradients refractory to the MV maneuvers described.

4.4. Venoarterial extracorporeal membrane oxygenation and ventilation of the lungs

Protective and ultraprotective MV settings can lead to hypercarbia. In patients on VV ECMO, this concern is mitigated significantly because of the ECMO circuit's ability to effectively clear CO_2. In the patient on VA ECMO, however, alveolar hypoventilation may be a therapeutic tool.

Patients on VA ECMO have a unique physiology where the pulmonary circulation (Q_p) is unlinked from, and is necessarily lower than, the systemic circulation (Q_s) because a significant amount of the total CO (Q_T) is shunted through the VA ECMO circuit (Q_{ecmo}). This decoupling of the pulmonary circulation from total cardiac output may lead to unusual ventilation and perfusion conditions in the lung. In patients on VA ECMO, the decrease in Q_p can be expected to decrease pulmonary arterial pressures (P_{pa}). This decrease in pulmonary perfusion should increase areas of relative dead space if ventilation is held constant. However, in the lung injured patient, pulmonary perfusion is likely to be heterogeneous worsening V/Q matching and increasing both shunt and dead space. This decreased Q_p and P_{pa} requires some additional considerations when selecting a ventilation strategy for patients on VA ECMO.

Patients on VA ECMO with "normal" alveolar ventilation but a relatively low flow through the pulmonary vascular system (low Q_p) may be at risk for significant localized pulmonary hypocapnia and alkalosis. In a rat lung model, hypocapnia, independently of pH, directly impaired alveolar fluid reabsorption [80]. Hypocapnia also has direct bronchoconstricting effects, demonstrated to decrease lung compliance in small studies of human subjects [81]. Although both impaired alveolar fluid reabsorption and bronchoconstriction have been noted to be reversible with a return to normocapnia, there is increasing evidence that hypocapnia is not innocuous and may exert directly harmful effects to the lungs [53]. Conversely, there is animal data to suggest that therapeutic hypercapnia may attenuate pulmonary inflammation and reduce free radical injury; there is also some support for the therapeutic use of hypercapnea [82, 83]. These positive effects need to be balanced against the increase in PVR and RV afterload that can be caused by hypercarbia. Therefore, while lung protective ventilation is recommended in patients receiving ECMO, the benefit of avoiding localized hypocarbia may make ultraprotective ventilation more enticing. Future studies into the therapeutic benefit of hypercapnia in these patients will be needed to offset the downsides of increased RV afterload.

4.5. Venoarterial extracorporeal membrane oxygenation and arterial blood gas measurements

Arterial blood gas measurements are not normally representative of pulmonary function for patients on VA ECMO. For patients who are on VV ECMO, oxygenated blood from the ECMO circuit is mixed with deoxygenated venous blood prior to entering the right ventricle. Therefore, the patient's lungs increase the oxygen content and clear CO_2 for all of the blood entering the patient's arterial circulation equally. If the ECMO flow is increased on VV ECMO, the oxygen content of all of the patient's blood is increased. Similarly, when native pulmonary CO_2 clearance improves all of the patient's arterial blood will reflect these changes.

For patients on VA ECMO, oxygenated blood from the ECMO circuit is returned to the patient distal to their native pulmonary circulation. Depending the patient's native cardiac output (Q_p), this effectively "isolates" the lung from interrogation via arterial blood gases. It is not unusual, for example, for a patient on VA ECMO to have Q_p equal to 20% of Q_s (with the other 80% coming from Q_{ecmo}). Pulmonary function would then accounts for, at most, 20% of the oxygen content found in the peripheral arterial blood. However, even this estimate may be misleading, as ECMO blood may not mix uniformly with blood ejected from the native heart at the site where it is sampled by as arterial blood gas. As a result, arterial blood gas analysis in a patient on VA ECMO may provide more information about the patient's native cardiac function then native pulmonary function. In other words, the arterial blood gas reflects the patient's native cardiac output (Q_p) relative to Q_{ecmo} more than the effects of pulmonary oxygenation or ventilation. Consequently, making decisions about MV based on arterial blood gas analyses in patients on VA ECMO should be done cautiously.

Ironically, when cardiac output improves in patients on VA ECMO it is normal to find a worsening PaO_2 on arterial blood gas measurement. While this should not occur in patients with satisfactory lung function, as Q_p increases in a patient with poor native lung function (and represents and increasingly higher percentage of Q_s) a lack of oxygenation from the native lung would be unmasked. At that point, it may become necessary to either escalate MV settings or transition to veno-venoarterial ECMO. Conversely, when arterial blood gases indicate a very high PaO_2 (approximating the PaO_2 found in the arterial limb of the ECMO circuit), it may indicate worsening cardiac function rather than improving lung function.

5. Conclusion

The primary goal of mechanical ventilation in patients on ECMO should be optimization of respiratory variables to permit healing from the pathologic state. Much of the data used to establish guidelines for mechanical ventilation strategies in ECMO patients is derived from studies of patients with ARDS. Similar to ARDS, the prevention of VALI remains of central importance to pulmonary recovery for patients on ECMO. Furthermore, by mitigating hypercarbia, ECMO may lift some of the previously encountered limits on MV permitting ultraprotective ventilation to be used.

Hemodynamic effects of MV are important considerations for patients on ECMO. Many patients on both VV and VA ECMO for ARDS have significant RV compromise and may benefit from optimized RV preload and afterload by closely attending to intrathoracic pressures and pulmonary lung volumes [84].

Finally, it is important to consider the possibility that patients on ECMO may not require invasive MV support at all. There has been at least one case report of a patient undergoing VA ECMO support without the need for mechanical ventilation and only minimal analgosedation [85]. Although additional data will need to be obtained before definitive guidelines can help improve the quality of MV during ECMO, it is important to consider that, for some patients, the best strategy for mechanical ventilation is to remove it entirely.

Author details

David Stahl MD* and Victor Davila MD

*Address all correspondence to: david.stahl@osumc.edu

Department of Anesthesiology, The Ohio State University, Columbus, OH, USA

References

[1] Morris, A.H., et al., *Randomized clinical trial of pressure-controlled inverse ratio ventilation and extracorporeal CO_2 removal for adult respiratory distress syndrome.* Am J Respir Crit Care Med, 1994. 149(2 Pt 1): p. 295–305.

[2] Zapol, W.M., et al., *Extracorporeal membrane oxygenation in severe acute respiratory failure. A randomized prospective study.* JAMA, 1979. 242(20): p. 2193–6.

[3] Davies, A., et al., *Extracorporeal membrane oxygenation for 2009 influenza A (H1N1) acute respiratory distress syndrome.* JAMA, 2009. 302(17): p. 1888–95.

[4] Brodie, D. and M. Bacchetta, *Extracorporeal membrane oxygenation for ARDS in adults.* N Engl J Med, 2011. 365(20): p. 1905–14.

[5] The Acute Respiratory Distress Syndrome Network. N Engl J Med, 2000. 342(18): p. 1301–8. http://www.nejm.org/doi/full/10.1056/NEJM200005043421801#t=article.

[6] Amato, M.B., et al., *Effect of a protective-ventilation strategy on mortality in the acute respiratory distress syndrome.* N Engl J Med, 1998. 338(6): p. 347–54.

[7] Kuchnicka, K. and D. Maciejewski, *Ventilator-associated lung injury.* Anaesthesiol Intensive Ther, 2013. 45(3): p. 164–70.

[8] Oeckler, R.A. and R.D. Hubmayr, *Ventilator-associated lung injury: a search for better therapeutic targets.* Eur Respir J, 2007. 30(6): p. 1216–26.

[9] Chiumello, D., et al., *Lung stress and strain during mechanical ventilation for acute respiratory distress syndrome.* Am J Respir Crit Care Med, 2008. 178(4): p. 346–55.

[10] Gattinoni, L., et al., *Ventilator-induced lung injury: the anatomical and physiological framework.* Crit Care Med, 2010. 38(10 Suppl): p. S539–48.

[11] Whitehead, T. and A.S. Slutsky, *The pulmonary physician in critical care * 7: ventilator induced lung injury.* Thorax, 2002. 57(7): p. 635–42.

[12] Uhlig, S., *Ventilation-induced lung injury and mechanotransduction: stretching it too far?* Am J Physiol Lung Cell Mol Physiol, 2002. 282(5): p. L892–6.

[13] *Extracorporeal Life Support Organization (ESLO) Guidelines for Adult Respiratory Failure v1.3.* December 2013; Available from: http://www.elso.org/Portals/0/IGD/Archive/

FileManager/989d4d4d14cusersshyerdocumentselsoguidelinesforadultrespiratoryfai-
lure1.3.pdf.

[14] Schmidt, M., et al., *Mechanical ventilation during extracorporeal membrane oxygenation.* Crit Care, 2014. 18(1): p. 203.

[15] Marhong, J.D., et al., *Mechanical ventilation during extracorporeal membrane oxygenation. An international survey.* Ann Am Thorac Soc, 2014. 11(6): p. 956–61.

[16] Schmidt, M., et al., *Mechanical ventilation management during extracorporeal membrane oxygenation for acute respiratory distress syndrome: a retrospective international multicenter study.* Crit Care Med, 2015. 43(3): p. 654–64.

[17] Brower, R.G., et al., *Higher versus lower positive end-expiratory pressures in patients with the acute respiratory distress syndrome.* N Engl J Med, 2004. 351(4): p. 327–36.

[18] Meade, M.O., et al., *Ventilation strategy using low tidal volumes, recruitment maneuvers, and high positive end-expiratory pressure for acute lung injury and acute respiratory distress syndrome: a randomized controlled trial.* JAMA, 2008. 299(6): p. 637–45.

[19] Mercat, A., et al., *Positive end-expiratory pressure setting in adults with acute lung injury and acute respiratory distress syndrome: a randomized controlled trial.* JAMA, 2008. 299(6): p. 646–55.

[20] Briel, M., et al., *Higher vs lower positive end-expiratory pressure in patients with acute lung injury and acute respiratory distress syndrome: systematic review and meta-analysis.* JAMA, 2010. 303(9): p. 865–73.

[21] Esteban, A., et al., *Characteristics and outcomes in adult patients receiving mechanical ventilation: a 28-day international study.* JAMA, 2002. 287(3): p. 345–55.

[22] Terragni, P.P., et al., *Tidal volume lower than 6 ml/kg enhances lung protection: role of extracorporeal carbon dioxide removal.* Anesthesiology, 2009. 111(4): p. 826–35.

[23] Terragni, P.P., et al., *Tidal hyperinflation during low tidal volume ventilation in acute respiratory distress syndrome.* Am J Respir Crit Care Med, 2007. 175(2): p. 160–6.

[24] Bein, T., et al., *Lower tidal volume strategy (approximately 3 ml/kg) combined with extracorporeal CO_2 removal versus 'conventional' protective ventilation (6 ml/kg) in severe ARDS: the prospective randomized Xtravent-study.* Intensive Care Med, 2013. 39(5): p. 847–56.

[25] Peek, G.J., et al., *Efficacy and economic assessment of conventional ventilatory support versus extracorporeal membrane oxygenation for severe adult respiratory failure (CESAR): a multicentre randomised controlled trial.* Lancet, 2009. 374(9698): p. 1351–63.

[26] *Extracorporeal Membrane Oxygenation for Severe Acute Respiratory Distress Syndrome (EOLIA) Study Protocol NCT01470703.*

[27] Frank, J.A., et al., *Low tidal volume reduces epithelial and endothelial injury in acid-injured rat lungs.* Am J Respir Crit Care Med, 2002. 165(2): p. 242–9.

[28] Bein, T., et al., *Pumpless extracorporeal removal of carbon dioxide combined with ventilation using low tidal volume and high positive end-expiratory pressure in a patient with severe acute respiratory distress syndrome.* Anaesthesia, 2009. 64(2): p. 195–8.

[29] Hager, D.N., et al., *Tidal volume reduction in patients with acute lung injury when plateau pressures are not high.* Am J Respir Crit Care Med, 2005. 172(10): p. 1241–5.

[30] Mauri, T., et al., *Long-term extracorporeal membrane oxygenation with minimal ventilatory support: a new paradigm for severe ARDS?* Minerva Anestesiol, 2012. 78(3): p. 385–9.

[31] Viitanen, A., M. Salmenpera, and J. Heinonen, *Right ventricular response to hypercarbia after cardiac surgery.* Anesthesiology, 1990. 73(3): p. 393–400.

[32] Maung, A.A. and L.J. Kaplan, *Airway pressure release ventilation in acute respiratory distress syndrome.* Crit Care Clin, 2011. 27(3): p. 501–9.

[33] Afshari, A., et al., *Aerosolized prostacyclin for acute lung injury (ALI) and acute respiratory distress syndrome (ARDS).* Cochrane Database Syst Rev, 2010(8): p. Cd007733.

[34] Nielsen, N.D., et al., *Apneic oxygenation combined with extracorporeal arteriovenous carbon dioxide removal provides sufficient gas exchange in experimental lung injury.* Asaio J, 2008. 54(4): p. 401–5.

[35] Kallet, R.H., et al., *Lung collapse during low tidal volume ventilation in acute respiratory distress syndrome.* Respir Care, 2001. 46(1): p. 49–52.

[36] Santa Cruz, R., et al., *High versus low positive end-expiratory pressure (PEEP) levels for mechanically ventilated adult patients with acute lung injury and acute respiratory distress syndrome.* Cochrane Database Syst Rev, 2013. 6: p. Cd009098.

[37] *Strategies for Optimal Lung Ventilation in ECMO for ARDS: The SOLVE ARDS Study (SOLVE ARDS) Study Protocol NCT01990456.*

[38] Gattinoni, L., et al., *Lung recruitment in patients with the acute respiratory distress syndrome.* N Engl J Med, 2006. 354(17): p. 1775–86.

[39] Hodgson, C., et al., *Recruitment manoeuvres for adults with acute lung injury receiving mechanical ventilation.* Cochrane Database Syst Rev, 2009(2): p. Cd006667.

[40] Fan, E., et al., *Recruitment maneuvers for acute lung injury: a systematic review.* Am J Respir Crit Care Med, 2008. 178(11): p. 1156–63.

[41] Grasso, S., et al., *Inhomogeneity of lung parenchyma during the open lung strategy: a computed tomography scan study.* Am J Respir Crit Care Med, 2009. 180(5): p. 415–23.

[42] Toth, I., et al., *Hemodynamic and respiratory changes during lung recruitment and descending optimal positive end-expiratory pressure titration in patients with acute respiratory distress syndrome.* Crit Care Med, 2007. 35(3): p. 787–93.

[43] Kallet, R.H., *Patient-ventilator interaction during acute lung injury, and the role of sponta-neous breathing: part 2: airway pressure release ventilation.* Respir Care, 2011. 56(2): p. 190–203; discussion 203–6.

[44] Kollisch-Singule, M., et al., *Mechanical breath profile of airway pressure release ventilation: the effect on alveolar recruitment and microstrain in acute lung injury.* JAMA Surg, 2014. 149(11): p. 1138–45.

[45] Putensen, C., et al., *Spontaneous breathing during ventilatory support improves ventilation-perfusion distributions in patients with acute respiratory distress syndrome.* Am J Respir Crit Care Med, 1999. 159(4 Pt 1): p. 1241–8.

[46] Yoshida, T., et al., *The impact of spontaneous ventilation on distribution of lung aeration in patients with acute respiratory distress syndrome: airway pressure release ventilation versus pressure support ventilation.* Anesth Analg, 2009. 109(6): p. 1892–900.

[47] Grasso, S., et al., *ECMO criteria for influenza A (H1N1)-associated ARDS: role of transpul-monary pressure.* Intensive Care Med, 2012. 38(3): p. 395–403.

[48] Talmor, D., et al., *Mechanical ventilation guided by esophageal pressure in acute lung injury.* N Engl J Med, 2008. 359(20): p. 2095–104.

[49] [cited 2016 February 29]; EPVent 2- A Phase II Study of Mechanical Ventilation Directed by Transpulmonary Pressures (EPVent2) Study Protocol NCT01681225]. Available from: https://clinicaltrials.gov/ct2/show/NCT01681225.

[50] Aboab, J., et al., *Effect of inspired oxygen fraction on alveolar derecruitment in acute respira-tory distress syndrome.* Intensive Care Med, 2006. 32(12): p. 1979–86.

[51] Santos, C., et al., *Pulmonary gas exchange response to oxygen breathing in acute lung injury.* Am J Respir Crit Care Med, 2000. 161(1): p. 26–31.

[52] Meineri, M., A.E. Van Rensburg, and A. Vegas, *Right ventricular failure after LVAD implantation: prevention and treatment.* Best Pract Res Clin Anaesthesiol, 2012. 26(2): p. 217–29.

[53] Laffey, J.G., D. Engelberts, and B.P. Kavanagh, *Injurious effects of hypocapnic alkalosis in the isolated lung.* Am J Respir Crit Care Med, 2000. 162(2 Pt 1): p. 399–405.

[54] Shekerdemian, L. and D. Bohn, *Cardiovascular effects of mechanical ventilation.* Arch Dis Child, 1999. 80(5): p. 475–80.

[55] Brewer, L.M., et al., *Measurement of functional residual capacity by modified multiple breath nitrogen washout for spontaneously breathing and mechanically ventilated patients.* Br J Anaesth, 2011. 107(5): p. 796–805.

[56] Brewer, L.M., D.G. Haryadi, and J.A. Orr, *Measurement of functional residual capacity of the lung by partial CO_2 rebreathing method during acute lung injury in animals.* Respir Care, 2007. 52(11): p. 1480–9.

[57] Chiumello, D., et al., *Bedside selection of positive end-expiratory pressure in mild, moderate, and severe acute respiratory distress syndrome.* Crit Care Med, 2014. 42(2): p. 252–64.

[58] Lambermont, B., et al., *Comparison of functional residual capacity and static compliance of the respiratory system during a positive end-expiratory pressure (PEEP) ramp procedure in an experimental model of acute respiratory distress syndrome.* Crit Care, 2008. 12(4): p. R91.

[59] Suarez-Sipmann, F., et al., *Use of dynamic compliance for open lung positive end-expiratory pressure titration in an experimental study.* Crit Care Med, 2007. 35(1): p. 214–21.

[60] Hickling, K.G., *Best compliance during a decremental, but not incremental, positive end-expiratory pressure trial is related to open-lung positive end-expiratory pressure: a mathematical model of acute respiratory distress syndrome lungs.* Am J Respir Crit Care Med, 2001. 163(1): p. 69–78.

[61] Stahl, C.A., et al., *Dynamic versus static respiratory mechanics in acute lung injury and acute respiratory distress syndrome.* Crit Care Med, 2006. 34(8): p. 2090–8.

[62] Cressoni, M., et al., *Compressive forces and computed tomography-derived positive end-expiratory pressure in acute respiratory distress syndrome.* Anesthesiology, 2014. 121(3): p. 572–81.

[63] Stahl, D.L., et al., *Case scenario: power of positive end-expiratory pressure: use of esophageal manometry to illustrate pulmonary physiology in an obese patient.* Anesthesiology, 2014. 121(6): p. 1320–6.

[64] Duke, G.J., *Cardiovascular effects of mechanical ventilation.* Crit Care Resusc, 1999. 1(4): p. 388–99.

[65] Jardin, F. and A. Vieillard-Baron, *Is there a safe plateau pressure in ARDS? The right heart only knows.* Intensive Care Med, 2007. 33(3): p. 444–7.

[66] Wiesen, J., et al., *State of the evidence: mechanical ventilation with PEEP in patients with cardiogenic shock.* Heart, 2013. 99(24): p. 1812–7.

[67] Gattinoni, L., E. Carlesso, and M. Cressoni, *Selecting the 'right' positive end-expiratory pressure level.* Curr Opin Crit Care, 2015. 21(1): p. 50–7.

[68] Mekontso Dessap, A., et al., *Acute cor pulmonale during protective ventilation for acute respiratory distress syndrome: prevalence, predictors, and clinical impact.* Intensive Care Med, 2015.

[69] Argenziano, M., et al., *Randomized, double-blind trial of inhaled nitric oxide in LVAD recipients with pulmonary hypertension.* Ann Thorac Surg, 1998. 65(2): p. 340–5.

[70] Adhikari, N.K., et al., *Inhaled nitric oxide does not reduce mortality in patients with acute respiratory distress syndrome regardless of severity: systematic review and meta-analysis.* Crit Care Med, 2014. 42(2): p. 404–12.

[71] Roberts, J.D., Jr., et al., *Inhaled nitric oxide and persistent pulmonary hypertension of the newborn. The Inhaled Nitric Oxide Study Group.* N Engl J Med, 1997. 336(9): p. 605–10.

[72] Liu, L.L., et al., *Special article: rescue therapies for acute hypoxemic respiratory failure.* Anesth Analg, 2010. 111(3): p. 693–702.

[73] Ichinose, F., J.D. Roberts, Jr., and W.M. Zapol, *Inhaled nitric oxide: a selective pulmonary vasodilator: current uses and therapeutic potential.* Circulation, 2004. 109(25): p. 3106–11.

[74] Dzierba, A.L., et al., *A review of inhaled nitric oxide and aerosolized epoprostenol in acute lung injury or acute respiratory distress syndrome.* Pharmacotherapy, 2014. 34(3): p. 279–90.

[75] Hill, N.S., I.R. Preston, and K.E. Roberts, *Inhaled therapies for pulmonary hypertension.* Respir Care, 2015. 60(6): p. 794–802; discussion 802–5.

[76] Torbic, H., et al., *Inhaled epoprostenol vs inhaled nitric oxide for refractory hypoxemia in critically ill patients.* J Crit Care, 2013. 28(5): p. 844–8.

[77] Lamarche, Y., et al., *Preliminary experience with inhaled milrinone in cardiac surgery.* Eur J Cardiothorac Surg, 2007. 31(6): p. 1081–7.

[78] Laflamme, M., et al., *Preliminary experience with combined inhaled milrinone and prostacyclin in cardiac surgical patients with pulmonary hypertension.* J Cardiothorac Vasc Anesth, 2015. 29(1): p. 38–45.

[79] Pasero, D., et al., *Inhaled nitric oxide versus sodium nitroprusside for preoperative evaluation of pulmonary hypertension in heart transplant candidates.* Transplant Proc, 2013. 45(7): p. 2746–9.

[80] Myrianthefs, P.M., et al., *Hypocapnic but not metabolic alkalosis impairs alveolar fluid reabsorption.* Am J Respir Crit Care Med, 2005. 171(11): p. 1267–71.

[81] Cutillo, A., et al., *Effect of hypocapnia on pulmonary mechanics in normal subjects and in patients with chronic obstructive lung disease.* Am Rev Respir Dis, 1974. 110(1): p. 25–33.

[82] Laffey, J.G., et al., *Therapeutic hypercapnia reduces pulmonary and systemic injury following in vivo lung reperfusion.* Am J Respir Crit Care Med, 2000. 162(6): p. 2287–94.

[83] Ni Chonghaile, M., B. Higgins, and J.G. Laffey, *Permissive hypercapnia: role in protective lung ventilatory strategies.* Curr Opin Crit Care, 2005. 11(1): p. 56–62.

[84] Repesse, X., C. Charron, and A. Vieillard-Baron, *Acute cor pulmonale in ARDS: rationale for protecting the right ventricle.* Chest, 2015. 147(1): p. 259–65.

[85] van Houte, J., et al., *Non-intubated recovery from refractory cardiogenic shock on percutaneous VA-extracorporeal membrane oxygenation.* Neth Heart J, 2015. 23(7–8): p. 386–8.

Extracorporeal Membrane Oxygenation Support for Complex Percutaneous Coronary Interventions in Patients without Cardiogenic Shock

Vladimir I. Ganyukov, Roman S. Tarasov and
Dmitry L. Shukevich

Abstract

It has been shown that extracorporeal membrane oxygenation (ECMO) may provide cardiopulmonary support during percutaneous coronary interventions (PCI) in patients with refractory cardiogenic shock. Current guidelines consider ECMO and implantable left ventricular assist devices in selected non-ST-segment elevation acute coronary syndrome (NSTE-ACS) patients. High-risk PCI remains a viable revascularization strategy for those patients who are not suitable for surgery or those refusing it. However, such a subset of patients is considered to be at an extremely high risk of PCI complications as there is a risk of hemodynamic collapse during balloon inflations or complex procedures, particularly, if coronary dissection with vessel closure or no reflow occurs. This chapter is devoted to the use of ECMO support for high-risk complex PCI in NSTE-ACS patients without cardiogenic shock based on the theoretical rationale, observational retrospective single-center studies and clinical case examples.

Keywords: ECMO, high-risk PCI, multivessel disease, non-ST-elevation acute coronary syndrome, stable hemodynamics patients

1. Introduction

In this chapter, we will try to justify the use of extracorporeal membrane oxygenation (EC-MO) support for high-risk complex percutaneous coronary interventions (PCI) in non-ST-segment elevation acute coronary syndrome (NSTE-ACS) patients without cardiogenic shock based on the theoretical rationale, observational retrospective single-center studies and clinical case examples.

Cardiogenic shock complicates up to 8% of ST-segment-elevation (MI) and up to 3% of non-ST-segment-elevation myocardial infarctions. For cardiogenic shock patients, who fail pharmacological treatment, mechanical circulatory support devices can be introduced to augment myocardial performance and systemic perfusion. It has been shown that ECMO may provide cardiopulmonary support during PCI in patients with refractory cardiogenic shock [1–6]. Nichol et al. reviewed 84 studies of 1494 patients with cardiogenic shock, cardiac arrest or both, who were treated with PCI supported by ECMO, and showed an overall survival of 50% [3]. A similar more recent analysis found 49% survival rate either in the setting of mechanical circulatory support devices or ECMO and concluded that, in the current era, roughly half of the patients, who need a mechanical circulatory support device for refractory cardiogenic shock, survive, and roughly half of these survivors require an implantable ventricular assist device [4]. As there are no large randomized controlled trials with the use of ECMO for cardiogenic shock patients, the opinion of European experts on revascularizing this patient setting with ECMO support is not clear: "In younger patients with no contraindication for cardiac transplantation, left ventricular assist device therapy can be implemented as a bridge to transplantation. In patients not eligible for transplant, left ventricular assist devices may be inserted as a bridge to recovery or with the goal of destination therapy" [2]. At the same time, there is not enough evidence regarding safety and efficacy of ECMO during PCI in high-risk patients with NSTE-ACS without cardiogenic shock. Therefore, current guidelines consider ECMO and implantable left ventricular assist devices in selected NSTE-ACS patients [7].

Based on the United States registry data, there were ~0.4 million NSTE-ACS discharges in 2010 [8], which makes approximately1250 discharges per 1 million of the population per year. Additionally, it is well known that NSTE-ACS prognosis is unfavorable. Despite the fact that hospital mortality rate in NSTE-ACS is lower than in ST-segment-elevation myocardial infarctions, mortality at 6 months is comparable and, furthermore, mortality at 4 years is two-fold higher [9–11]. Based on our experience, we have had the evidence of an extremely poor prognosis in NSTE-ACS patients with multivessel disease that often undergo high-risk PCI [12]. Thus, this is a significant medical and social issue.

What do we know about NSTE-ACS with multivessel disease? First of all, this patient settings make up to 50% of all NSTE-ACS patients [13]. Secondly, no contemporary randomized clinical trials comparing PCI with coronary artery bypass surgery (CABG) in patients with NSTE-ACS and multivessel disease are available. Therefore, the selection of the optimal revascularization modality continues to be controversial. What is the right way to revascularize patients with NSTE-ACS and multivessel disease? Should we use CABG or PCI? Should we perform a complete or target vessel procedure? Should we choose stand-alone revascularization or a staged approach? When is it suitable to perform the procedure in relation to perioperative antithrombotic therapy and very high-risk NSTE-ACS? What is the place of staged (PCI-CABG) strategy? Currently, all these questions do not have answers apart from the point of view on complete revascularization: a complete revascularization strategy for significant lesions should be pursued in NSTE-ACS with multivessel disease patients [7]. This statement is based on the results of several trials which demonstrated, on the one hand, the benefit of an early complete revascularization approach irrespective of the possibility to identify the culprit lesion and; on the other hand, data show a poor 1-year outcome in NSTE-ACS patients with multivessel disease, who had a residual SYNTAX Score >8 [14–17].

There are limitations for CABG and PCI revascularization. Surgeons refuse CABG for high STS score or EuroScore II patients [18–21]. Factors associated with surgical mortality after CABG surgery include acute coronary syndrome, low left ventricular ejection fraction (EF), obesity, prior CABG and significant comorbidity (diabetes mellitus, cerebrovascular disease, peripheral artery disease, chronic obstructive pulmonary disease and renal failure) [22]. The rejection could be also based on the difficulties in balancing ischemic and bleeding risks (P2Y12 inhibitors loading) [23, 24].

The reason for PCI refusal is a high risk of death or major complications during or after PCI. At present, variables that contribute to a higher risk during PCI have been well defined by 2015 SCAI/ACC/HFSA/STS clinical expert consensus statement [1] and can be categorized into three major groups: (1) patient specific, (2) lesion specific and (3) clinical presentation specific. The statement demonstrates patient-specific (age, left ventricular function, symptoms of heart failure, diabetes mellitus, chronic kidney disease, prior myocardial infarction, peripheral vascular disease) and lesion-specific data (multivessel or left main disease, saphenous vein grafts) for high-risk PCI. There is no doubt that the clinical setting (acute coronary syndrome, cardiogenic shock) can increase a risk of PCI-related adverse events. A PCI is more high risk if we deal with a combination of factors, i.e., a large amount of myocardium at risk, complex PCI, low global left ventricular function, comorbidities and, finally, if we deal with acute coronary syndrome. For instance, if we are treating a complex coronary stenosis that affects a large amount of the left ventricle (Jeopardy score ≥ 8/12 [25] or the last patent coronary vessel) in patient with ejection fraction less than 40%, it can result in a quick hypotension or cardio-vascular collapse. All of these factors may lead to a high incidence of death and major complications during and after PCI and require a personalized approach to treatment. One of the right ways to exclude a risk of hemodynamic compromise during and after a complex high-risk procedure is to use percutaneous mechanical circulatory support devices as an adjunct to PCI. Unfortunately, there are no risk calculators to assess the immediate need for mechanical circulatory support devices during PCI and this requires further investigation.

There are a lot of hemodynamically stable NSTE-ACS patients with multivessel disease in a real clinical practice. A surgical revascularization is not always feasible due to the criticality of the patient status (which is associated with a high mortality risk). Because of high surgical risk, CABG intervention could be refused either by the heart team or by a patient. Therefore, high-risk PCI remains a viable revascularization strategy for those patients who are not suitable for surgery or those refusing it. However, such a subset of patients is considered to be at an extremely high risk of PCI complications as there is a risk of hemodynamic collapse during balloon inflations or complex procedures, particularly, if coronary dissection with vessel closure or no reflow occurs. Nowadays, the development of cardiac support devices has allowed a safer approach for high-risk patients.

The next part of this chapter will discuss the number of NSTE-ACS patients with multivessel disease and the results of their treatment based on the single-center registry data reflecting real clinical practice.

2. Single-center experience in the management of NSTE-ACS patients with multivessel disease

We have observed NSTE-ACS patients consecutively admitted to our hospital in 2012. All patients had multivessel coronary disease (stenoses of two or more significant epicardial arteries and /or large branches (≥2.5 mm) ≥70% and / or stenosis of the left main coronary artery (LMCA) ≥50%). In general, NSTE-ACS patients (n = 150) had a high risk of adverse cardiovascular outcomes (mean GRACE Score 135±47.6, 40% patients had GRACE ≥140) and a significant surgical risk: mean EuroScore II was 5.7±6.4. Significant LMCA stenosis was diagnosed in 16% of patients and mean SYNTAX Score was 21.3 ± 9.9. Diabetes mellitus was presented in every fourth patient, 45% had a history of myocardial infarction, and peripheral artery disease was observed in 42% of patients of the study population (**Table 1**).

NSTE-ACS patients	n =150
Mean age	61.6 ± 9.8 (35–82)
Male	89 (58.9%)
Mean left ventricular ejection fraction	55.9 ± 11.2 (21–73)
Mean GRACE Score	135 ± 47.6 (63–328)
GRACE ≥140	60 (40%)
LMCA stenosis ≥50%	24 (16%)
Chronic kidney disease	14 (9.3%)
Diabetes mellitus	36 (24%)
Prior myocardial infarction	68 (45.3%)
Arterial hypertension	134 (89.3%)
Peripheral artery disease	64 (42.6%)
Prior stroke	9 (6%)
EuroScore II	5.7 ± 6.4
SYNTAX Score	21.3 ± 9.9

Table 1. Baseline characteristics of the study population.

After coronary angiography all the cases were discussed by the multidisciplinary team and were divided into three groups depending on the treatment strategy: (1) PCI (n = 91, 60.6%); (2) CABG (n = 40, 26.6%) and (3) pharmacological treatment (n = 9, 6%). In addition, 10 patients

(6.6%) required PCI followed by CABG. The mean hospital stay was 15.3±4.2 days (from 10 to 32 days). There was a conversion of treatment strategies for some patients. As a result, the treatment groups were made as follows: PCI/CABG/pharmacological treatment: 107 (71.3%)/25 (16.6%)/18 (12%), respectively. The comparison of clinical and demographic characteristics of the patient groups is presented in **Table 2**.

Variables	PCI* (n = 107)	CABG (n = 25)	Pharmacological treatment (n = 18)	$p \leq 0.05$ (PCI vs. CABG)	$P \leq 0.05$ (PCI vs. pharmaco)	$P \leq 0.05$ (CABG vs. pharmaco)
Mean age	60.5 ± 9.9	62.1 ± 7.9	67.4 ± 10.2		0.05	
Male	66 (61.7%)	17 (68%)	6 (33%)		0.04	0.05
Mean left ventricular ejection fraction	56.4 ± 10.8	56.3 ± 10.8	51.9 ± 14.1			
Mean GRACE Score	130.4 ± 41.7	133.7 ± 49.3	180.5 ± 72.9		0.004	0.02
LMCA ≥ 50%	9 (8.4%)	9 (36%)	6 (33%)	0.0005	0.009	
Chronic kidney disease	10 (9.3%)	2 (8%)	2 (11.1%)			
Diabetes mellitus	25 (23.4%)	5 (20%)	6 (33%)			
Prior myocardial infarction	44 (41.1%)	12 (48%)	12 (67%)			
Arterial hypertension	94 (87.9%)	23 (92%)	17 (94.4%)			
Peripheral artery disease	40 (37.4%)	15 (60%)	9 (50%)	0.06		
Prior stroke	4 (3.7%)	2 (8%)	3 (16.6%)			
EuroScore II	5.2 ± 6.0	5.0 ± 5.4	9.8 ± 8.4		0.03	0.03
SYNTAX Score	18.7 ± 8.8	26 ± 10.8	29.5 ± 7.6	0.001	0.001	

Table 2. Baseline characteristics of the groups.

The largest number of conversion strategy cases (*n* = 15) have been reported among patients who were initially selected for CABG. Seven patients were moved to the PCI group and eight patients to the pharmacological treatment group. The main reason for the strategy conversion was an extremely high risk of surgery associated with older age, female sex, severe concomitant diseases, obesity, reduced global contractility of the left ventricle, valvular pathology and a poor condition of the distal parts of the coronary arteries. It is important that hospital mortality in patients initially planned for CABG, but finally having received only pharmacological treatment was extremely high (20%). If any strategy of revascularization (PCI or CABG) was substituted with a pharmacological treatment, every third of such cases was associated with in-hospital mortality.

There were significant differences between the CABG and PCI groups in the incidence of LMCA stenosis (36% vs. 8.4%, respectively, *p* = 0.009) and peripheral artery disease (60% vs. 37%, respectively, *p* = 0.06). Patients receiving pharmacological treatment compared with the

PCI and CABG groups had older age (67.4 ± 10.2 years), higher number of females (67%) and a high risk of adverse cardiac outcomes (mean GRACE Score 180.5±72.9), significantly greater SYNTAX Score (29.5±7.6) and EuroScore II (9.8±8.4), which reflected the greatest risk of surgical and endovascular treatment.

During the first day after admission to hospital, 62.6% (n = 94), patients underwent revascularization (93 PCI and 1 CABG). Thus, in the first day of hospitalization PCI was performed for 86.9% of patients of the PCI group (93 of 107), whereas only 4% of CABG-group patients underwent CABG in this period (1 of 25). The absolute majority of the patients remaining free of revascularization in the first day received PCI within 7 days, whereas CABG was performed during 2–3 weeks after hospital admission.

Variables	PCI* (n = 107)	CABG (n = 25)	Pharmacological treatment (n = 18)	NSTE-ACS (n = 150)	$p \le 0.05$ (PCI vs. CABG)	$p \le 0.05$ (PCI vs. pharmaco)	$p \le 0.05$ (CABG vs. pharmaco)
Death	10 (9.3%)	2 (8%)	6 (33.3%)	18 (12%)	–	0.015	–
Myocardial infarction	16 (15%)	1 (4%)	5 (27.7%)	22 (14.7%)	–	–	–
Stroke	3 (2.8%)	0	1 (5.5%)	4 (2.7%)	–	–	
Revascula rization (all)	35 (32.7%)	1 (4%)	6 (33.3%)	42 (28%)	0.008	–	–
Revascula rization (elective)	27 (25.2%)	1 (4%)	5 (27.8%)	33 (22%)	0.04	–	–
Combined endpoint (death + non-fatal MI)	18 (16.8%)	2 (8%)	6 (33.3%)	26 (17.3%)	–	–	–

Table 3. Long-term out comes of various treatment strategies.

The study endpoints included significant adverse events such as death, myocardial infarction, stroke and unplanned revascularization, which occurred during the follow-up period (15.3 ± 4.2 days and 27.6 ± 3.5 months). A comparative analysis of the hospital outcomes showed the worst results in the pharmacological treatment group. Hospital mortality among patients, who did not receive revascularization, was 27.7% (n = 5), compared with 5.6% and 8% in the PCI and CABG groups, respectively.

Long-term outcomes (27.6 ± 3.5 months) of the study are presented in **Table 3**. Twelve percent mortality was observed in the long-term follow-up in the overall patient population. The pharmacological treatment group kept leadership in the number of deaths. Mortality and the incidence of the combined endpoint (death + non-fatal MI) in patients who did not receive revascularization in the hospital period significantly exceeded mortality in the PCI and CABG groups. It is important to note that 33% of patients in the pharmacological treatment group received revascularization in the long-term follow-up period. This might have prevented a dramatic mortality increase in this group.

Myocardial infarction in the long-term follow-up period was predominantly due to the complicated hospital period in the pharmacological treatment group and a significant number of post-PCI myocardial infarctions. In the long-term follow-up period, the general incidence of repeat revascularizations was 28%. The majority of these cases (78.6%) were elective as part of the staged procedure in patients with multivessel coronary artery disease.

It is important that hospital mortality (15.3 ± 4.2 days) in the pharmacological treatment group was 27.7% and 30% among the patients converted to pharmacological treatment. The outcomes in the pharmacological therapy group could have been improved by increasing the availability of early revascularization. There are the two most important treatment strategies for these patients: early CABG or PCI with left ventricular assist device, which can be used for severe patients, representing a very high risk for CABG.

In summary, the results of the presented study showed that the majority of NSTE-ACS patients with multivessel disease required PCI. Nevertheless, for a significant number of patients, CABG is an optimal revascularization strategy. An essential proportion of patients, who require CABG, do not receive it in the early hospital period due to a high surgical risk, and this leads to poorer hospital outcomes among acute coronary syndrome patients. Patients of the pharmacological treatment group have the highest rate of hospital mortality. This fact suggests a need to increase the availability of early CABG or PCI with left ventricular assist device in high-risk PCI patients. A rationale for the choice of ECMO as support for a high-risk PCI in NSTE-ACS patients will be presented in the next section of this chapter.

3. Why did we choose ECMO to support a high-risk PCI in patients without cardiogenic shock?

To rule out the risk of hemodynamic compromise during and after the high-risk PCI, we can use percutaneous mechanical circulatory support devices. There has been a significant increase in the utilization of mechanical circulatory support devices from 1.3% of all PCIs in 2004 to 3.4% in 2012 (p trend < 0.001) in patients undergoing PCI in the United States [26]. Historically, the intra-aortic balloon pump (IABP) has long been used as a percutaneous hemodynamic support [27, 28]. Nowadays, a number of new devices have become available and have entered clinical practice. These include left ventricle to aorta assist devices, such as Impella (microaxial flow pumps); left atrial to the iliofemoral arterial system bypass pumps, specifically the TandemHeart; and extracorporeal membrane oxygenation [1].

The IABP provides modest ventricular unloading and enhances cardiac output, but does increase mean arterial pressure and coronary blood flow. A trigger from electrocardiographic rhythm or arterial pressure ensures balloon inflation and deflation. Based on the BSIC-I randomized trial, Perera et al. [29] concluded that routine elective use of IABP did not reduce the incidence of major adverse cardiac and cardiovascular events following high-risk PCI. There was no difference between the two groups in the 6-month mortality rate (IABP 4.6% vs. no IABP 7.4%; $p = 0.32$). These results do not support a strategy of routine IABP placement before PCI in all patients with severe left ventricular dysfunction and extensive coronary disease.

The Impella moves blood from the left ventricle to the aorta, thereby unloading the left chambers of the heart and increasing the cardiac output. A sufficient right ventricular performance or additional right ventricular assist devices are necessary to maintain left ventricular preload and hemodynamic support during Impella pumping [1]. Only 14-F (CP device) or 21-F cannula (5.0 and LD devices) can provide an output of 5 L/min. The biggest experience to date has been gained with the Impella 2.5 device which can provide the flow rate only up to 2.5 L/min. CE mark approves the use of Impella up to 6 days. The PROTECT II study represents the largest prospective, randomized trial comparing hemodynamic support with Impella 2.5 ($n = 226$) versus IABP ($n = 226$), initiated prior to planned high-risk PCI in symptomatic patients with complex three-vessel disease or unprotected LMCA coronary artery disease, and severe ventricular dysfunction [30]. Although Impella provided better hemodynamic support with a maximum decrease in the cardiac power output from the baseline (0.04 ± 0.24 W for Impella 2.5 in comparison with 0.14 ± 0.27 W for IABP ($p = 0.001$)) and was required for a shorter duration, no significant difference in 30-day major adverse event rate was observed between the two groups (35.1% for Impella vs. 40.1% for IABP; $p = 0.227$). However, at 90 days, a strong trend toward lower major adverse event rate was observed in Impella 2.5L supported patients in comparison with IABP (40.6% vs. 49.3%; $p = 0.066$). Cohen et al. have published the article [31], analyzing the use of percutaneous left ventricular assist device to support high-risk PCI. The authors performed retrospective observational analysis of 339 patients included in the USpella registry, who were supported for high-risk PCI with a micro-axial rotational pump (Impella 2.5). There were patients who have met the eligibility criteria for the Impella arm of the PROTECT II trial [2]. In-hospital outcomes of the USpella registry patients were compared with the results of 216 patients treated in the Impella arm of the PROTECT II randomized trial. The authors concluded that despite a higher risk in the registry patients, clinical outcomes appeared to be favorable and consistent compared with the randomized trial.

The TandemHeart pumps blood from the left atrium to the iliofemoral arterial system through a transseptally placed cannula, thereby bypassing the left ventricle. The device reduces left ventricular preload, left ventricular workload, filling pressures and myocardial oxygen demand [1]. The TandemHeart provides an option of including an oxygenating membrane within its circuit. CE mark approves the use of the TandemHeart up to 30 days. No contemporary comparable large-scale randomized clinical trials of high-risk PCI with the TandemHeart device are available. Several observational studies have reported centers' experience of elective implantation of the TandemHeart device prior to high-risk PCI [32–34]. Although these latter small studies confirmed that the TandemHeart is technically feasible and may provide excellent hemodynamic support, the device use continues to be associated with significant complications such as stroke, limb ischemia and bleeding around the cannulation site. More recently, in 54 patients with extensive CAD (mean SYNTAX Score 33), undergoing high-risk PCI with the TandemHeart device for support, Alli et al. [35] reported 97% of success and 13% of major vascular complications, with survival rates at 30 days and at 6 months, as high as 90% and 87%, respectively. Finally, a small study compared the Impella 2.5 versus the Tandem-Heart to support high-risk PCI [36]. The 30-day major adverse cardiac event rate (death, myocardial infarction and target lesion revascularization) was 5.8% and was similar between the two groups with 99% of the PCI success rate in the both groups.

ECMO uses a centrifugal pump to drive blood from a patient through an oxygenator system before returning to the patient's arterial system. Cannulation sites include the femoral artery and the femoral vein (venoarterial ECMO) or the internal jugular vein/right atrium and the common femoral vein (venovenous ECMO). In addition to blood oxygenation, venoarterial ECMO can provide systemic circulatory support, augment cardiac output and unload both the right and left ventricles. The advantages of ECMO include the possibility of cannulation at the bedside. Currently, we have very few data on the use of ECMO to support high-risk PCI without cardiogenic shock as adjunct modality. The data are limited to single report. Galassi et al. [37] reported the successful use of ECMO for a high-risk NSTE-ACS patient with low ejection fraction (<20%) who underwent three-vessel total occlusive antegrade revascularization by PCI. Tomasello et al. [38] demonstrated a single-center experience of ECMO support for complex high-risk elective PCIs. Twelve patients underwent elective high-risk PCI with ECMO support. All PCI procedures were successful and no in-hospital major adverse cardiac or cardiovascular events were observed. At 6 months, neither death nor MI was observed. Two patients (17%) required further revascularization, and one patient required chronic hemodialysis. The authors concluded that elective high-risk PCI supported by ECMO is a viable therapeutic alternative for patients with severe coronary artery disease and left ventricular dysfunction, who are at a very high risk for CABG and able to ensure good immediate and mid-term outcome.

Our single-center registry data showed extremely poor prognosis if the revascularization for high-risk multivessel NSTE-ACS was refused [10]. As shown in the previous part of this chapter, hospital mortality rate is 28% if we choose a pharmacological strategy versus 5.5% for PCI and 8% for CABG. The pharmacological strategy group patients were refused any kind of revascularization and, of course, there were predictors of high-risk PCI (the mean SYNTAX Score 32, the mean GRACE Score 180 and unprotected left main stenosis in 33% of patients, all patients had signs of high-risk NSTE-ACS). At that moment we asked ourselves: What can we do with such multivessel high-risk NSTE-ACS patients? Could we help such patients with PCI supported by ECMO?

Why did we choose ECMO support for high-risk PCI in patients without cardiogenic shock? As compared with other devices, IABP provides a relatively modest augmentation of cardiac output (0.3–0.5 L/min). Conversely, the TandemHeart and ECMO may provide up to 3.5 and 5 L/min of cardiac support, respectively, whereas the Impella catheter can increase the cardiac output up to 2.5, 3.8 or 5 L/min, according to the selected size. Notably ECMO, TandemHeart and Impella 5L devices, often required a surgical cut-down, whereas IABP, Impella 2.5L and

3.8L could be exclusively managed percutaneously. In comparison with other ventricular assist devices, ECMO has the advantage to provide a more comprehensive circulatory support as it is responsible for both cardiac pump function and pulmonary gas exchange. For example, with ECMO, even if we deal with a cardiac arrest, a patient is still alive, and we can continue the high-risk PCI procedure. Importantly, the TandemHeart provides an option of including an oxygenating membrane within its circuit, thus, creating an ECMO-type circuit. However, despite their encouraging results, the expensive cost of both TandemHeart and Impella devices represents a major problem to extend their use.

It is believed that ECMO is limited by its complexity and the need for perfusion expertise and is rarely used in the cath-labs. These restrictions are not significant for Russian cath-lab teams as there is a widespread use of Prostar XL devices and 24/7 on-duty anesthesiologist (a member of the cath-lab team) who can provide ECMO perfusion. On the other hand, usually, these NSTE-ACS patients without cardiogenic shock do not need immediate revascularization, which means that a calm perfusion preparation and performing PCI on an elective basis is possible. Additionally, one of the main limitations of ECMO is that the left ventricle is not decompressed and this leads to a higher left ventricular wall stress. Theoretically, this has negative consequences on myocardial protection that can be decreased by a combination of ECMO and Impella (IABP) support [1, 39].

Thus, based on our single-center real-life registry data, there are up to 12% of the hemodynamically stable multivessel disease NSTE-ACS patients who were refused any kind of revascularization and had extremely poor prognosis with pharmacological approach [10]. PCIs for this setting have an extremely high risk of hemodynamic collapse so they need to be performed with hemodynamic support. A number of devices have been used for this purpose but we consider ECMO to be the best device. ECMO is able to provide the cheapest complete circulatory support (both oxygenation and circulatory support). However, randomized trials are necessary to establish effectiveness of percutaneous mechanical circulatory support devices in adjunction with high-risk PCI. Since 2012, we have begun to perform PCI with ECMO support for extremely high-risk multivessel NSTE-ACS patients who have been refused any form of revascularization. To evaluate the results, we decided to compare them with the outcomes of CABG for multivessel NSTE-ACS patients. The next part of this chapter will show the analysis of our single-center retrospective observation.

4. Extracorporeal membrane oxygenation support for complex high-risk percutaneous coronary interventions in patients without cardiogenic shock: a single-center experience

PCI with ECMO support and high-risk CABG for NSTE-ACS patients with multivessel disease will be presented in this section. It was a single-center registry, which compared 30-day outcomes of PCI with ECMO support and CABG in high-risk NSTE-ACS patients.

Variables	PCI + ECMO (n = 22)	CABG (n = 53)	p
Demographic			
Age	64.2 ± 9.7	63.5 ± 7.5	0.4
Male	68.2% (15)	66% (35)	0.4
Body mass index	31.9 ± 6	27.1 ± 4.7	0.0002
Clinical			
Diabetes	31.8% (7)	15% (8)	0.05
Arterial hypertension	100% (22)	90.5% (48)	0.07
Hypercholesterolemia	81.8% (18)	39.6% (21)	0.0007
Prior MI	40.9% (9)	50.9% (27)	0.2
Prior stroke	9.1% (2)	7.5% (4)	0.4
Prior CABG	0	1.9% (1)	0.3
Chronic obstructive pulmonary disease	9.1% (2)	1.9% (1)	0.08
Peripheral artery disease	63.6% (14)	30.2% (16)	0.004
Glomerular filtration rate	91.5 ± 31.7	75.2 ± 28.4	0.05
Left ventricular ejection fraction, %	38.8 ± 12.7	53.6 ± 10	0.0001
GRACE	148 ± 22.9	95.6 ± 16.4	0.0001
EuroScore II, %	4.7 ± 3.7	3.61 ± 1.9	0.05
Angio			
Multivessel disease	100% (22)	100% (53)	0.5
Unprotected LMCA	81.8% (18)	39.6% (21)	0.0007
Mean LMCA stenosis %	78.1 ± 21.5	69.7 ± 18.1	0.1
Right dominance	68.2% (15)	92.4% (49)	0.02
SYNTAX Score	34±9.7	30±8.2	0.04
Jeopardy Score	11.2±1.7	8.4±1.9	0.0001

*Cockroft–Gault formula.

Table 4. Baseline characteristics and angiographic data.

High-risk CABG was based on a high-risk logistic EuroSCORE II (>5) and included one of the following: obesity (body mass index (BMI) > 30); severe concomitant disease (diabetes, cerebrovascular disease, peripheral vascular disease, chronic obstructive pulmonary disease and renal dysfunction); and dual antiplatelet therapy within the past 24 h.

High-risk PCI was defined as (1) the presence of impaired left ventricular function (ejection fraction < 30% on echocardiography); (2) a large amount of myocardium affected by stenosed vessels (Jeopardy Score ≥ 8), characterized by LMCA stenosis or by a target vessel that provided collateral supply to the occluded second vessel that, in turn, supplied > 40% of the myocardium; and, additionally, technical difficulties with the PCI procedure; and (3) intervention for bifurcation and/or left main and/or chronic total occlusion.

The study included 75 patients (PCI + ECMO, n = 22; and CABG, n = 53). All patients had multivessel disease with Syntax Score >25. PCI + ECMO group had more patients with obesity, hypercholesterolemia, diabetes, low ejection fraction, unprotected LMCA and peripheral artery disease, compared with the CABG group. In addition, the PCI group had a higher risk of the deterioration in the following scores: GRACE, EuroScore II, SYNTAX Score and Jeopardy Score. Thus, PCI + ECMO group had a potentially poorer prognosis (**Table 4**).

For PCI + ECMO, 21–23 Fr venous cannula was inserted in the right common femoral vein to the right atrium using a surgical technique. The 17–18 Fr arterial cannula was placed in the iliac artery. The mean cardiopulmonary support flow was 2.2–2.7 L/min/m². The mean bypass duration was 95.4 ± 25.2 min. The medications during PCI included unfractionated heparin and acetylsalicylic acid. The loading dose of clopidogrel before PCI received 42% of patients. The remaining 58% of patients had a loading dose of clopidogrel immediately after the surgical cannulation wound closure.

ECMO began immediately prior to PCI. We used the "RotaFlow System," developed by the MAQUET Getinge Groupe, Hirrlingen, Germany. The study endpoints were the success of the intervention, death, myocardial infarction, stroke, repeated revascularization and bleeding, as well as the combined endpoint of death, myocardial infarction, stroke and revascularization.

The mean revascularization waiting time was about 2 weeks in the both groups. In all the cases, the revascularization was successful in the both groups. Most of the CABG patients (94.3%) had a complete revascularization compared with 54.5% in the PCI + ECMO group (p = 0.0001). The mean length and diameter of implanted stents were 49 ± 16.7 mm and 3.5 ± 0.5 mm, respectively.

There were two fatal cases (9.1%) in the PCI + ECMO group and four patients died (7.5%) in the CABG group at 30-day follow-up (p = 0.2). Two patients (3.8%) of the CABG group had myocardial infarction as a complication of the postoperative period. One of these cases led to death. A major bleeding was observed in seven patients (13.2%) in the CABG group versus two patients (9.1%) in the PCI + ECMO group (p = 0.3). There were no significant differences in the incidence of endpoints at 30-day follow-up (**Table 5**).

Variables	PCI + ECMO (n = 22)	CABG (n = 53)	p
Successful revascularization	100% (22)	100% (53)	0.5
MACE	9.1% (2)	9.4% (5)	0.15
Death	9.1% (2)	7.5% (4)	0.2
Myocardial infarction	0	3.8% (2)	0.2
Repeated revascularization	0	0	0.5
Stroke	0	0	0.5
Major bleeding (TIMI)	9.1% (2)	13.2% (7)	0.3

Table 5. Thirty-day outcomes of revascularization.

The present study included patients with high risk of adverse outcomes for any kind of revascularization (CABG and PCI). The main hypothesis of the study was that PCI + ECMO may be an alternative strategy of revascularization for NSTE-ACS patients at a high risk for CABG.

All the patients had an extremely severe diffuse coronary artery disease with LMCA stenoses, bifurcation lesions and chronic total occlusions (CTO) and underwent challenging PCI with ECMO support, which allowed to carry out a successful revascularization in stable hemodynamic conditions.

Despite the fact that CABG is a preferred method of revascularization for complex multivessel coronary disease patients, PCI with ECMO as a hemodynamic support can be successfully performed in a high-risk cohort of NSTE-ACS patients. Therefore, PCI with ECMO support may increase revascularization availability for this severe group of patients with a very high risk of in-hospital fatal outcomes, reaching 27% in the absence of the procedure.

The present study had several limitations. First of all, it was not randomized and the groups were not comparable. Nevertheless, the PCI +ECMO patients group had a more severe clinical and angiographic status, which made it possible to test PCI with ECMO as a method of revascularization in extremely high-risk cohort of NSTE-ACS patients. Second of all, a small number of patients included in the study did not allow to make definitive conclusions. Thus, in order to answer the question on the role of ECMO for high-risk PCI NSTE-ACS patients, randomized trials are required.

5. Clinical case examples of high-risk PCI supported by ECMO in NSTE-ACS patients

5.1. Clinical case example 1

The first case is presenting a successful antegrade recanalization of a 67-year-old male who survived cardiopulmonary resuscitation after non-ST-segment-elevation myocardial infarction. The patient experienced a cardiac arrest due to ventricular fibrillation after admission to hospital and he was stabilized after 25 min of cardiopulmonary resuscitation. After the resuscitation no neurological symptoms were detected. Coronary angiography revealed CTO in three vessels with severe coronary calcifications (**Figure 1A–C**); the patient was not considered to be a surgical candidate due to his poor clinical condition (very low EF <20% and ACS at presentation) and to his angiographic characteristics (very small coronary arteries without visualization of distal coronary segments). ECMO (ECMO for the circulatory failing heart system in real clinical patient setting after epidural anesthesia and surgical cannulation of the femoral vein and artery; the pump maintained a minimum flow of 2.0 L/min/m²) and PCI, with the use of new composite dual coil guidewire Fielder XTR (Asahi Intecc Co., Japan) 48h after acute MI, were used to fully recanalize the left anterior descending artery (LAD), circumflex artery (CX) and right coronary artery (RCA). Excellent angiographic results were

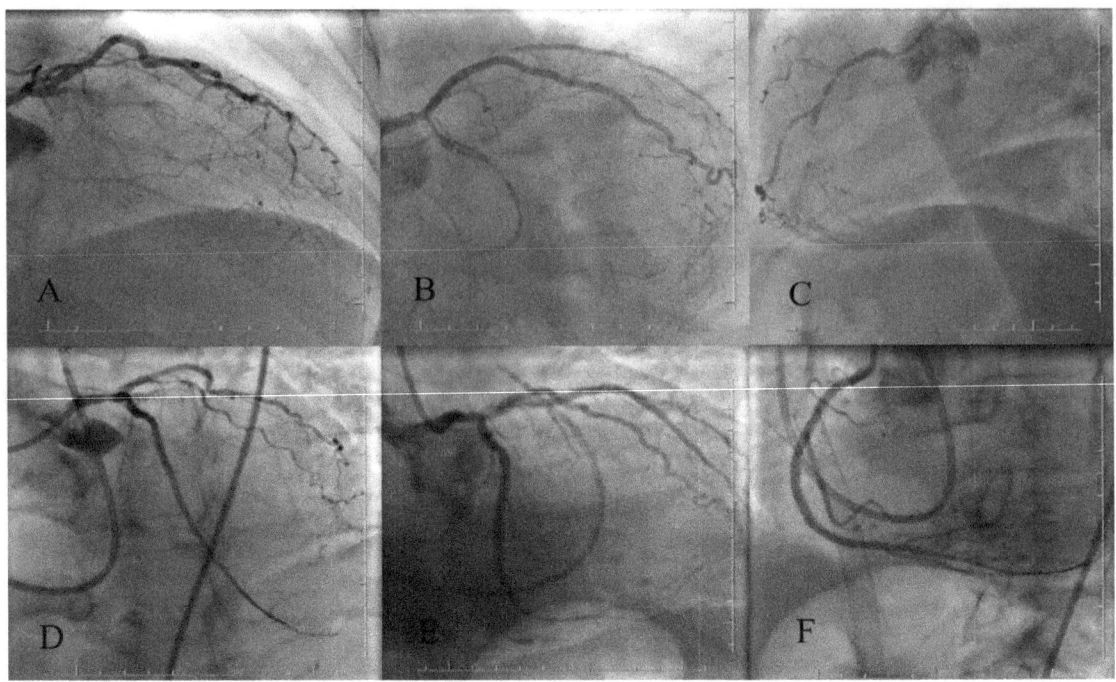

Figure 1. A successful antegrade recanalization of three CTOs in the NSTE-ACS patient supported by ECMO.

obtained by the use of three, two and four drug eluting stents (DES) in the LAD, CX, and RCA, respectively (**Figure 1D–F**), and ECMO was terminated at the end of the procedure.

In the search of technical solutions to improve the results of PCI in CTO, intracoronary guide wires represent, probably, the most advanced class of devices. The recent setup of the so-called "composite core, dual coil" guidewires can be considered an absolute turning point, especially when the complexity of CTO, patient clinical conditions and the use of an antegrade technique might limit procedural success.

To the best of our knowledge, this is the first case presentation of a three-CTO PCI executed in a single procedure and supported by ECMO in a patient in critical clinical condition. Percutaneous coronary intervention was considered the last remaining option to improve the outcome, and ECMO was used to guarantee circulatory assistance during the procedure. Indeed, CTO lesions and a critical hemodynamic patient condition due to ACS are considered the worst revascularization scenario taking into account that these patients are not suitable for cardiac surgery. Nevertheless, based on the excellent results of CTO revascularization already demonstrated in less complex clinical conditions, we believe that, by minimizing the risk of intra-procedural adverse events with the use of ECMO, revascularization of CTOs is possible even in the case of severe clinical conditions, by offering a patient an opportunity of revascularization therapy, the survival could be improved. Notably, the patient did not have any periprocedural adverse events, the EF improved up to 32% at 1-week follow-up, and he was discharged 9 days after the procedure.

5.2. Clinical case example 2

The second case is presenting a successful high-risk multivessel PCI of a 58-year-old NSTE-ACS patient with a hemodynamic support by ECMO. The patient was presented with high-risk ACS (GRACE = 173). Coronary angiography revealed a three-vessel disease with significant severe thrombotic LMCA stenosis (85%) and RCA stenosis (75% of prox. part and 90% of mid. part) (SYNTAX Score = 23) (**Figure 2A** and **B**). The patient was obese with a body mass index of 35 kg/m^2. According to the echocardiography assessment, left ventricular ejection fraction was 50%. Before the admission to hospital, the patient received a loading dose of clopidogrel (300 mg) and acetylsalicylic acid (250 mg). At the time of angiography, the patient had severe chest pain associated with hemodynamic instability (hypotension, brady-cardia), requiring analgesia and cardiotonic infusion. There was a very high risk for emergency CABG (hemodynamic instability, dual antiplatelet therapy, obesity), and the multidisciplinary team decided to carry out multivessel PCI supported by ECMO. Using artificial lung ventilation and multicomponent anesthesia, the puncture of the common femoral artery and the common femoral vein with closure device placement of ("Pro-Star" system) was performed (**Figure 3**). A venous cannula was positioned in the right atrium and an arterial cannula in the infrarenal part of the aorta. The pump maintaining a flow of 2.4–2.7 L/min was used. The middle and proximal RCA stenting was performed in ECMO conditions. Two DES were implanted with a diameter of 4 mm and a length of 22 mm (**Figure 2C** and **D**). As the next step kissing-predilation of LMCA-LAD and LMCA-IMA was performed. DES with a diameter of 4 mm and a length of 23 mm was implanted to LMCA-LAD. At the end of PCI T-provisional technique with kissing-dilatation of LMCA-LAD (balloon catheter 4.5–20 mm) and LMCA-IMA (balloon catheter 3.5–20 mm) was used (**Figure 2E** and **F**). ECMO was terminated at the end of the procedure. The arterial and vein cannulas were removed. The vascular access was successfully closed with the "Pro-Star" system. The patient was transferred to the intensive care unit. The patient was extubated when awake. The hemodynamics remained stable and

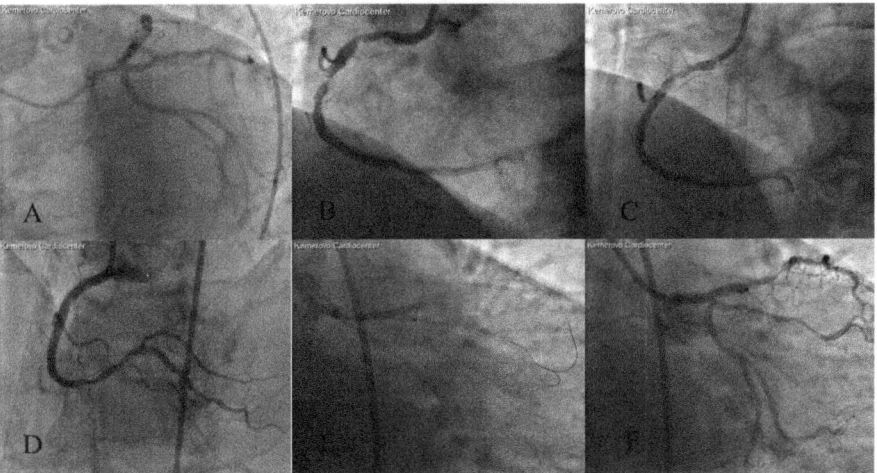

Figure 2. High-risk multivessel PCI with hemodynamic support by ECMO in the NSTE-ACS patient.

ischemia did not recurred. After 10 days, the patient was discharged from the clinic. Therefore, the use of ECMO allowed to perform a high-risk multivessel PCI in the NSTE-ACS patient in stable hemodynamic conditions.

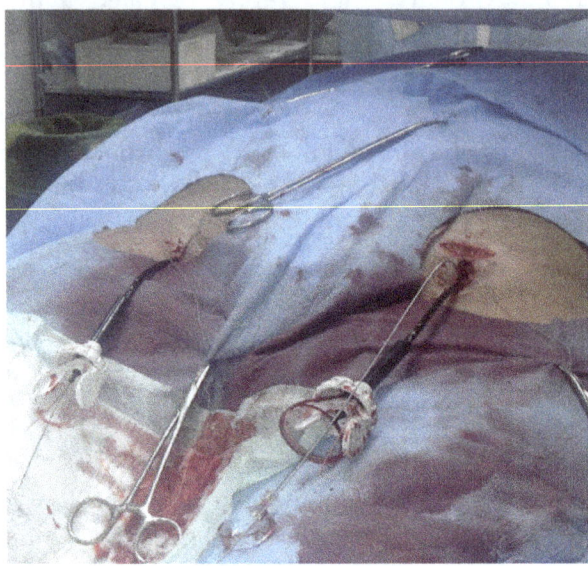

Figure 3. Using the "Pro-Star" system for arterial and venous vascular access closure.

Thus, these clinical cases showed efficacy and safety of high-risk PCI with ECMO support in the treatment of NSTE-ACS patients, unsuitable for CABG and having extremely poor prognosis in the absence of revascularization. It is possible to use ECMO cannulas with a surgical or a puncture method and the Pro-Star system as a vascular access closure device. A local anesthesia in combination with an epidural block or total intravenous anesthesia can be used.

6. Conclusions

The current status of ischemic heart disease patients is characterized by an increase in the prevalence of advanced coronary disease, poor distal targets, severe comorbidities, reopera-tion, advanced age or impaired left ventricular function, which make surgical revasculariza-tion unattractive. PCI may be an alternative for these so-called high-risk PCI patients. Given aging population, increasing morbidity, technical advantages of percutaneous revasculariza-tion and improved quality of medical care, the number of such patients will grow.

Multivessel NSTE-ACS patients are one of the high-risk PCI groups based on such predictors as advanced complex coronary disease, a large amount of myocardium at risk, low global left ventricular function, comorbidities and high GRACE Score. The prevalence of multivessel NSTE-ACS (up to 50% of all NSTE-ACS patients [13]) and extremely poor prognosis with a pharmacological approach (hospital mortality rate of 28% [12]) make the issue of these patients treatment very important. PCI supported by ECMO is an unexplored strategy for this patient setting. Current recommendations suggest performing PCI with ECMO support for cardiogenic shock or cardiac arrest patients [1, 2]. There are limited data on the use of ECMO for high-risk PCI as well as for complex PCI in NSTE-ACS patients without cardiogenic shock [37, 38]. However, elective application of the device has a theoretical rationale, showed encouraging results based on the results of our single-center retrospective observation and was demonstrated by the presented clinical case examples.

There are two main unresolved issues related to the use of percutaneous mechanical circulatory support devices for high-risk elective PCI that will represent a challenge for the future progress. When should we use them? Which device is the best? The expert consensus statement suggested a schema for the support device use in high-risk PCI, which provides a clear solution only in the case of a combination of two risk factors: severe left ventricular dysfunction and an anticipated technically challenging PCI [1]. One of these makes it necessary to use the approach with IABP/Impella as a backup, which creates issues in case there is a need for emergency complete circulatory support. Clearly, the main disadvantage of this scheme is that it does not take into account an important adverse prognostic factor such as acute coronary syndrome. Thus, there is a necessity to further investigate the risk calculators to assess the online need for mechanical circulatory support devices during high-risk PCI. Finally, device selection is a matter of a personalized approach and the results of subsequent large randomized comparative studies.

Thus, in the current chapter, we attempted to provide the rationale for the hypothesis that a very high-risk complex PCI facilitated by ECMO can provide successful myocardial revascularization in patients ineligible for CABG. PCI with ECMO support is a feasible approach for high-risk interventions in hemodynamically stable NSTE-ACS patients with multivessel disease who were refused any kind of revascularization. Further research is needed to define precise indications for the use of ECMO and its priority role in high-risk PCI patients.

Author details

Vladimir I. Ganyukov[1*], Roman S. Tarasov[2] and Dmitry L. Shukevich[3]

*Address all correspondence to: ganyukov@mail.ru

1 Laboratory of Interventional Cardiology, State Research Institute for Complex Issue of Cardiovascular Diseases, Kemerovo, Russia

2 Laboratory of Reconstructive Surgery, State Research Institute for Complex Issue of Cardiovascular Diseases, Kemerovo, Russia

3 Laboratory of Critical Conditions, State Research Institute for Complex Issue of Cardiovascular Diseases, Kemerovo, Russia

References

[1] Rihal CS, Naidu SS, Givertz MM, et al. 2015 SCAI/ACC/HFSA/STS clinical expert consensus statement on the use of percutaneous mechanical circulatory support devices in cardiovascular care (endorsed by the American Heart Association, the Cardiological Society of India, and Sociedad Latino Americana de Cardiología Intervencionista; affirmation of value by the Canadian Association of Interventional Cardiology—Association Canadienne de Cardiologie d'intervention). J Am Coll Cardiol. 2015; 65(19):2140–2141.

[2] Windecker S, Kolh P, Alfonso F, et al. Task Force Members, 2014 ESC/EACTS Guidelines on myocardial revascularization: the Task Force on Myocardial Revascularization of the European Society of Cardiology (ESC) and the European Association for Cardio-Thoracic Surgery (EACTS) Developed with the special contribution of the European Association of Percutaneous Cardiovascular Interventions (EAPCI). Eur Heart J. 2014; 35 (37):2541–2619.

[3] Nichol G, Karmy-Jones R, Salerno C, et al. Systematic review of percutaneous cardiopulmonary bypass for cardiac arrest or cardiogenic shock states. Resuscitation. 2006; 70:381–394.

[4] Takayama H, Truby L, Koekort M, et al. Clinical outcome of mechanical circulatory support for refractory cardiogenic shock in the current era. J Heart Lung Transplant. 2013; 32:106–111.

[5] Tsao NW, Shih CM, Yeh JS, et al. Extracorporeal membrane oxygenation-assisted primary percutaneous coronary intervention may improve survival of patients with acute myocardial infarction complicated by profound cardiogenic shock. J Crit Care. 2012; 27(5):530.e1–e11.

[6] Sheu JJ, Tsai TH, Lee FY, et al. Early extracorporeal membrane oxygenator-assisted primary percutaneous coronary intervention improved 30-day clinical outcomes in patients with ST-segment elevation myocardial infarction complicated with profound cardiogenic shock. Crit Care Med. 2010; 38(9):1810–1817.

[7] Patrono C, Collet J-Ph, Mueller Ch, et al. 2015 ESC Guidelines for the management of acute coronary syndromes in patients presenting without persistent ST-segment elevation. Eur Heart J. DOI:10.1093/eurheartj/ehv320.

[8] Mozaffarian D, Benjamin EJ, Go AS, et al. Heart Disease and Stroke Statistics—2015 Update: A Report from the AmericanHeart Association. Circulation. 2015; 131:e29–e322.

[9] Terkelsen CJ, Lassen JF, Nørgaard BL, et al. Mortality rates in patients with ST-elevation vs. non-ST-elevation acute myocardial infarction: observations from an unselected cohort. Eur Heart J. 2005; 26(1):18–26.

[10] Eagle KA, Goodman SG, Avezum A, et al. Practice variation and missed opportunities for reperfusion in ST-segment-elevation myocardial infarction: findings from the Global Registry of Acute Coronary Events (GRACE). Lancet. 2002; 359:373–377.

[11] Steg PG, Goldberg RJ, Gore JM, et al. Baseline characteristics, management practices, and in-hospital outcomes of patients hospitalized with acute coronary syndromes in the Global Registry of Acute Coronary Events (GRACE). Am J Cardiol. 2002; 90:358–363.

[12] Barbarash LS, Ganyukov VI, Popov VA, et al. Hospital results of treatment of acute coronary syndrome without ST-segment elevation in multivessel coronary artery disease, depending on the method and strategies of revascularization. Kardiologicheskij Vestnik. 2013; 8 (2):17–23.

[13] Stone GW, Maehara A, Lansky AJ, et al. A prospective natural-history study of coronary atherosclerosis. N Engl J Med. 2011; 364:226–235.

[14] Fox KA, Poole-Wilson PA, Henderson RA, et al. Randomized Intervention Trial of unstable Angina I. Interventional versus conservative treatment for patients with unstable angina or non-ST-elevation myocardial infarction: the British Heart Foundation RITA 3 randomised trial. Randomized intervention trial of unstable angina. Lancet. 2002; 360:743–751.

[15] Wallentin L, Lagerqvist B, Husted S, et al. Outcome at 1 year after an invasive compared with a non-invasive strategy in unstable coronary-artery disease: the FRISC II invasive randomised trial. Lancet. 2000; 356:9–16.

[16] Farooq V, Serruys PW, Bourantas CV, et al. Quantification of incomplete revascularization and its association with five-year mortality in the SYNergy between percutaneous coronary intervention with TAXus and cardiac surgery (SYNTAX) trial validation of the residual SYNTAX score. Circulation. 2013; 128:141–151.

[17] Genereux P, Palmerini T, Caixeta A, et al. Quantification and impact of untreated coronary artery disease after percutaneous coronary intervention: the residual SYNTAX (SYNergy between PCI with TAXus and cardiac surgery) score. J Am Coll Cardiol. 2012; 59:2165–2174.

[18] Chalmers J, Pullan M, Fabri B, et al. Validation of EuroSCORE II in a modern cohort of patients undergoing cardiac surgery. Eur J Cardiothorac Surg. 2013; 43(4):688–694.

[19] Grant SW, Hickey GL, Dimarakis I, et al. How does EuroSCORE II perform in UK cardiac surgery; an analysis of 23 740 patients from the Society for Cardiothoracic Surgery in Great Britain and Ireland National Database. Heart. 2012; 98(21):1568–1572.

[20] Shahian DM, O'Brien SM, Filardo G, et al. Society of Thoracic Surgeons Quality Measurement Task Force. The Society of Thoracic Surgeons 2008 cardiac surgery risk models: part 3: valve plus coronary artery bypass grafting surgery. Ann Thorac Surg. 2009; 88(1 Suppl):S43–S62.

[21] Shahian DM, O'Brien SM, Filardo G, et al. Society of Thoracic Surgeons Quality Measurement Task Force. The Society of Thoracic Surgeons 2008 cardiac surgery risk models: part 1: coronary artery bypass grafting surgery. Ann Thorac Surg. 2009; 88(1 Suppl):S2–S22.

[22] Fukui T, Tabata M, Morita S, Takanashi S. Early and long-term outcomes of coronary artery bypass grafting in patients with acute coronary syndrome versus stable angina pectoris. J Thorac Cardiovasc Surg. 2013; 145:1577–1583.

[23] Chu MW, Wilson SR, Novick RJ, et al. Does clopidogrel increase blood loss following coronary artery bypass surgery? Ann Thorac Surg. 2004; 78:1536–1541.

[24] Solodky A, Behar S, Boyko V, et al. The outcome of coronary artery bypass grafting surgery among patients hospitalized with acute coronary syndrome: the Euro Heart Survey of acute coronary syndrome experience. Cardiology. 2005; 103:44–47.

[25] Califf RM, Phillips HR, Hindman MC, et al. Prognostic value of a coronary artery jeopardy score. J Am Coll Cardiol. 1985; 5:1055–1063.

[26] Khera R, Cram P, Vaughan-Sarrazin M, et al. Use of mechanical circulatory support in percutaneous coronary intervention in the United States. Am J Cardiol. 2016; 117:10–16.

[27] Lapid JD, Madras PN, Jones RT, et al. Theoretical and experimental analysis of the intra-aortic balloon pump. Trans Am Soc Artif Intern Organs. 1968; 14:338–343.

[28] Voudris V, Marco J, Morice MC, et al. "High-risk" PTCA with preventive intra-aortic balloon counterpulsation. Cathet Cardiovasc Diagn. 1990; 19(3):160–164.

[29] Perera D, Stables R, Thomas M, et al. BCIS-1 Investigators. Elective intra-aortic balloon counterpulsation during high-risk percutaneous coronary intervention: a randomized controlled trial. JAMA. 2010; 304 (8):867–874.

[30] O'Neill WW, Kleiman NS, Moses J, et al. A prospective, randomized clinical trial of hemodynamic support with Impella 2.5 versus intra-aortic balloon pump in patients undergoing high-risk percutaneous coronary intervention: the PROTECT II study. Circulation. 2012; 126:1717–1727.

[31] Cohen MG, Matthews R, Maini B, et al. Percutaneous left ventricular assist device for high risk percutaneous coronary interventions. Real world versus clinical trial experience. Am Heart J. 2015; 170:872–879.

[32] Vranckx P, Meliga E, De Jaegere PP, et al. The TandemHeart, percutaneous transseptal left ventricular assist device: a safeguard in high-risk percutaneous coronary interventions. The six-year Rotterdam experience. EuroIntervention. 2008; 4:331–337.

[33] Aragon J, Lee MS, Kar S, et al. Percutaneous left ventricular assist device: "Tandem-Heart" for high-risk coronary intervention. Catheter Cardiovasc Interv. 2005; 65:346–352.

[34] Vranckx P, Schultz CJ, Valgimigli M, et al. Assisted circulation using the TandemHeart during very high-risk PCI of the unprotected left main coronary artery in patients declined for CABG. Catheter Cardiovasc Interv. 2009; 74:302–310.

[35] Alli OO, Singh IM, Holmes DR, et al. Percutaneous left ventricular assist device with TandemHeart for high-risk percutaneous coronary intervention: the Mayo Clinic experience. Catheter Cardiovasc Interv. 2012; 80 (5):728–734.

[36] Kovacic JC, Nguyen HT, Karajgikar R, et al. The Impella Recover 2.5 and TandemHeart ventricular assist device are safe and associated with equivalent clinical outcomes in patients undergoing high-risk PCI. Catheter Cardiovasc Interv. 2013; 82(1):E28–E37.

[37] Galassi AG, Ganyukov V, Tomasello SD, et al. Successful antegrade revascularization by the innovation of composite core dual coil in a three-vessel total occlusive disease for cardiac arrest patient using extracorporeal membrane oxygenation. Eur Heart J. 2014; 35(30):2009.

[38] Tomasello SD, Boukhris M, Ganyukov V, et al. Outcome of extracorporeal membrane oxygenation support for complex high-risk elective percutaneous coronary interventions: a single-center experience. Heart Lung. 2015; 44(4):309–313.

[39] Pozzi M, Quessard A, Nguyen A, et al. Using the Impella 5.0 with a right axillary artery approach as bridge to long-term mechanical circulatory assistance. Int J Artif Organs. 2013; 36(9):605–611.

Appendices

Appendix A.

The GRACE (2.0) Acute Coronary Syndrome Risk Calculator

The GRACE (Global Registry of Acute Coronary Events) 2.0 Acute Coronary Syndrome (ACS) Risk Calculator is a tool to help clinicians assess the future risk of death or myocardial infarction (MI), as a guide to treatment options, in a patient with ACS. It includes clinical findings at admission that have been shown to have predictive power for adverse events. These factors include age, pulse rate, systolic blood pressure, renal function, congestive heart failure, ST-segment deviation, cardiac arrest and elevated biomarkers, which together provide more than 90% of the accuracy of the complete multivariable prediction model. Outputs are given in terms of probability of dying (as a percentage) while in hospital, and at 6 months and 1 and 3 years after admission. The combined risk of death or MI at 1 year is also given. The GRACE Score at 6 months is also provided as guidelines have categorized patients into low (≤108 GRACE Score), medium (109–140 GRACE Score) and high risk (>140 GRACE Score) [7].

The updated calculator is derived from the original GRACE Score. The work on the updated calculator was supported by the British Heart Foundation, the Chief Scientist in Scotland and an educational grant from AstraZeneca to the University of Edinburgh. Professors Frederick

A. Anderson, Jr. and Gordon FitzGerald of the Center for Outcomes Research, University of Massachusetts Medical School, analyzed the GRACE population risk factors and created the algorithms. The algorithms were implemented, and the app and website were created by AS&K Communications.

GRACE is an international observational program of outcomes for patients who were hospitalized with ACS in a period of 10 years from 1999. GRACE includes nearly 250 hospitals in 30 countries, and enrolled a total of 102,341 patients. Participating physicians receive confidential quarterly reports showing their outcomes side by side with the aggregate outcomes of all participating hospitals. The GRACE Risk Score has been extensively validated prospectively and externally.

The GRACE 2.0 ACS Risk Calculator is available online on the Internet (http://www.grace-score.org). To calculate the GRACE risk for any patient with documented or suspected ACS, enter the patient data by selecting from the ranges given or by using the yes/no toggle switches. Press "Calculate" to obtain risk of event probabilities or "Reset" to clear all entered data. On the results screen, use "Edit input" to change individual parameters for the same patient or "New calculation" to reset the calculator and start over. The results are given first as a probability (expressed as a percentage) of either death alone, or death/MI, occurring up to given time points after admission. The original GRACE Score is also provided for 6-month results (**Figure A1**).

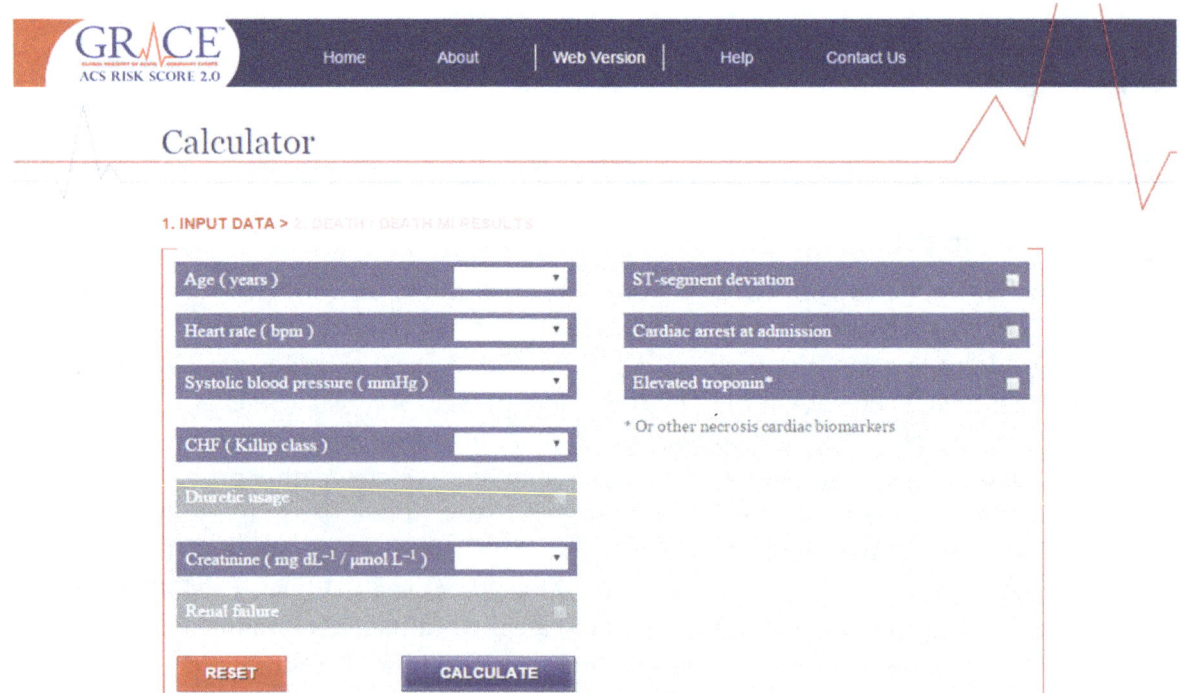

Figure A1. The Global Registry of Acute Coronary Events 2.0 Acute Coronary Syndrome Risk Calculator (http://www.gracescore.org).

Appendix B.

The SYNTAX Score calculator

The SYNTAX Score is an angiographic tool used to characterize the coronary vasculature and predict outcomes of coronary intervention based on anatomical complexity. The SYNTAX Score was developed in connection with the SYNTAX (The SYNergy between percutaneous coronary intervention with TAXus and cardiac surgery) trial, which compared percutaneous coronary intervention (PCI) using Taxus Express paclitaxel-eluting stents (Boston Scientific Corporation, Natick, MA) to cardiac surgery in complex, high-risk patients with left main and/or three-vessel disease. A heart team (cardiac surgeon and interventional cardiologist) assessed each patient for suitability for both revascularization modalities, and consequently calculated the patient's SYNTAX Score based on coronary lesion complexity prior to the revascularization procedure. The Syntax Score and related materials were developed under the direction of the SYNTAX Steering Committee, and it was made possible by the support from Boston Scientific Corporation and Cardialysis BV.

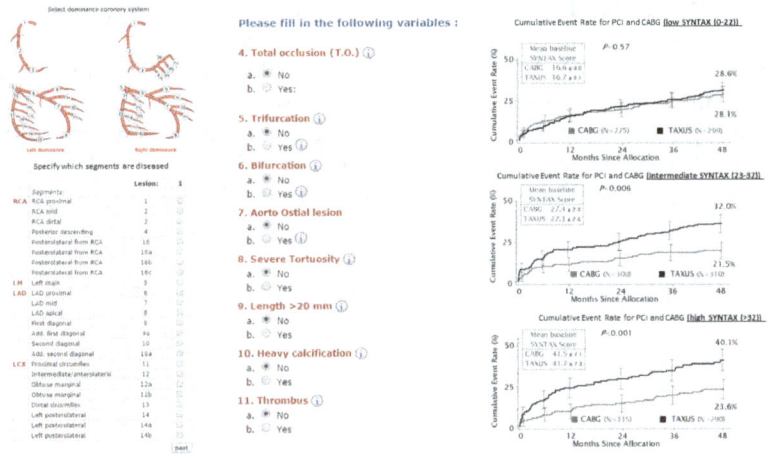

Figure B1. The SYNTAX Score Calculator (http://www.syntaxscore.com).

A computer program calculates the SYNTAX Score after answering a set of interactive, self-guided questions. The online SYNTAX Score calculator consists of 11 questions. Two questions determine the coronary artery dominance and diffuse disease/small vessels and will be asked only once per patient. The remaining questions refer to detailed adverse lesion characteristics and will be repeated for each lesion separately. The SYNTAX Score calculates a point value for each lesion, which will be summed to generate the patient's overall SYNTAX score. For patients with three-vessel disease and/or left main disease (SYNTAX trial population), the cumulative MACCE outcomes by SYNTAX score will be illustrated on a Kaplan–Meier curve. The patient's name, ID number and date of birth can be added, and the SYNTAX score document can be saved or printed for the patient's file. The SYNTAX Score Calculator is available online on the Internet (http://www.syntaxscore.com) (**Figure B1**).

10

Practical and Theoretical Considerations for ECMO System Development

Nodar Khodeli, Zurab Chkhaidze,
Jumber Partsakhashvili, Otar Pilishvili and
Dimitri Kordzaia

Abstract

Extracorporeal membrane oxygenation (ECMO) is a well-established therapy for the temporary substitution for the heart and/or lungs in patients with acute cardiac or pulmonary failure. Recently, the development of portable systems has allowed for implementation of therapy outside of the intensive care units. ECMO can even be initiated in out-of-hospital situations to allow for patient stabilization and subsequent transfer to an appropriate hospital. This chapter will focus on the authors' development of a perfusion system based on a new double chamber pump. This unique design will, in theory, allow for a more complete and effective circulatory support to allow for myocardial and pulmonary recovery. The evolution from bench-top to animal testing will be described. The theoretical issues—including the advantages and disadvantages of roller and centrifugal pump designs—will also be discussed.

Keywords: blood pump, pulsatile flow, resuscitation, circulatory support

1. Introduction

The use of extracorporeal membrane oxygenation (ECMO), as a therapy for acute cardiopulmonary failure, as a form of "substitute" for the full circulation has undergone extensive development over the years. ECMO is a method of temporary replacement for cardiac and/or pulmonary function in cases of failure to wean from cardiopulmonary bypass after open-heart surgery, or cardiac arrest, or acute respiratory failure. As a result, ECMO has the ability to provide a broad spectrum of support options for patients with severe combined heart–lung, or isolated cardiac or pulmonary diseases. The therapy is based on the temporary replacement of native vital organs (heart and lungs) with artificial analogs (blood pumps and oxygenators) in the clinical scenarios of a critical impairment or temporary absence of their functions [1, 2].

Historic milestones of ECMO development track closely the rapid development of other similar medical technologies over the past 50 years—specifically, the development of a number of clinically useful portable extracorporeal biocompatible blood pumps and membrane oxygenators. As with other developing medical technologies, the initial applications clinically tended to be in extremely high-risk or near-futile cases in which the chances of meaningful survival, even with technical success, was rare. Therefore, as with new methods for external blood circulation (extracorporeal support), membrane oxygenation was used in cases of dying patients and the outcomes, predictably, were poor [3]. Consequently, successful cases were uncommon. Hence, prior to the creation of modern membrane oxygenators, ECMO was rarely used. In subsequent years, the indications for the use of oxygenators widened and ECMO used became more common in children after cardiac surgery and in newborns with severe respiratory distress.

Regarding the terminology, according to the nomenclature of Extracorporeal Life Support Organization (ELSO-1989) a modern term—extracorporeal life support (ECLS) is often used instead of the term extracorporeal membrane oxygenation (ECMO). It is believed that ECLS simultaneously involves the use of other methods of circulatory support—ventricular assist device (VAD) as well as extracorporeal circulation (ECC) circuits [4].

In recent years, despite considerable expense, there is a trend toward a significant increased used of ECLS clinically. Annually published ELSO registry data from the 36,000 patients worldwide treated with ECLS as of 2008, more than 26,000 (72%) survived. Among the patients requiring extracorporeal cardio-pulmonary resuscitation (ECPR) 26% survived.

By 2012, nearly 51,000 patients had been treated with ECLS. Thirteen thousand patients were treated with ECLS for the purpose of circulatory support during the cardiac arrest or cardiogenic shock. Accordingly, in cases of ECPR, a 40% survival rate was observed in newborns, 49% in children, and 39% in adult patients [5, 6].

2. Types of pumps for extracorporeal perfusion

Depending on the clinical application, ECLS support differs in the manner in which the patient is connected to the artificial system, the configuration of bypass circuit, the character of pulse wave, and whether "arterial" or "venous" blood enters into the machine. The components of technical devices themselves also vary considerable as well. In order to understand the essence of the ECLS therapy, it is necessary to consider the configuration of partial (or in some cases full) blood bypass using an artificial pump and the integrated blood oxygenator [7, 8].

Thus, for the treatment of acutely and potentially reversible respiratory, cardiac, or combined failure, refractory to standard therapy, the usage of veno-venous (VV) or veno-arterial (VA),

ECMO is indicated. While VV ECMO is used in cases of severe respiratory failure, VA ECMO is mainly used with severe heart failure. The differences between them lie in the blood bypass configuration and how the system is "connected" to the patient.

In cases of veno-venous support:

• The blood intake is drained out from the inferior vena cava through a cannula, typically, inserted into the femoral vein. As for the pumping, it is returned into the right atrium by a separate cannula, inserted through the right internal jugular vein or the contralateral femoral vein;

• With a dual-lumen cannula, inserted through the right internal jugular vein (often requiring ultrasound or fluoroscopic guidance), intake of the blood may be performed from the right atrium, pumped it through the second inflow of the catheter with flow directed across the tricuspid valve into the right ventricle.

In cases of veno-arterial support:

• The blood intake is carried out from the right atrium by means of cannula inserted through the right internal jugular vein or either femoral vein, and actively pumping into the arterial system via either the right common carotid artery (in neonates), the axillary artery, or by direct cannulation of the ascending aorta;

• Alternatively, peripheral arterial return can be provided via the femoral artery.

Each of the described methods has its own indications, advantages, and disadvantages. But, in general, veno-venous bypass is used in case of respiratory insufficiency while veno-arterial can be used for either respiratory or cardiac insufficiency [9, 10].

For cardiac arrest and cardiogenic shock developing in the hospital or in an out-of-hospital situation, the complete setup of machine is similar. The system can be assembled as a mobile, portable ECLS system is used for the ECPR [11]. Teams experienced with emergency cardio-pulmonary resuscitation are required to successfully use these devices. The purpose of using ECLS during cardiac arrest (ECPR), first of all, is the restoration of blood circulation in the patient. In these instances, artificial pump replace the ejecting function of the heart. In extreme conditions, when surgical venous and arterial cut-downs cannot be performed, percutaneous cannulation of large peripheral vessels (in most cases cannulation of the femoral artery and vein) can be performed. Such configurations of ECLS implementation (veno-arterial), require, by definition, a membrane oxygenator with heat exchanger, in addition to the main blood pumping components [12–15].

When connecting an artificial perfusion system to a living body, an interdependent bio-technical system is created. In other words, complex of biological to mechanical (bio-object) system is created for the purpose of the functional support (temporary or permanent replacement of the function) of vital organs. To understand the processes taking place within this complex system, it is necessary to consider all the parameters of the operation of the artificial components of the system, their technical characteristics affecting the bio-object and disadvantages, causing certain morphological and functional changes within the extra and intra-corporeal system [10, 11].

Advanced extracorporeal life support (ECLS) systems consist of three main components: the pumping unit, the unit for gas exchange and blood flow temperature support, and the monitoring unit. Each of them, individually, has evolved through a long path of development and formation, with each becoming specific components of the perfusion system. This applies to blood pumps as well, which are key parts of the perfusion system.

From a technical point of view, all the pumping equipment designed for pumping liquids are divided into two main classes: dynamic (so-called continuous current) and volumetric (so-called shifting volume). In dynamic pumps, liquid entered into them and then get ejected in a continuous fashion. The driving force in them becomes inertia. For volumetric pumps—pumping process is based on the alternate filling in with liquid of the operating chamber and ejecting the liquid. For dynamic pumps, there is a characteristics double conversion of energy. On the first stage, mechanical energy is converted into kinetic energy, and on the second stage, the kinetic energy is converted then into potential energy. As for volumetric pumps—liquid is transferred, under pressure at its surface, with periodic changes in the pump chamber volume, which is alternately intercommunicating with the inlet and outlet of the pump. There is only a single energy conversion. It means that mechanical energy is directly converted into potential energy. Both classes of pumps are divided into main subgroups (**Tables 1** and **2**).

	VV ECMO	VA ECMO
Advantages	• The ability to avoid arterial cannulation	• Provides cardiopulmonary support
	• The ability to use a single cannula	• Reduces preload right ventricle (RV) and left ventricle (LV)
	• Provides direct pulmonary oxygenation	
	• Improves coronary oxygenation	• No risk of blood recirculation
	• Reduces the risk of neurological disorders	• Better oxygen delivery
	• May improve cardiac output	
Disadvantages	• Adequate oxygenation may be not achieved	• Increases LV post-load
	• There is no direct support for the heart	• Reduces pulse pressure
	• High risk of recirculation	• Coronary perfusion from the left ventricle
		• Stunning
		• Certain artery cannulation
		• Ischemia during peripheral arterial cannulation

Table 1. Comparison of the advantages and disadvantages according to the configuration.

The basic requirements for blood pumps were generally formulated at the beginning of the second half of the twentieth century. Therefore, at various stages of development of the extracorporeal circulation systems industry, pumps were developed and used.

Dynamic	Volumetric
• Centrifugal	• Piston drive
• Axial	• Membrane
• Vortex	• Screw
• Auger	• Peristaltic
• Jet	• Air driven (pneumatic)

Table 2. Classification of pumping equipment for pumping over fluids.

These pumps belonged to most of the above-mentioned sub-groups with various names assigned to each design (roller, finger, rotor, rotating in a liquid, centrifugal, axial, etc.). Over time, the requirements and details were continually refined and depended on the type of perfusion system as well as their particular purpose.

Hence, we believe that a modern extracorporeal blood pump should have:

- Maximum biocompatibility (biochemical and hemocompatibility);
- Maximum atraumaticity (not to injure the plasma and formed elements—that is, blood cells);
- The ability to pump up to 10 l/min of blood;
- Minimum of dilution (to have a minimum amount of filling blood chambers);
- Discharging (outlet) mode, continuous, as well as pulse (controlled pulse flow, from the predetermined, an internal asynchronous rhythm as well as from ECG or pressure curve— cardio-synchronized counter pulsation);
- Compact and transportable (with minimum size and weight) control system and power supply (battery powered for several hours of continuous use).

Based on these requirements, today, the most commonly used ECLS systems are equipped with either a volumetric peristaltic (shifting volume, for convenience are referred to as roller) pumps, or with dynamic centrifugal pumps [16–18].

2.1. The peristaltic (roller) pumps

According to the latest classification of blood pumps, proposed at the 94th Annual Congress of the American Association of Thoracic Surgery (Toronto 2014), peristaltic (roller) pumps should be attributed functionally to extracorporeal blood pumps as for mono- or biventricular support; for mechanical short-term circulatory support [up to 4 h on the recommendations of US Food and Drug Authority (U.S. FDA)], as a bridge for the heart recovery.

The operating principle of such a pump is based on the fact that the rollers pinch the tube with a fluid and push the liquid forward while moving along the tube. Usually, it consists of a flexible tube, several (usually two or three) rollers, and the surface (track) against which the rollers compress the tube. There are some designs without a bearing surface as the tube is clamped down on the roller due to the tension applied to the roller.

According to the implementation of the housing roller, pumps can be monobloc (Cased pump) and modular (Close-coupled pump). For the monobloc pumps, the drive, the reducer (gear), and control elements are all within a single unitary case housing. In a modular pump, the modules are also connected to each other, but there is no housing. Capacity of the roller pump depends on the rotational speed of the shaft and the number of rollers. The number of rollers also determines evenness of the fluid flow.

The peristaltic pumps, in contrast to other types of pumps, are not equipped with valves or seals. When in use, the pumped blood is in contact only with the inner surface of the tube. Tubes for roller pump, the most important element of the entire pump, determine: system pressure, volume of inflow, capacity, and durability of the pump. The process of the pump service is minimal, as far as only tubes are changed. Its main hydrodynamic characteristics are as follows:

- Ability to set totally or partially occlusive;

- Positive displacement—pushes blood by "squeezing" raceway;

- Automatically calculated blood flow (stroke volume × revolutions per minute);

- Blood flow is not dependent on resistance.

These pump properties, as well as high reliability and simplicity of operation, have resulted in widespread adoption clinically. In addition, it has been successfully used in ECMO systems.

2.2. The centrifugal pump

The centrifugal pump (rotating in the direction of flow) using the same classification system as roller pumps (Toronto 2014) considers extracorporeal or paracorporeal blood pumps. Centrifugal pumps can be used for uni- or bi-ventricular bypass for mechanical circulatory support for cases that require short-term therapy (up to 9 h according to US Food and Drug Authority—U.S. FDA—recommendations) as a stage for the heart recovery.

A centrifugal pump consists of housing with a tapered shape. Positioned inside is a rigidly fixed wheel consisting of two disks with blades fixed between them. They are bent away from the radial direction in the opposite direction in which the wheel is directed to rotate. Pump connection with inlet and outlet connectors to main lines is used to direct blood flow.

The operating principle of centrifugal pumps is as follows: an impeller rotates in the case filled with fluid (i.e., blood). The result from rotation is a centrifugal force that causes flow of the fluid from the center of the wheel to the peripheral areas. This flow creates a high pressure that begins to displace fluid in the outlet pipe. Lowering the pressure in the center of the impeller makes fluid to enter the pump through the inlet. Thus, the work for continuous fluid supply is performed [19].

Centrifugal pumps may have a different number of impellers, the shape and number of blades, the slope and volume of the housing cone, the number of rotor rotations per minute (1000–4000 rpm), and so on. But, regardless, the operating principles of centrifugal pumps remain the same—the fluid shifts are performed by the centrifugal force caused by rotating the impeller in the fluid. This last fact is extremely important from the point of view of a blood trauma. However, technological advances and the introduction of new coating materials for the surfaces that are in direct contact with blood, significantly reduced the risk of a blood trauma. The innovation in coating surfaces has resulted in a large number of structurally modified centrifugal pumps (Roto Flow (Jostra); Sorin (Revolution); Delphin (Sarns); Centri-Mag (Levitronix); Capiox (Terumo); BioMedicus, BP-80 Biopump (Medtronic); Nikkiso (Nikkiso), etc) into clinical practice. In spite of such developments, the hydrodynamic characteristics of these pumps are not significantly different from each other and they generally have the following characteristics:

- Unlike roller pumps, they are totally non-occlusive

- Passive displacement—Cones or impellers create kinetic energy using centrifugal force of fluid constrained vortexing

- Revolutions per minute are proportional to resistance

- Blood flow is inversely proportional to resistance

- Priming volume 30–60 ml

- Blood flow rate 5–10 lpm

- Minimal surface area

- Low blood transit time

- No stagnant areas

Considering the above-mentioned pump characteristics, operation, and management of these pumps require specific conditions, namely

➤ They are preload and after-load dependent, that is, an increase in downstream resistance decreases forward flow delivered to the patient.

  ○ This has both favorable and unfavorable consequences.

  ○ Flow is not determined by rotational rate alone, so a flow meter must be incorporated in the arterial outflow to quantify pump flow.

➤ When the pump is connected to the patient's arterial system but is not running, blood will flow backward through the pump and out of the patient unless the arterial line is clamped.

  ○ This can cause reverse flow (left to right shunt), exsanguination of the patient or aspiration of air into the arterial line (e.g. from around the purse string sutures);

- o Thus, whenever the centrifugal pump is not running, the arterial line MUST be clamped!

➤ Blood flow is dependent on:

- o Revolutions per minute's (within limitation as increased rotational rates can result in over pressurization and cavitation);

- o After-load;

- o Pre-load.

Over the years, there has been a vast accumulated experience in the experimental and clinical use of these pumps in a variety of perfusion systems. Each pump has specific advantages over other types of blood pumps. However, each of them is also characterized by the specific disadvantages that are manifested in the course of their operation—especially during prolonged and long-term applications. Complications, inherent to the specifics of each pump, are associated with the peculiarities of their construction and therefore are hard to overcome.

2.3. Disadvantages and complications inherent to used pumps

The literature relating the history of the blood pump development shows a difficult, controversial path, passed by researchers from the second quarter of the last century to the present day. Trying to reproduce the work of the heart by the means of artificial analog has been initially implemented in two directions:

- The maximal work of artificial pump is according to the basic parameters of native heart operation (these systems were known for high complexity, difficult to manage, technological inaccessibility, and high prices)—hence, widespread clinical implementation has not been reached (mainly concerns pumps, shifting volume);

- The complete detachment from the morphological and physiological identity in favor of the simplicity of design, practicality, physiological adequacy, and affordability (such designs had been intensively developed and attained clinical application), while continuing to improve on all of the basic characteristics as described above.

Technical advances along with the introduction of new materials and technologies into clinical practice have led to the rapid development of industries focusing on artificial perfusion. A major area of this focus has been regarding therapies directed to advancing ECMO and ECPR. There are generalized advantages of different pump designs and perfusion benefits achieved as well as the complications and potential disadvantages related to their design. While analyzing the advantages related to the clinical application of roller and centrifugal pumps, we should note the existence of "old" deficiencies and complications, inherent in these pumps. This is interdependence of blood inflow and outflow parameters, lack of counter pulsation, potential for blood trauma, and other problems reflect the inherent limitations of all extracorporeal systems [20].

These theoretical disadvantages limit, to some extent, the effectiveness of such perfusion systems and the clinical applications in which they are being used. In situations, when the perfusion system is used for the treatment of respiratory insufficiency, the main function of oxygenating blood is performed by a membrane oxygenator. The blood pump then functions in an auxiliary role by serving as a means of transporting blood inside the complex bio-technological system. With veno–veno perfusion, non-pulsatile blood flow, implemented by the pump, is quite acceptable, when the oxygenation (and elimination of carbon dioxide) function of the impaired lung is replaced. A significant disadvantage of such bypass scheme is the risk of blood recirculation, which can partially reduce by modifying bypass circuit. Recirculation is where the inflow and outflow cannulas are physically close to one another and the suction of the outflow cannula actively drains the inflow. An example would be dual-lumen cannula, draining the blood from the right atrium with one lumen and with the other lumen, directed across the tricuspid valve into the right ventricle pumping the blood in which any misdirection of inflow blood is aspirated back into the drainage lumen.

The needs of the pump are greatly increased during combined cardiopulmonary insufficiency, when in addition to the needs of gas exchange replacement (i.e., lung function), the need for cardiac pumping function is also required. In such patients, the veno-arterial bypass configuration, pumping oxygenated blood directly into the aorta (or a major branch—such as the iliac, axillary, or femoral arteries) is used. This configuration allows for replacing the oxygenation function of the injured lung and simultaneously reducing the pre-load of the right heart. However, at the same time, due to the necessity of continuous shifting of the blood volume into the aorta, the after-load of the left ventricle myocardium is increased. This is an important downside of the VA support, particularly evident in patients with left ventricular myocardial dysfunction. The solution was found while using intra-aortic balloon pump (IABP) using counter pulsation in the thoracic aorta and reducing post-load of the left heart.

2.4. Extracorporeal cardio-pulmonary resuscitation (ECPR)

Since the beginning of the twentieth century, ECLS has been intensively for circulatory support in the cases of cardiogenic shock or cardiac arrest. ECLS can be applied in a variety of clinical settings—such as in out-of-hospital conditions. In cases within the hospital setting, determination the indications for use, implanting the ECLS system, and managing its operation is provided by qualified hospital staff. In out-of-hospital conditions, these activities are performed by specially trained teams of medical and technical personnel, emergently called to the scene of a witnessed cardiopulmonary arrest [21–23]. In cases where conventional cardio-pulmonary resuscitation (CPR) is ineffective, an essential component of success is the speed and quality of the initiation ECLS machine and restoring systemic circulation. This more aggressive approach to extracorporeal cardio-pulmonary resuscitation (ECPR) has no other alternatives. According to recent literature, this approach is considered to be the most effective, as is quite justified from etiological and pathogenic points of view. This is confirmed by encouraging outcome data, accordingly, successful ECPR cases exceeds 60% on average, while same outcomes of the standard CPR varies—often within the range of 15% [6, 24].

The bypass configuration during ECPR is veno-arterial, but there can be used different cannulation sites. In order to connect the perfusion system, options include the femoral vessels (arterial and/or vein), jugular vein and carotid artery (inflow connection) or a combination thereof (mixed connection). Moreover, the careful selection of the cannula to ensure adequate, smooth, and even flow of blood to the pump from the venous bed and then pumping, according to the predefined hemodynamic requirements to a particular arterial tissue bed is essential. Modern venous cannula and technique of great vessel cannulation allow for delivery of up to 70% of the circulating blood volume (CBV) through the common jugular vein from the right atrium. At the drainage location of the end of venous cannula (when it is located not in the right atrium, but in the lumen of a vein), the prevention of the suction of the venous walls should be considered, which is achieved by controlling the value "pressure gradient," in addition to using special cannulas to avoid such "suction events." Depending on specific ECPR method, in most cases for returning blood (particularly in terms of out-of-hospital conditions), the femoral artery is used. In the case of veno-arterial ECMO oxygenated blood is pumped into the aorta in a retrograde manner. Therefore, depending on position of the end of the cannula, oxygenated blood is mainly returned to the distal part of a patient's body, and the brain and ventricular myocardium are still in more unfavorable perfusion condition. In such cases, we speak of uneven redistribution of oxygenated blood at the level of the aorta and its branches, called the "Harlequin Effect." Thus, in theory, the optimal location for the location of the end of the cannula should be considered as the ascending aorta or arch.

Depending on the specific ECPR approach, important is the providing the appropriate system for safe, quick, and easy to initiate therapy. Requirements for the system include portability, mobility, flexibility, minimum weight, a complete set components, and ease of management. Obviously, affordability is also important. The basic unit of this system, of course, remains the blood pump. Modern devices in most cases are equipped with centrifugal pumps. The relatively small size, a small amount of filling, reliable control, and monitoring of the entire system all increase the chances of clinical success and a good outcome. However, considering the fact that centrifugal pumps rotate in the flow and belong to a class of dynamic pumps, they are capable of producing only a continuous, steady stream of flow. Therefore, realizing 70% of the blood flow, it can be effective even in cases of asystole. However, in cases of successful ECPR and restoration of cardiac activity, operation of the pump in continuous mode can increase the after-load of left ventricular myocardium hence limiting adequate cardiac recovery, worsening ischemia (or other pressure and/or volume overload variables). It is necessary to take into account the nature and localization of the pathological process (zone of ischemia) caused by the cardiogenic shock, especially if it covers the area of the heart and the left atrial septum. In such cases, the overall outcome of ECPR may be worsened and impact patient outcomes. Regardless, during the period of therapy in the case of ECPR, the phases of therapy can be divided into two periods—each requiring maintenance of different blood inflow and pumping options:

- I—The period before the restoration cardiac activity

- II—The period after the restoration of cardiac activity

In period I of extracorporeal resuscitation, the recovery of hemocirculation using continuous blood flow in the cardiovascular system is far preferable to blood flow, implemented by external heart massage (providing not more than 5% of cerebral blood flow). Artificial perfusion with oxygenated blood, in which the desired temperature mode, the acid-base balance (ABB) and drug saturation can be easily maintained, is able to provide adequate tissue and organ blood flow. In case of a high-end location of the aortic cannula, the adequate coronary perfusion is also possible. Such perfusion is able to support the required electrical activity of the myocardium and the restoration of sinus rhythm, sometimes even without defibrillation.

In period II of ECPR, after the restoration of cardiac activity, the pump must carry out support for the systemic circulation. The goal should be maximum unloading of the myocardium for the gradual, smooth and simultaneous recovery of the myocardium, weakened by "disaster". In other words, the perfusion mode should ensure that pumping of a certain volume of blood from the right atrium to the aorta not to impede the emptying of the natural ventricular. Left ventricular ejection must continue—as because stagnation of blood in the cavity can result, even in the setting of adequate anticoagulation, clotting of blood which when ejected can be fatal. Therefore, unloading of the myocardium of both ventricles in terms of volume and pressure must be considered as the best option. Such perfusion therapies, for example, are characteristic for the pulsating types of left ventricular assist devices (LVADs) with the pumps serving to shift the volume. A pump operating in counter pulsation mode, taking up a blood from the right atrium, will unload right heart in terms of volume. By pumping this volume back into the aorta, it also bypasses the left heart, also unloading it in terms of volume, while at the same time contributing to additional after-load reduction of the right heart. Finally, if the volume of blood is pumped into the aorta during diastole (provided the aortic valve is closed), there will be additional after-load reduction of the left ventricle—and much like the function of an IABP, coronary perfusion with oxygenated blood will also increase [25–28].

2.4.1. Pulse wave properties at extracorporeal circulation

Probably, the largest and longest standing debates between the experts about the advantages and disadvantages of the blood flow are the nature of extra-corporeal blood flow/wave properties. Specifically, it is the comparison of non-pulsatile, continuous flow with a pulsatile flow synchronized with the cardiac cycle of native heart flow. The main argument supporting non-pulsatile flow is the significant decrease of the pulsatile flow from the aorta and its major branches to the thin peripheral arteries—arterioles, and then the eventual elimination, or "smoothing out" of the pulse wave as it reaches the capillaries. According to this logic, if the transcapillary flow in normal physiological conditions has a continuous, non-pulsatile nature, then in case of artificial continuous flow (i.e., ECMO), cell and accordingly tissue blood flow should not be affected. On the other hand, supporters of pulsatile flow, in case of the artificial perfusion, insist on the need of maintaining the pulsatile wave, especially in the central part of the cardiovascular system. Numerous investigations suggest that besides the large arteries, arterioles, particularly those in kidneys, contain baroreceptors. In addition, the baroreceptors of the aortic arch trigger neural and humoral reactions that impact the regulation of circulating blood volume and arterial blood pressure by increasing sympathetic tone and activating the renin–angiotensin system and vasopressin release. The large main arteries provided with baroreceptors instantly and quite sensitively react to the slightest pressure changes within this system and participate in the redistribution of blood volume, depending on the needs of the body. In the process of blood flow redistribution, little to no function is performed by the arterioles, which are called "taps" of the vascular system or "resistance vessels." About 50–60% of the total resistance to blood flow is contributed to by these vessels. Arterioles determine the systemic blood flow at the regional and microcirculatory level. Total vascular resistance at different parts of the body contribute to the systemic diastolic blood pressure, changes it a certain level as the result of common neurogenic and humoral changes of the tone of these vessels. Differently directed changes of the tone of different regional arterioles provide volumetric blood flow redistribution between regions—this complex feedback mechanism controls the microcirculation. The cardiovascular system (especially the large, main arterial vessels), which are evolutionary adapted to such neuro-humoral regulation, if not receiving the normal physiologic (or even pathophysiologic) baro-excitation, results in the adverse operating conditions. Thus, in a continuous flow, they react adversely to the non-physiological artificial perfusion. This results in repeatedly described situations of inadequate peripherial circulation, secondary impairment of the microcirculation, impairment of organ blood flow, the accumulation of toxic metabolites, and buffer shifts with homeostasis dysfunction. However, clinicians over the years have learned to correct these shifts timely, both by means of medications and fluid (crystalloid and colloid) as well as the use of technical devices (i.e., dialysis and renal replacement therapies). But, despite all attempts and various degrees at correction of these biochemical abnormalities, the damages continue to exist as they are believed to be related to the non-physiological flow of artificial perfusion [29–31].

In cases of ECLS, carried out during cardiac arrest or cardiogenic shock, there are additional reasons to employ synchronized pulsatile flow. Specifically, the need of reduce both pre- and after-load in the weakened ventricular myocardium. To do this, blood, taken by the pump from the right atrium, should be returned, provided with the required kinetic energy, to the aorta during diastole (after closing aortic valve—critical to preventing LV distention). None of the above-discussed structures of the pumps, which are commonly used clinically are able to carry out such a specific counter pulsation. Therefore, we can conclude that despite certain clinical successes of the different ECLS methods, the technology is far from perfect and there is a critical need for improvement of blood pumps. Given this, the goal of the researchers is the creation of universal extracorporeal pump is understandable. The structure of such pump, regardless of the nature of the blood flow, should allow for the desired pumping of flow both in non-pulsatile mode as well as in a controlled counter pulsatile mode [32].

2.5. Description of blood pump with own design

Since 2000, our team has been developing paracorporeal blood pumps for perfusion in ECLS systems. Currently, many of our pump designs are protected by national patents. These pumps, which are handmade, are tested in systems of cardiopulmonary bypass, ECMO systems, portable systems to be used for ECPR and in retrofit systems for the perfusion of isolated organs and organ systems "in situ."

After the bench testing, the systems are tested in various experimental models on animals. In addition to blood pumps, the complete circuit of these systems generally includes the parts and accessories for single-use perfusion sets for cardiopulmonary bypass: oxygenator with heat exchanger, the arterial filter, a set of flexible connecting tubes from PVC or silicone, various fittings, taps, etc. The blood pump itself belongs to the class of volume shifting pumps. With regard to the sub-group, it is a hybrid between membrane and pneumatic pumps. It is equipped with two chambers, connecting tubes (lines) for blood and air, external electronic clamps of the tube-lines, the pulsator, and a control system.

In the design of the pump, in order to separate the functions of filling and ejection, we have chosen a two-chamber circuit in which both chambers perform the opposite function at the same time. At the time, when in one of the chambers experiences blood inflow through the inlet branch conduit and it is filled, the blood from other chamber is ejected through the outlet branch conduit and the chamber is emptied. This allows controlling parameters of inlet and outlet separately. This is in contrast to similar parameters in roller or centrifugal pumps and is a significant distinguishing feature of this pump.

The second distinctive feature is the absence of any parts, moving in the flow, hence minimizing affecting blood cells and traumatizing them. So, compressed air (pressure) was chosen for pumping in the capacity of the substance imparting kinetic energy to the blood.

In the pump, running on a pneumodrive (actuator), compressed air, or a vacuum is applied to the rigid chamber from the branch pipes of the compressor with the receivers of positive and negative pressure (**Figures 1–3**). Each of the branch pipes is provided with an electrically operated stop-cock, consisting of external electronic clamps (EEC) on the tubing lines. Thus, each rigid clamp has four holes with branch pipes provided with the EEC. Accordingly, both chambers together have eight such branch pipes. In the filling cycle (diastole) of one of the chambers, two of them are open and two are closed. At this time, in the other chamber, there is a pump cycle, and again, two EEC are open and two are closed. Consequently, in each phase of the pump operation, four of the eight EECs are open, and four are closed.

1 Casing of the first chamber.

1a Bag of the first chamber.

2 Casing of the second chamber.

2a Bag of the second chamber.

3 The blood inlet branch-pipe of the first chamber.

4 The blood inlet branch-pipe of the second chamber.

5 The blood outlet branch-pipe of the first chamber.

6 The blood outlet branch-pipe for second chamber.

7 The common outlet tubing-line of the pump.

8 The common inlet tubing-line of the pump.

9 Sensors of filling and emptying the bags.

10 EEC of the blood inlet branch-pipe of the first chamber.

11 EEC of the blood inlet branch-pipe of the second chamber.

12 EEC of the blood outlet branch-pipe of the first chamber.

13 EEC of the blood outlet branch-pipe of the second chamber.

14, 15 Vacuum line EECs of the chambers.

16, 17 Pneumatic pressure line EECs.

18 Compressor of the positive and negative pressure.

19 Pressure receiver.

20 Vacuum receiver.

21, 22 Pneumatic pressure lines.

23, 24 Vacuum lines.

25 Pulsator.

26 Control system.

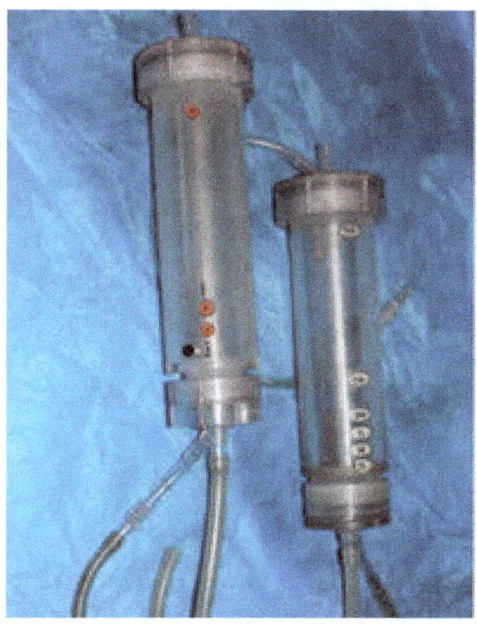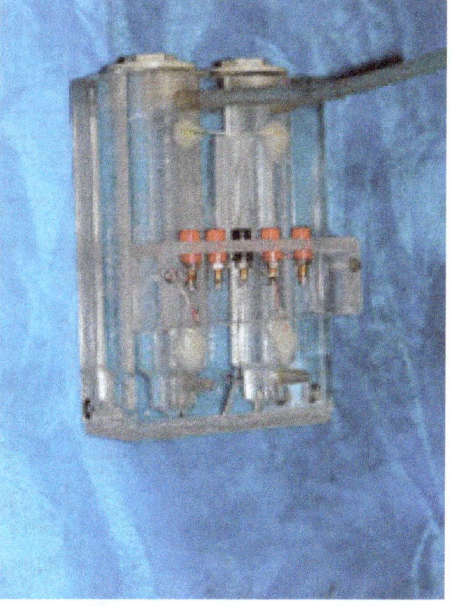

Figure 1. Variety of pumps developed with our design.

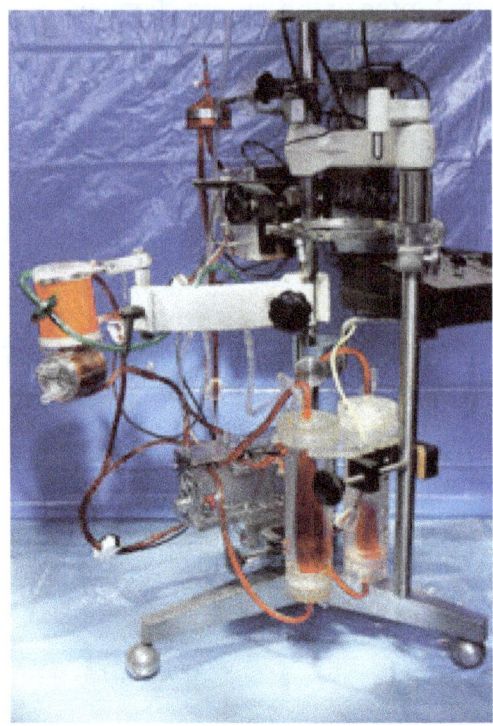

Figure 2. The external view of the pump.

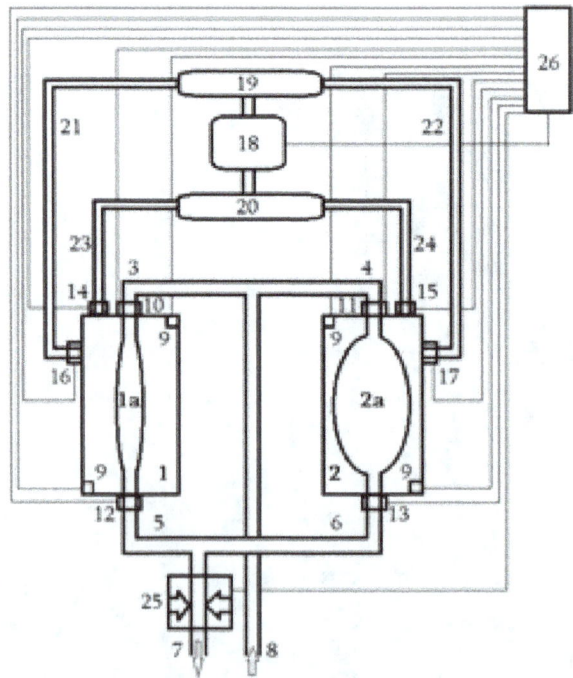

Figure 3. Scheme of the two-chamber pump.

In order to keep the components separate (i.e., blood from the air), the principle of a saccular chamber "Bag in Can" was chosen. This consists of an outer housing—"Can", which is a cylindrically shaped casing and is made of a transparent rigid material that can withstand pressures up to 3 atm (303.9 kPa). The inner, elliptically shaped, chamber—"bag", it is a thin-walled, elastic, biologically compatible (polyurethane) blood bag. Inlet and outlet conduits of the blood chamber are located at the poles of ellipsoidal bag and are mounted in the branch pipes of the rigid housing. Blood enters directly, via the inlet branch-pipe, directly into the blood chamber from the one end. After passing through the bag, it is pumped out through the outlet-branch pipe of the rigid housing, located at its opposite end.

Another feature of the pump is that each of the blood chambers filling (storage) and emptying (systole—pumping) functions is integrated. Thus, the filling (diastole) process, as well as emptying, is multi-cyclic. This means that filling (or discharging) chamber can store blood volume, equal to a few cardiac outputs. Accordingly, this increases the amount pump can store as a whole. This feature becomes evident when the pump is in a pulsatile mode. This mode of operation allows, depending on the specific requirements of the clinical situation, the blood to be stored in the blood pump for a certain number of native heart cycles with an arbitrary frequency of pulse cycles of the pump. In addition, it is possible to change the volume and pressure of each pump ejection and arbitrarily. In other words, the pump construction maintains one of the most important characteristics of myocardium—the ability to adapt to the amount of blood inflowing in accordance with the Starling law (in terms of volume and pressure changes).

Each chamber is equipped with electronic sensors for filling and emptying the blood storage "bags" (i.e., bladders). With these sensors, it is possible to set the desired maximum and minimum blood bag filling volume in each chamber. When blood volume exceeds the set value, the sensors are instantly activated and the give impulse to the control system that switches the chambers and changes their function—from filling to ejection.

Both chambers are functionally integrated into a single pump and reservoir unit, acting both —as a blood accumulator (reservoir) and a hydraulic pump. Thus, only changing the chambers of a certain size to the chambers of another leads to creation of the pump with different capacity and identical hydrodynamic characteristics to those, described above. Inlet branching conduits of both chambers are interconnected with a free end connected to the inflow (venous) bloodline of the patient. The outlet branch conduit of the chambers is also interconnected—with a free end serving as the outflow back to the patient.

Finally, one of the most important parts of the pump is pulsator. It is located at the connection between outlet tubing of the pump and the oxygenator. The principle of pulsator function is very simple—external clamping of the silicone tubing-line. However, management of this pulsator allows achieving the desired effects of adequate circulatory support, namely

- Carry out pulsation mode in cases of native heart asystole;

- Change the clamping frequency—pump pulsation frequency;

- Change the duration of clamping—the time of "diastole" of the pump;

- Change the duration of time between clamping—the time of "systole";

- Synchronize pulsation of the pump in accordance with an electrocardiogram or pulse wave in cases even minimal cardiac activity;

- Change the timing ratio of "systole" and "diastole" of the pump in the counter pulsation mode to match the native cardiac cycle.

Although, in terms of universality of the pump, it should be noted that it has the ability to perform not only the pulsatile flow, which attempts to match physiologically arterial flow, but also non-pulsatile flow—a characteristic of the venous bed. It is this feature, which we realized in a number of experiments in the settle of liver transplantation that demonstrated adequate protection of the recipient patient in the anhepatic phase.

By choosing appropriate pump chamber sizes (i.e., volume), it can be adapted to both—perfusion applications (chamber volume up to 1000 ml) for large experimental animals (calves, donkeys—some weighing up to 100 kg), as well as medium-sized experimental animals (dogs, sheep, pigs—weighing 45 kg). We have successfully tested circuits for small experimental animals (rabbit, rat—weighing less than 3 kg) with the chamber volume up to 50 and 20 ml.

2.5.1. Description of the pump operation

The priming volume of the pump chambers may vary depending on the type and size of the experimental animal and the planned experimental model. For example, in the model ECPR on the sheep (up to 40 kg), we used blood pump with the chamber volume up to 200 ml. The total volume of priming of the entire system with the oxygenator and arterial filter was 750 ml.

I phase

In the first chamber, after the activation of the blood level sensor, the EEC closes the inlet branch-pipe for blood—a vacuum line then opens the tubing conduit for pressure and blood release. The pumping begins. Simultaneously, by a signal from the level sensor in the second chamber, the EEC closes the outlet branch-pipe for blood—the pneumatic pressure tubing conduit then opens the inlet branch-pipe for the blood and the vacuum line. Thus, the second chamber begins filling.

II phase

When blood reaches a certain volume level, the sensor switches the position of tubing conduit of the EECs. Thus, the chambers change their functions instantly: Empty changes to filling, and filling starts pumping. By changing the position of the volume level sensor in the circuit, filling level of blood chambers and therefore, the filling level of the pump system may be changed.

Since the chambers function cyclically, all their work can be divided into two opposite phases: the filling phase and the emptying phase (**Figures 4** and **5**). The compressor (#18) is switched on after priming the blood circuit pump. The receivers (#19, #20) provide excess pressure and vacuum relief valves. Thus, in phase I in the casing of the chamber (#1), the air is supplied from the control system by the EEC (through line #21), under pressure from the receiver (#19). In this chamber under the action of an impulse from the control system, the branch conduits (#10 and #14) are closed and branch conduits (#12 and #16) are opened. Thus, the chamber (#1a) begins to pump blood through the outlet branch conduit (#12) and the outlet tubing-line (#5) to the common output line (#7). The pulsator (#25) is located on this tubing line, and it is also controlled from the general control panel. At the same time, automatically, by remote control impulses in the chamber (#2), the branch conduits (#13 and #17) are closed and the other branch pipes (#11 and #15) are opened. In the chamber casing, the vacuum is supplied through the line (#24) from the receiver (#20). The blood chamber (#2a) begins to fill with blood from the common inflow tubing-line (#8). After reaching a certain filling or emptying blood level, level sensors (#9) are switching over all and EECs of the branch conduits are changed to the opposite position and the chambers then change (reverse) functions and phase II begins.

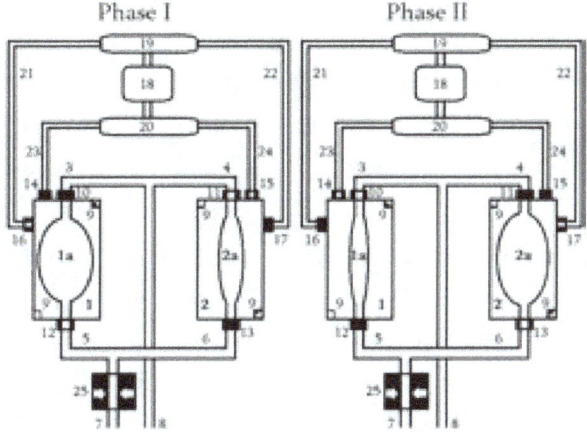

Figure 4. Phases of the pump operation.

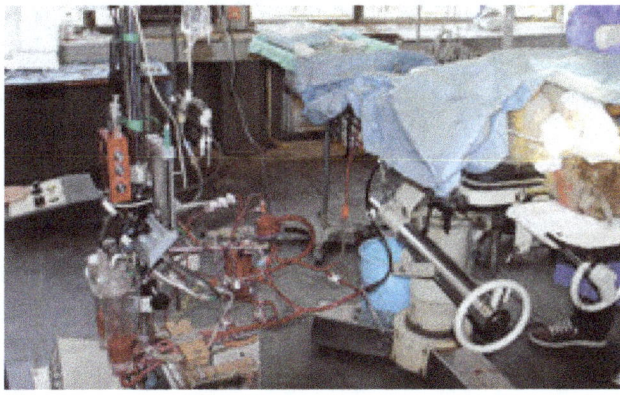

Figure 5. Process of the experiment on animal.

Kind of pump Specifications	Rotary (roller) pump	Centrifugal pump	Our pump on the pneumatic actuator
Design features and capabilities (resources)			
Manufacturer (Brand)	CAPIOX (Terumo)	LIFEBRIDGE (Sorin), CARDIOHELP (Maquet)	Prototype
The volume of the blood chamber (SV—stroke volume)	Variable SV for different-sized patients	Filling volume up to ≈ 50 ml	Filling volume up to ≈ 150–300 ml
Managing the power component	Electric drive	Electric drive	Pneumatic actuator
Use	As a system of cardiopulmonary bypass during cardiopulmonary resuscitation	As a system of cardiopulmonary bypass during cardiopulmonary resuscitation, preferable for long-term extracorporeal support	As a system of cardiopulmonary bypass during cardiopulmonary resuscitation, as well as in preservation of organs in situ
Maximum capacity	Up to 10 l/min	Up to 8 l/min	Up to 10 l/min
Realizable value of the system pressure	60/40 mm.Hg	60/40 mm.Hg	120/80 mm.Hg
Advantages			
Duration of conducted safe perfusion	Limitation in time several (3–4) hours	Possible long-term perfusion	Possible long-term perfusion
Discharge flow characteristics	Excessive positive or negative pressure	Provides positive and negative pressure (poor)	Provides positive and negative pressure (as close as possible to the created native myocardium)
Specifications filling flow	–	–	Adaptation to the venous return
Opportunities	It provides systemic circulation	Higher bypass for right or left ventricles	Maximum bypass the right or left ventricle
The nature of the pulse wave	The possibility of a weak pulsation	The possibility of a weak pulsation	The ability to flow as a non-pulsed and clear counterpulsation
Disadvantages			
Possibility of reverse flow along arterial line	No blood return	Potentially exists	Potentially exists
Embolism	Potentially massive air embolism	Protection against massive air embolism	Protection against massive air embolism
Damage to the blood cells	Hemolysis	Slight hemolysis	No hemolysis

Kind of pump Specifications	Rotary (roller) pump	Centrifugal pump	Our pump on the pneumatic actuator
The possibility of damage to blood contact details	The destruction of tubes	The destruction of rotor blades	–
Additional requirements	Tubing-line occlusion control is required	–	An additional compressor with vacuum supply control is required
Additional accessories	The volume of ejected blood is automatically calculated	The flowmeter is required	The flowmeter is required
Possibility of circuit disruption from excessive line pressure buildup	Possible of circuit disruption and termination and termination	No possibility	No possibility
Cost	Low	High	Low

Table 3. Comparison of blood pumps used commonly and pump developed by us.

Prototype pumps are made by hand. Bench testing has shown that the main hydrodynamic parameters and efficiency, safety, and reliability are similar to clinically used, commercially available, pumps (**Table 3**).

During bench testing, a dual-chamber pump with a chamber volume of 350 ml was placed at the same level as a volume of liquid, attempting to match clinical flow. Perfusion was carried out in two different modes of blood flow—non-pulsatile and pulsatile. Blood flow was measured in the output tubing-line of pump.

In the non-pulsatile flow mode:

- Pressure in the receiver #20: 1.5 atm;
- Vacuum in the receiver #19:0.7 atm;
- Flow through lines #21, #22: up to 6 1/min;
- Flow through lines #23, #24:1 to 4 1/min;
- Total flow in the line #7: upto 10 1/min.

In the pulsatile flow mode:

- Pressure in the receiver #20: 1.5 atm
- Vacuum in the receiver #19: 0.7 atm
- Flow through lines #21, #22:8 1/min
- Flow through lines #23, #24: upto 2 1/min
- Total flow in the line #7 (after pulsator):10 1/min

2.5.2. Experimental studies on animals

The pump was tested in several acute experiments on the animal models in the various perfusion setting:

- Heart–lung bypass (HLB) machine

- ECLS system for ECPR

- Perfusion preservation of isolated donor organs and complexes of organs "in situ"

The dual-chamber pump passed a long-standing test as a heart–lung bypass machine in 68 different experiments on dogs and sheep. In these experiments, the main pump circuit was connected via a standard configuration in cases of an open-chest model, simulating various cardiac surgery scenarios. The pump provided adequate heart–lung bypass for 2–6 h, both with the non-pulsatile and pulsatile flow without difficulty. Hemodynamic parameters were maintained within physiological limits, and therefore, the main parameters of physiology of animals during extra-corporeal perfusion did not require significant correction.

In the ECLS configuration, which was designed for ECPR on sheep, the pump was tested in 14 experimental models of cardiac arrest. A portable, mobile version of the pump and the entire perfusion system complete set with autonomous energy supply was used in these experiments. The effects of extra-corporeal perfusion in a number of experiments on models, within 10 min of cardiac arrest, confirmed the following:

- Successful recovery of the cardiac contraction (in case of non-pulsatile and pulsatile mode);

- Stable rehabilitation of cardiac activity with prolonged perfusion (in a synchronized mode counter pulsation).

In addition, in some experiments on rabbits, the pumps have been tested using a portable system for extra-corporeal isolated preservation of donor organs and organ complexes "in situ." The standard conserving solutions, as well as whole blood at various temperatures, were used as preservatives.

3. Conclusions

In the design of the dual-chamber pump, with saccular chambers modelling the concept of a "Bag in Can," there are incorporated a full range of opportunities for achieving the desired range of physiologic perfusion parameters similar to that of a healthy native heart. The dual-chamber design, with inter-changing chamber functions, allows for separate control of the different parameters for the filling and emptying functions, thus allowing for optimization of blow independently. In other words, the design allows the pump to be filled with a smooth, non-pulsatile flow, while simultaneously ejecting with physiologic pulsatile flow. The pump design provide minimal trauma of the blood cells due to lack of internal valves and, most importantly, the absence of the rotating parts in the path of flow. Changing only the chamber unit with a different size "bag," while leaving other components of the unit unchanged allows for a full range of volumetric hemo-circulatory pump characteristics. In other words, the pump can be easily adapted for extra-corporeal perfusion experimental on animals of different sizes. Consequently, in a clinical setting, it can be used, with only minor changes, for infants, children, and as well as for adults. The pump can perform non-pulsatile blood flow—characteristic for the venous bed while also providing pulsatile flow—characteristic of flow in the aorta and large arteries. Moreover, it can be easily switched from pulsatile flow to non-pulsatile perfusion, depending on the specific necessities, at any time. Finally, counter pulsation during pump operation during ECPR allows continuous unloading of the work of the heart, hence contributing to the actual recovery of the weakened and injured myocardium. Prolonged and stable rehabilitation of cardiac activity in a synchronized counter–pulsation mode can also be accomplished.

In addition, in experiments on rabbits, the pumps have been successfully tested using a portable system for isolated perfusion and preservation of donor organs and organ complexes "in situ."

Acknowledgements

The authors of the chapter would like thank Dr. Michael Firstenberg for his expertise and great input in refining the text.

Author details

Nodar Khodeli[1*], Zurab Chkhaidze[1], Jumber Partsakhashvili[1], Otar Pilishvili[2] and Dimitri Kordzaia[1]

*Address all correspondence to: nkhodeli@gmail.com

1 Tbilisi State University, Tbilisi, Georgia

2 Israel Georgian Medical Research Clinic Helsicor, Tbilisi, Georgia

References

[1] Makdisi G, Wang IW. Extra corporeal membrane oxygenation (ECMO) review of a lifesaving technology. J Thorac Dis. 2015;7(7):166–176. doi:10.3978/j.issn. 2072-1439.2015.11.45

[2] Passaroni AC, Silva MAM, Yoshida WB. Cardiopulmonary bypass: development of John Gibbon's heart-lung machine. Rev Bras Circ Cardiovasc. 2015;30(2):235–245. doi: 10.5935/1678-9741.20150021 (Cardiopulmonary bypass: development of John Gibbon's

heart-lung machine Cardiopulmonary bypass: development of John Gibbon's heart-lung machine)

[3] Cobb LA, Eliastam M, Kerber RE, Melker R, Moss AJ. Report of the American Heart Association task force on the future of cardiopulmonary resuscitation. Circulation. 1992;85:2346–2355. doi:10.1161/01.CIR.85.6.2346

[4] Cave DM, Gazmuri RJ, Otto CW, Nadkarni VM, Cheng A, Brooks S, Daya M, Sutton RM, Branson R, Hazinski MF. 2010 American Heart Association guidelines for cardiopulmonary resuscitation and emergency cardiovascular care science. Circulation. 2010;122:720–728. doi:10.1161/CIR.0000000000000259

[5] Jacobs I, Nadkarni V, Bahr J. Cardiac arrest and cardiopulmonary resuscitation outcome reports: update and simplification of the Utstein templates for resuscitation registries. Resuscitation. 2004;63(3):233–249. doi:10.1016/j.resuscitation.2004.09.008

[6] Paden ML, Conrad SA, Rycus PT, Thiagarajan RR. Extracorporeal life support organization registry report 2012. ASAIO J. 2013;59(3):202–10. doi:10.1097/MAT.0b013e3182904a52.

[7] Gazmuri RJ, Weil MH, Terwilliger K, Shah DM, Duggal C, Tang W. Extracorporeal circulation as an alternative to open-chest cardiac compression for cardiac resuscitation. Chest. 1992;102(6):1846–1852. doi:10.1378/chest.102.6.1846

[8] Twomeya D, Dasa M, Subramaniana H, Dunning J. Is internal massage superior to external massage for patients suffering a cardiac arrest after cardiac surgery? Interact Cardiovasc Thorac Surg. 2008;7(1):151–157. doi:10.1510/icvts.2007.170399

[9] Thiagarajan RR, Laussen PC, Rycus PT, Bartlett RH, Bratton SL. Extracorporeal membrane oxygenation to aid cardiopulmonary resuscitation in infants and children. Circulation. 2007;116:1693–1700. doi:10.1161/CIRCULATIONAHA.106.680678

[10] MacLaren G, Combes A, Bartlett RH. Contemporary extracorporeal membrane oxygenation for adult respiratory failure: life support in the new era. Intensive Care Med. 2011;38(2):210–220. doi:10.1007/s00134-011-2439-2

[11] Dembitsky WP, Moreno-Cabral RJ, Adamsn RM, Daily PO. Emergency resuscitation using portable extracorporeal membrane oxygenation. Ann Thorac Surg. 1993;55(1): 304–309. doi:10.1016/0003-4975(93)90542-P

[12] Foerster K, D'Inka M, Beyersdorf F, Benk, Nguyen-Thanh T, Mader I, Fritsch B, Ihling C, Mueller K, Heilmann C, Trummer G. Prolonged cardiac arrest and resuscitation by extracorporeal life support: favourable outcome without preceding anticoagulation in an experimental setting. Perfusion. 2013;28(6):520–528. doi:10.1177/0267659113495081

[13] Arlt M, Philipp A, Voelkel S, Rupprecht L, Mueller T, Hilker M, Graf BM, Schmid C. Extracorporeal membrane oxygenation in severe trauma patients with bleeding shock. Resuscitation. 2010;81(7):804–809. doi:10.1016/j.resuscitation.2010.02.020

[14] Shin JS, Lee SW, Han GS, Jo WM, Choi SH, Hong YS. Successful extracorporeal life support in cardiac arrest with recurrent ventricular fibrillation unresponsive to standard cardiopulmonary resuscitation. Resuscitation. 2007;73(2):309–313. doi: 10.1016/j.resuscitation.2006.09.011

[15] Chkhaidze Z, Khodeli N, Pilishvili O, Partsakhashvili D, Jangavadze M, Kordzaia D. New model of veno-venous bypass for management of anhepatic phase in experimental study on dogs. Transpl Proc. 2013; 45: 1734–1738. doi:10.1016/j.transproceed. 2012.10.049

[16] Partsakhashvili D., Chkhaidze Z., Khodeli N., Pilishvili O., Jangavadze M., Kordzaia D. Experimental liver autotransplantation with novel scheme of veno-venous bypass as a model of liver denervation and delymphatization. Transpl Proc. 2013;45:1739–1742. doi:10.1016/j.transproceed.2012.10.048

[17] Wassenberg PAJ. The Abiomed BVS 5000 biventricular support system. Perfusion. 2000;15(4):369-371. doi:10.1177/026765910001500413.

[18] Jaggy C, Lachat M, Leskosek B, et al. Affinity pump system: a new peristaltic pump for cardiopulmonary bypass. Perfusion. 2000;15:77–83. doi:10.1177/026765910001500111

[19] Park M, Mendes PV, Hirota AS, dos Santos EV, Costa ELV, Azevedo LP. Blood flow/ pump rotation ratio as an artificial lung performance monitoring tool during extracorporeal respiratory support using centrifugal pumps. Rev Bras Ter Intensiva. 2015;27(2):178–184. doi:10.5935/0103-507X.20150030

[20] Wakisaka Y, Taenaka Y, Chikanari K, Nakatani T, Tatsumi E, Masuzawa T, Nishimura T, Takewa Y, Ohno T, Takano H. Long-term evaluation of a nonpulsatile mechanical circulatory support system. Artif Organs. 1997;21(7):639–644. doi:10.1111/j. 1525-1594.1997.tb03714.x

[21] Fink R, Al-Obaidi M, Grewal S, Winter M, Pepper J. Monocyte activation markers during cardiopulmonary bypass. Perfusion. 2003;18(2):83–86. doi: 10.1191/0267659103pf645oa

[22] Holmberg M, Holmberg S, Herlitz J. Effect of bystander cardiopulmonary resuscitation in out-of-hospital cardiac arrest patients in Sweden. Resuscitation. 2000;47(1):59–70. doi:10.1016/S0300-9572(00)00199-4

[23] Charapov I, Eipe N. Cardiac arrest in the operating room requiring prolonged resuscitation. Can J Anesth. 2012;59(6):578–585. doi:10.1007/s12630-012-9698-4

[24] Mongero LB, Beck JR, Charette KA. Managing the extracorporeal membrane oxygenation (ECMO) circuit integrity and safety utilizing the perfusionist as the "ECMO Specialist". Perfusion. 2013;28(6):555–556. doi:10.1177/0267659113498993

[25] Chen YS, Lin JW, Yu HY, Ko WJ, Jerng JS, Chang WT. Cardiopulmonary resuscitation with assisted extracorporeal life-support versus conventional cardiopulmonary resuscitation in adults with in-hospital cardiac arrest: an observational study and

propensity   analysis.   Lancet.   2008;372(9638):554–561.   doi:10.1016/
S0140-6736(08)60958-7

[26] Anastasiadis K, Westaby S, Antonitsis P, Argiriadou H, Karapanagiotidis G, Pigott D,
      Papakonstantinou C. Minimal extracorporeal circulation circuit standby for "off-
      pump" left ventricular assist device implantation. Artif Organs. 2010; 34(12):1156–1158.
      doi:10.1111/j.1525-1594.2009.00983.x

[27] Haneya A, Philipp A, Puehler T, Camboni D, Hilker M, Hirt SW, Schmid C. Successful
      use of a percutaneous miniaturized extracorporeal life support system as a bridge and
      assistance to left ventricular assist device implantation in a patient with severe
      refractory   cardiogenic   shock.   Perfusion.   2012;27(1):18–20.   doi:
      10.1177/0267659111419887

[28] Liu Y, Tao L, Wang X, Cui H, Chen X, Ji B. Beneficial effects of using a minimal
      extracorporeal circulation system during coronary artery bypass grafting. Perfusion.
      2012;27(1):83–89. doi:10.1177/0267659111424636

[29] Farrar DJ. The thoratec ventricular assist device: a paracorporeal pump for treating
      acute and chronic heart failure. Semin Thorac Cardiovasc Surg. 2000;12(3):243–250. doi:
      10.1053/stcs.2000.19620

[30] Slaughter MS, Pagani FD, Rogers JG, Miller LW, Sun B, Russell SD, Starling RC, Chen
      L, Boyle AJ, Chillcott S, Adamson RM, Blood MS, Camacho MT, Idrissi KA, Petty M,
      Sobieski M, Wright S, Myers TJ, Farrar DJ. Clinical management of continuous-flow
      left ventricular assist devices in advanced heart failure. J Heart Lung Transpl.
      2010;29(4):1–39. doi:10.1016/j.healun.2010.01.011

[31] Iijima T, Bauer R, Hossmann KA. Brain resuscitation by extracorporeal circulation after
      prolonged cardiac arrest in cats. Intensive Care Med. 1993;19(2):82–88. doi:10.1007/
      BF01708367

[32] Trummer G, Foerster K, Buckberg GD, Benk C, Mader I, Heilmann C, Liakopoulos O,
      Beyersdorf F. Superior neurologic recovery after 15 minutes of normothermic cardiac
      arrest using an extracorporeal life support system for optimized blood pressure and
      flow. Perfusion. 2014;29(2):130–138. doi:10.1177/0267659113497776

11

Weaning Strategy from Veno-Arterial Extracorporeal Membrane Oxygenation (ECMO)

Nadia Aissaoui, Christoph Brehm,
Aly El-Banayosy and Alain Combes

Abstract

Background: Significant advances in extracorporeal technology have led to the more widespread use of veno-arterial extracorporeal membrane oxygenation (VA ECMO) for cardiac failure. However, procedures for weaning from VA ECMO are not standardized. High death rate after successful weaning shows that many questions remain unresolved in this field.

Objectives: In this review, we discuss data from the literature and propose a strategy to optimize the weaning process.

Data synthesis and conclusions: It is especially important that the VA ECMO is not removed while the patient is still recovering from the condition that necessitated the use of VA ECMO implantation. Damaged organs need to recover before attempting weaning and the patient should be considered hemodynamically stable. The etiology of cardio-circulatory dysfunction must be compatible with myocardial recovery. Finally, weaning trials using echocardiographic and hemodynamic assessments are indispensable to assess the behavior of the ventricles and to determine whether the VA ECMO can be removed.

Keywords: ECMO, weaning, echocardiography, load conditions

1. Introduction

Veno-arterial extracorporeal membrane oxygenation (VA ECMO) is used to support patients with refractory cardiogenic shock [1, 2]. It has been successfully used as a bridge to myocardial recovery, cardiac transplantation, or implantation of a ventricular assist device in patients with overt cardiac failure of various causes, e.g., acute myocardial infarction, end stage dilated cardiomyopathy, viral or toxic myocarditis, complications of cardiac surgery, or cardiac arrest.

After a few days of mechanical assistance, the device can sometimes be successfully removed if the patient has partially or fully recovered from the condition that necessitated the use of ECMO. However, to date, only a few studies have reported strategies for weaning from VA ECMO [3, 4].

Moreover, weaning does not signify survival because 20–65% of patients weaned from VA ECMO support do not survive to hospital discharge.

This review will discuss the various factors influencing survival after weaning in addition to weaning strategies proposed in the literature. Based on this information, we will propose a strategy to optimize the weaning process.

2. Principles of VA ECMO

Patients with significantly impaired cardiac function (with or without impaired gas exchange) require venoarterial configuration for circulatory support. A venous cannula inserted into the right atrium drains blood from the patient into the pumping mechanism of the ECMO circuit. The blood is oxygenated through a membrane oxygenator and perfused in the aorta by a centrifugal pump via a second cannula [1, 2].

The typical configuration for VA ECMO involves femoral venous drainage and femoral arterial reinfusion. With this configuration, the reinfusion jet flows retrograde up the aorta and may meet resistance from antegrade flow generated by the left ventricle.

An ECMO circuit can be set up centrally through the right atrium and the ascending aorta, or peripherally through the femoral vein and the femoral or axillary artery. ECMO can support both heart and lung function and assists the two ventricles.

3. Indications for ECMO

The main indication for VA ECMO is medical cardiogenic shock, including that associated with acute myocardial infarction, fulminant myocarditis, acute exacerbation of severe chronic heart failure, drug intoxication, hypothermia, and acute circulatory failure due to intractable arrhythmia.

VA ECMO is also used in some particular situations for patients with postcardiotomy cardiac failure, after cardiac transplantation, or cardiac arrest requiring cardiopulmonary resuscitation [1, 2].

Furthermore, VA ECMO is starting to be used for patients with pulmonary embolism, sepsis associated cardiomyopathy, and pulmonary hypertension [1, 5].

4. Outcome of patients receiving VA ECMO

VA ECMO is used as a bridge to myocardial recovery and cardiac transplantation. It may also be used as "a bridge to a bridge", i.e., before implantation of a ventricular assist device [6]. No randomized controlled trials have compared VA ECMO to other mechanical support systems in patients with cardiogenic shock. However, several nonrandomized studies suggest that the early use of ECMO offers a survival advantage in such circumstances [1, 2, 5, 7–13]. The percentage of patients with refractory cardiogenic shock who are successfully weaned from ECMO varies from 31% to 76%, depending on the underlying cause of cardiogenic shock [7–14]. Patients successfully weaned from VA ECMO are defined as those having ECMO removed and not requiring further mechanical support because of recurring cardiogenic shock over the following 30 days [3].

However, 20–65% of patients weaned from ECMO do not reach survival to discharge [3, 7–11]. The most frequent reasons for death are cardiac and multisystem organ failure. These observations demonstrate the difficulties in predicting the future of patients after the removal of ECMO [8, 9].

5. Factors predicting death in weaned patients

Successful weaning from ECMO does not signify patient survival. Several studies have assessed the predictors of death after ECMO weaning in particular situations or settings, mainly in postcardiotomy shock and out-of-hospital cardiac arrest [10, 11, 15]. Markers associated with death after weaning include: door-to-VA ECMO implantation time (i.e., the elapsed time between cardiogenic shock and ECMO), cardiopulmonary resuscitation time, poor renal and liver function, high lactate levels, diabetes, obesity, and SOFA score [10, 11, 15]. These death-associated factors reflected the severity and the progression of multiorgan failure at the time of ECMO implantation. They should be considered prior to weaning from ECMO.

6. Factors predicting successful weaning from VA ECMO

Few studies have aimed to identify criteria to predict which patients can be successfully weaned from ECMO.

Fiser et al. studied 51 postcardiotomy patients receiving ECMO to identify factors that could predict when to discontinue ECMO [7]. They found that patients aged over 65 years or with ejection fractions of less than 30% after 48 hours of ECMO were less likely to survive after weaning.

Aissaoui et al. assessed the ability of clinical and echocardiographic variables to predict successful weaning in 51 patients receiving VA ECMO due to medical cardiogenic shock or postcardiotomy shock [3]. Among these 51 patients, 38 hemodynamically stable patients underwent at least one ECMO flow reduction trial, in which the flow rate was reduced to 1.5 L/min under clinical and Doppler echocardiography monitoring. Twenty patients were ultimately weaned from ECMO. High values of arterial systolic and pulse pressure, aortic velocity-time integral, LVEF, and lateral mitral annulus peak systolic velocity were associated with successful weaning. All patients weaned from ECMO had an LVEF ≥ 20–25%, an aortic velocity-time integral of ≥12 cm and a lateral mitral annulus peak systolic velocity of ≥6 cm/s under minimal ECMO support. In this study, successful weaning-associated factors are simple and easy-to-acquire echocardiographic variables evaluating LV systolic function (LVEF and lateral mitral annulus peak systolic velocity) and LV flow (aortic velocity-time integral) (**Figure 1**).

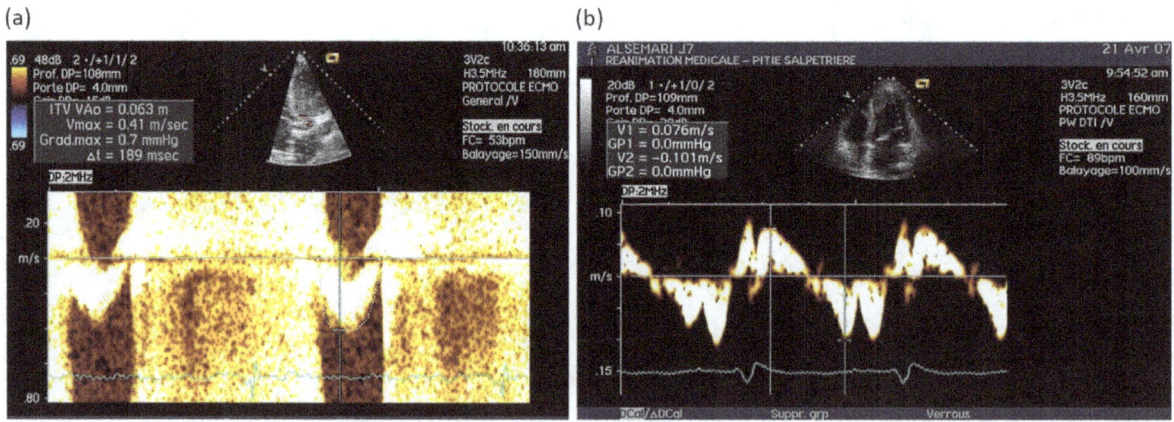

Figure 1. Echocardiographic variables measured by the Doppler method. A. Aortic velocity-time integration obtained by pulsed Doppler measured at the LV outflow tract. B. Lateral systolic peak obtained by spectral Doppler tissue imaging at the lateral mitral annulus.

Luyt et al. examined whether biomarkers could predict cardiac recovery in patients receiving VA ECMO [16]. They studied 41 consecutive patients with potentially reversible cardiogenic shock, and examined circulating concentrations of the N-terminal fragment of the B-type natriuretic peptide, troponin Ic, the midregional fragment of the proatrial natriuretic peptide, proadrenomedullin, and copeptin on days 1, 3, and 7 post-ECMO. There was no difference in the absolute values of these biomarkers or in their kinetics during the first week between patients who were weaned from ECMO and those who were not.

Thus, the current data suggest that echocardiography is an important tool to determine both the recovery of LV function and the readiness of patients for weaning from ECMO support, whereas early measurements of cardiac biomarkers are not useful for identifying those who will recover [17,18].

7. Appropriate conditions to attempt weaning from ECMO

According to the Extracorporeal Life Support Organization (ELSO) guidelines, hepatic function should have recovered prior to any attempt to wean patients from ECMO, irrespective of the findings of cardiac assessment [19].

In addition, it is unusual to attempt weaning in the first 72 hours after VA ECMO implantation because damaged organs need time to recover. However, the duration of ECMO may be shorter in cases of drug intoxication, and VA ECMO weaning can be attempted earlier [20–22]. In most previous studies, the mean duration of support was at least of 3.3 ± 2.9 days and was even 8.0 ± 6.0 days in one study [3, 9–11 , 23]. This time period is also necessary to allow the recovery of a potentially "stunned" myocardium [7]. In these studies, the mean duration of support was longer for patients successfully weaned from ECMO than those who were not [3, 11].

It is not necessary to wait for the recovery of renal function. Restoration of acute renal injury after cardiogenic shock can take up to four weeks after the improvement of cardiac output, by which time significant decreases in elevated filling pressures may have occurred [23, 24]. Other considerations include pre-ECMO status (age, comorbidities, cardiopulmonary resuscitation) and the etiology of cardio-circulatory dysfunction, which must be compatible with myocardial recovery (acute myocarditis, acute myocardial infarction, post-cardiotomy, drug intoxication, septic cardiomyopathy) [1, 2, 6].

VA ECMO should not be removed if the patient has not recovered from the condition which necessitated VA ECMO implantation (high volume overload and high doses of inotropic agents). Volume overload must be managed by diuretic or hemofiltration. Doses of inotropic agents should be decreased to a minimum. Furthermore, pulmonary edema must be resolved and pulmonary oxygenation of the blood must not be compromised [19]. The PaO_2/FiO_2 ratio should be more than 200 and the oxygen fraction delivered by the extracorporeal circuit should be 21% and that delivered by the ventilator circuits should be less than 60% [25]. These measurements should be made with an ECMO flow rate of less than 1 L/minute and a sweep gas flow rate of 1 L/minute. In case of persistent severe respiratory failure despite cardiac recovery, VA ECMO should be switched to VV ECMO [5].

Factors indicating cardiac recovery and thus patients who can be potentially weaned from ECMO include an increase in blood pressure, and return of pulsatility or an increase in the pulsatility of the arterial pressure waveform [19].

The patient should be considered hemodynamically stable, i.e., they should have a baseline mean arterial pressure (MAP) of >60 mmHg in the absence or at low doses of vasoactive agents, and a pulsatile arterial waveform maintained for at least 24 hours [3].

8. Utility of weaning trials

Weaning trials are essential to assess the behavior of the left ventricle during increases in preload, and to determine whether the ECMO can be removed.

Load conditions can be modified by varying the flow of the VA ECMO centrifugal pump. When ECMO flow is decreased, preload is increased, and afterload is decreased [18].

Aissaoui et al. varied ECMO flow and examined hemodynamic variables of the failed left ventricle in 22 patients receiving VA ECMO. With this approach, they found significant variations between patients who were successfully weaned and those who were not. Indeed, increased preload and decreased afterload were associated with increased systolic function in patients who survived weaning. These changes in systolic variables that occurred during modifications to ECMO flow identified a load-dependent contractile reserve, following the Frank-Starling law. The presence of this contractile reserve was associated with successful weaning [18].

A weaning trial is also very important to evaluate right ventricular (RV) function because the ECMO circuit creates negative pressure and drains venous blood from the right atrium. In these conditions, it is difficult to determine RV function in maximal ECMO flow [3, 4, 17, 18]. A reduction in ECMO flow results in an increase in preload and enables RV function to be assessed.

Cavarocchi et al. assessed the behavior of both ventricles during decreased ECMO support, volume loading and inotropic support in 21 patients [4]. They showed that a weaning trial involving left and right ventricle assessment by transesophageal echocardiography could accurately predict both successful weaning from ECMO and successful left VAD implantation without the occurrence of right ventricular heart failure. The assessment of RV function is very useful specifically in two cases: for patients receiving ECMO for postcardiotomy shock after heart transplantation and for those receiving ECMO prior to VAD implant surgery. Ideal candidates for LVAD placement are those who have isolated LV failure with reasonably recovered RV function. Failure to identify significant coexisting RV dysfunction may significantly increase the risk of postoperative morbidity and mortality in patients undergoing LVAD placement after ECMO, and requires prolonged use of inotropic agents, biventricular support, or extracorporeal support [26].

9. Strategies for carrying out ECMO weaning trials

Two echocardiographic strategies for carrying out an ECMO weaning trial have been reported in the literature: the first strategy involves trans-thoracic echocardiography (TTE) [3], and the second involves hemodynamic transesophageal echocardiography (hTEE) [4].

In the TTE study conducted by Aissaoui et al., an ECMO weaning trial was undertaken daily if: (1) the patient was considered hemodynamically stable, i.e., they had a baseline mean blood pressure of >60 mmHg in the absence or at low doses of vasoactive agents and a pulsatile arterial waveform maintained for at least 24 h; and (2) pulmonary oxygenation of the blood was not compromised [3]. The ECMO flow was decreased to 66% of the initial flow rate for 10–15 min. It was then decreased to 33% for 10–15 min and then to a minimum of 1–1.5 L/min for another 10–15 min.

If mean blood pressure dropped significantly and was constantly <60 mmHg during the trial, ECMO flow was returned to 100% of the initial flow and the trial was stopped. Doppler echocardiography was repeated at each ECMO flow rate. The removal of ECMO was considered if the patient had no end-stage cardiac disease, was partially or fully recovered from the initial cardiac dysfunction, tolerated the full weaning trial, and had a LVEF of >20–25% and aortic VTI of >10 cm under minimal ECMO support.

In the TEE study conducted by Cavarocchi et al., the weaning trial consisted of four stages and involved hemodynamic transesophageal echocardiography [4]. In the first stage, baseline LV and RV volume and function were assessed on full-flow ECMO support. During the second stage, ECMO flow was gradually decreased in increments of 0.5 L/min to half of the original flow rate (stage 2). Throughout the weaning protocol, LV and RV function and hemodynamic responses (heart rate and blood pressure) were monitored continuously to assess ventricular volume and function. If LV or RV distension or significant hypotension occurred, the weaning trial was stopped and the ECMO support was returned to full flow. Stage 3 consisted of monitoring hemodynamic responses during both volume challenge with 5% albumin (10 mL/kg) and a reduction of ECMO flow to a minimum rate of 1.2–1.5 L/min. Volume loading was used to achieve an appropriate preload. During the last stage (stage 4), left and right ventricular function was assessed during the infusion of inodilators (dobutamine and/or milrinone). These drugs were used to assess right ventricle function in patients with LV dysfunction under consideration for LVAD placement. The definitive removal of the ECMO was considered if both LV and RV functions recovered. If LV dysfunction persisted without RV failure, LVAD implantation was considered. An external right VAD placement was considered in cases of isolated, persistent RV dysfunction. If biventricular dysfunction remained, total artificial heart replacement was considered if the patient was a candidate for heart transplantation.

10. Transthoracic echocardiography *versus* transesophageal echocardiography

The weaning assessment requires repeated measurements to be recorded over several days. Echocardiographic variables of LV systolic function (LVEF and lateral mitral annulus peak systolic velocity), LV flow (aortic velocity-time integral), and right ventricular diameters can be used to predict successful weaning. These parameters are factors that are simple and easy-to-acquire with transthoracic echocardiography. For these reasons, the transthoracic approach is a good option because it can be repeated many times [17, 18]. In case of poor echogenicity, the transesophageal echocardiography can be used [4].

11. Hemodynamic assessment during the weaning attempt

Hemodynamic assessment can be useful during the weaning trial. In particular, the presence of volume overload can be determined from measurements of pulmonary capillary wedge pressure and central venous pressure. Such measurements also enable the assessment of cardiac output (cardiac index). Hemodynamic measurements should be performed at full flow, after reducing the ECMO flow to 50% and after stopping the pump.

For patients to be considered for VA ECMO weaning, hemodynamic variables with the pump off should be as follows: cardiac index >2.4 liters/min/m^2, mean blood pressure >60 mmHg, pulmonary capillary wedge pressure <18 mm Hg, and central venous pressure <18 mmHg [13]. The absence of volume overload can also be verified from this hemodynamic assessment. Systolic RV and LV function have to be evaluated by echocardiography.

12. Anticoagulation during the weaning attempt

ECMO weaning and weaning trials are associated with a risk of thromboembolic complications due to blood stagnation during the reduction of ECMO flow. The ELSO recommends that anticoagulant drugs should be continued during the trial, and that the blood lines and access cannulas should be periodically unclamped to avoid stagnation [19]. The activated partial thromboplastin time should be between 1.5 and 2.5 times the normal value [19, 27].

13. Aids to optimize weaning

Some teams assessed the ability of some medications to facilitate weaning from VA ECMO [28, 29].

The Levosimendan was assessed in six VA ECMO patients with the hypothesis that its remaining effects could favor the weaning from ECMO. This inodilator drug was infused in the patients 24 h before the planned weaning. In this small study, the use of Levosimendan was associated with an increased rate of successful weaning [28].

In an animal study, the author studied if thyroid hormone supplementation in refractory cardiogenic shock pigs improved abnormalities induced by ischemia-reperfusion, cardiac function, and rate of weaning from ECMO. They found that it improved cardiac function during VA ECMO [29, 30].

These strategies were reported for very small populations or animals and must be confirmed in larger series.

The use of an intra-aortic balloon pump may improve survival in ECMO patients [8, 11]. In a recent study conducted by Petroni et al., the use of an intra-aortic balloon pump in patients receiving VA ECMO restored pulsatility and decreased left ventricular afterload, and was associated with small left ventricular dimensions and low pulmonary artery pressure [31]. No study has assessed the value of intra-aortic balloon pumps during VA ECMO weaning.

14. Proposed weaning strategy

In light of all these data, we propose a strategy to optimize weaning from VA ECMO (**Figure 2**) [32].

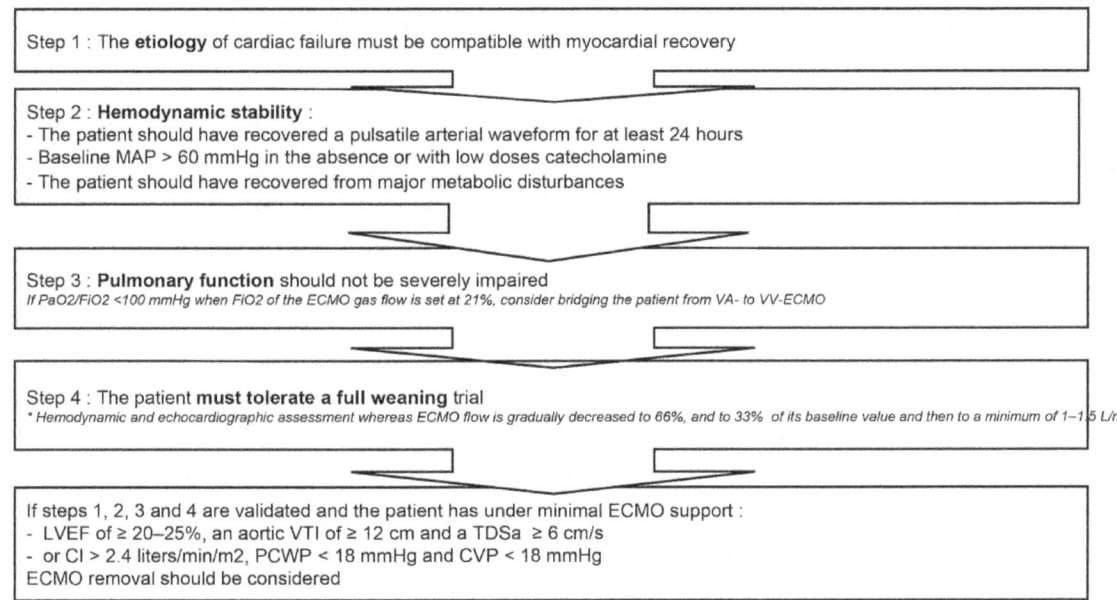

Figure 2. Recommendations for successful weaning from VA ECMO. MAP, mean arterial pressure; VTI, velocity-time integration; LVEF, left ventricular ejection fraction, TDS, tissue Doppler systolic velocity; RV, right ventricle, CI, cardiac index, PCWP, pulmonary capillary wedge pressure, CVP, central venous pressure.

First, some conditions should be gathered.

Hepatic function should first recover.

Patients with end-stage cardiac disease cannot be taken off ECMO. Indeed, the etiology of cardio-circulatory dysfunction must be compatible with myocardial recovery. Examples include acute myocarditis, acute myocardial infarction, post-cardiotomy, drug intoxication, and septic cardiomyopathy. The PaO_2/FiO_2 ratio should be more than 200.

Volume overload must be managed and doses of inotropic agents should be limited to a minimum.

The patient should be considered hemodynamically stable.

We advocate the use of transthoracic echocardiography over a transesophageal approach. Weaning trials are essential. The ECMO flow should be decreased progressively to a minimum of 1–1.5 L/min for at least 15 min.

The echographic evaluation has to take into account variables assessing LV systolic function (LVEF and lateral mitral annulus peak systolic velocity), LV flow (aortic velocity-time integral), and right ventricular diameters.

A hemodynamic assessment should be carried out to verify the absence of both volume overload and high capillary pressures.

Volume loading can be used to achieve appropriate preload and inotropic support to assess the RV during the weaning trial.

ECMO removal should be considered if the patient does not have end-stage cardiac disease, tolerates the full weaning trial, and has a LVEF of ≥20–25%, an aortic velocity-time integral of ≥12 cm and a lateral mitral annulus peak systolic velocity of ≥6 cm/s under minimal ECMO support.

15. Conclusion

Weaning from VA ECMO remains a difficult decision because it unfortunately does not signify survival for the patient. We proposed a strategy to optimize the weaning process. It is especially important that the ECMO is not removed while the patient is still recovering from the condition that necessitated the use of VA ECMO implantation. Damaged organs need to recover before attempting weaning and the patient should be considered hemodynamically stable. The etiology of cardio-circulatory dysfunction must be compatible with myocardial recovery. Then, weaning trials and echocardiographic and hemodynamic assessments during these tests are indispensable to assess the behavior of the ventricles and to determine whether the ECMO can be removed.

Author details

Nadia Aissaoui[1*], Christoph Brehm[2], Aly El-Banayosy[3] and Alain Combes[4]

*Address all correspondence to: nadia.aissaoui@egp.aphp.fr

1 Service de Réanimation Médicale, Hôpital Européen Georges Pompidou Assistance Publique–Hôpitaux de Paris and Université Paris Descartes, Paris, France

2 Department of Medicine, Division of Cardiology, Penn State College of Medicine, Heart and Vascular Institute, Penn State Milton S. Hershey Medical Center, Hershey, Pennsylvania, USA

3 INTEGRIS Baptist Medical Center, Oklahoma City, USA

4 Service de Réanimation Médicale, Institut de Cardiologie, Groupe Hospitalier Pitié-Salpêtrière and Université Paris 6, Paris, France

References

[1] Abrams D, Combes A, Brodie D. Extracorporeal membrane oxygenation in cardiopulmonary disease in adults. J Am Coll Cardiol. 2014;63:2769–78.

[2] Ghodsizad A1, Koerner MM, Brehm CE, El-Banayosy A. The role of extracorporeal membrane oxygenation circulatory support in the 'crash and burn' patient: from implantation to weaning. Curr Opin Cardiol. 2014;29:275–80.

[3] Aissaoui N, Luyt CE, Leprince P, Trouillet JL, Léger P, Pavie A, Diebold B, Chastre J, Combes A. Predictors of successful extracorporeal membrane oxygenation (ECMO) weaning after assistance for refractory cardiogenic shock. Intensive Care Med. 2011;37:1738–45.

[4] Cavarocchi NC, Pitcher HT, Yang Q, Karbowski P, Miessau J, Hastings HM, Hirose H. Weaning of extracorporeal membrane oxygenation using continuous hemodynamic transesophageal echocardiography. J Thorac Cardiovasc Surg. 2013;146:1474–9.

[5] Bréchot N, Luyt CE, Schmidt M, Leprince P, Trouillet JL, Léger P, Pavie A, Chastre J, Combes A. Venoarterial extracorporeal membrane oxygenation support for refractory cardiovascular dysfunction during severe bacterial septic shock. Crit Care Med. 2013;41:1616–26

[6] Marasco SF, Lukas G, McDonald M, McMillan J, Ihle B. Review of ECMO (extra corporeal membrane oxygenation) support in critically ill adult patients. Heart Lung Circ. 2008;17 Suppl 4:S41–7.

[7] Fiser SM, Tribble CG, Kaza AK, Long SM, Zacour RK, Kern JA, Kron IL. When to discontinue extracorporeal membrane oxygenation for postcardiotomy support. Ann Thorac Surg. 2001;71:210–4.

[8] Smedira NG1, Moazami N, Golding CM, McCarthy PM, Apperson-Hansen C, Blackstone EH, Cosgrove DM 3rd. Clinical experience with 202 adults receiving extracorporeal membrane oxygenation for cardiac failure: survival at five years. J Thorac Cardiovasc Surg. 2001;122:92–102.

[9] Luo XJ1, Wang W, Hu SS, Sun HS, Gao HW, Long C, Song YH, Xu JP. Extracorporeal membrane oxygenation for treatment of cardiac failure in adult patients. Interact Cardiovasc Thorac Surg. 2009;9:296–300.

[10] Chang WW, Tsai FC, Tsai TY, Chang CH, Jenq CC, Chang MY, Tian YC, Hung CC, Fang JT, Yang CW, Chen YC. Predictors of mortality in patients successfully weaned from extracorporeal membrane oxygenation. PLoS One. 2012;7:e42687.

[11] Rastan AJ1, Dege A, Mohr M, Doll N, Falk V, Walther T, Mohr FW. Early and late outcomes of 517 consecutive adult patients treated with extracorporeal membrane oxygenation for refractory postcardiotomy cardiogenic shock. J Thorac Cardiovasc Surg. 2010;139:302–11.

[12] Combes A, Leprince P, Luyt CE, Bonnet N, Trouillet JL, Leger P, Pavie A, Chastre. Outcomes and long term quality-of-life of patients supported by extracorporeal membrane oxygenation for refractory cardiogenic shock. Crit Care Med 2008;36:1404–11.

[13] Aziz TA, Singh G, Popjes E, Stephenson E, Mulvey S, Pae W, El-Banayosy A. Initial experience with CentriMag extracorporeal membrane oxygenation for support of critically ill patients with refractory cardiogenic shock. J Heart Lung Transplant. 2010;29:66–71.

[14] Chen YS, Chao A, Yu HY, Ko WJ, Wu IH, Chen RJ, Huang SC, Lin FY, Wang SS. Analysis and results of prolonged resuscitation in cardiac arrest patients rescued by extracorporeal membrane oxygenation. J Am Coll Cardiol. 2003;41:197–203.

[15] Leick J, Liebetrau C, Szardien S, Fischer-Rasokat U, Willmer M, van Linden A, Blumenstein J, Nef H, Rolf A, Arlt M, Walther T, Hamm C, Möllmann H. Door-to-implantation time of extracorporeal life support systems predicts mortality in patients with out-of-hospital cardiac arrest. Clin Res Cardiol. 2013;102:661–9.

[16] Luyt CE, Landivier A, Leprince P, Bernard M, Pavie A, Chastre J, Combes A. Usefulness of cardiac biomarkers to predict cardiac recovery in patients on extracorporeal membrane oxygenation support for refractory cardiogenic shock. J Crit Care. 2012;27:524.e7–14.

[17] Platts DG, Sedgwick JF, Burstow DJ, Mullany DV, Fraser JF. The role of echocardiography in the management of patients supported by extracorporeal membrane oxygenation. J Am Soc Echocardiogr 2012;25:131–41.

[18] Aissaoui N, Guerot E, Combes A, Delouche A, Chastre J, Leprince P, Leger P, Diehl JL, Fagon JY, Diebold B. Two-dimensional strain rate and Doppler tissue myocardial velocities: analysis by echocardiography of hemodynamic and functional changes of the failed left ventricle during different degrees of extracorporeal life support. J Am Soc Echocardiogr. 2012;25:632–40.

[19] ELSO Guidelines for Cardiopulmonary Extracorporeal Life Support Extracorporeal Life Support Organization, Version 1.3 November 2013 Ann Arbor, MI, USA. http://www.elsonet.org.

[20] Baud FJ1, Megarbane B, Deye N, Leprince P. Clinical review: aggressive management and extracorporeal support for drug-induced cardiotoxicity. Crit Care. 2007;11:207.

[21] Johnson NJ1, Gaieski DF, Allen SR, Perrone J, DeRoos F. A review of emergency cardiopulmonary bypass for severe poisoning by cardiotoxic drugs. J Med Toxicol. 2013;9:54–60.

[22] Masson R1, Colas V, Parienti JJ, Lehoux P, Massetti M, Charbonneau P, Saulnier F, Daubin C. A comparison of survival with and without extracorporeal life support treatment for severe poisoning due to drug intoxication. Resuscitation. 2012 ;83:1413–7.

[23] Durinka JB, Bogar LJ, Hirose H, Brehm C, Koerner MM, Pae WE, El-Banayosy A, Stephenson ER, Cavarocchi NC. End-organ recovery is key to success for extracorporeal membrane oxygenation as a bridge to implantable left ventricular assist device. ASAIO J. 2014;60:189–92.

[24] Khot UN1, Mishra M, Yamani MH, Smedira NG, Paganini E, Yeager M, Buda T, McCarthy PM, Young JB, Starling RC. Severe renal dysfunction complicating cardiogenic shock is not a contraindication to mechanical support as a bridge to cardiac transplantation. J Am Coll Cardiol. 2003;41:381–5.

[25] Richard C, Argaud L, Blet A, Boulain T, Contentin L, Dechartres A, Dejode JM, Donetti L, Fartoukh M, Fletcher D, Kuteifan K, Lasocki S, Liet JM, Lukaszewicz AC, Mal H, Maury E, Osman D, Outin H, Richard JC, Schneider F, Tamion F. Extracorporeal life support for patients with acute respiratory distress syndrome: report of a Consensus Conference. Ann Intensive Care. 2014;4:15. DOI: 10.1186/2110-5820-4-15.

[26] Aissaoui N, Morshuis M, Schoenbrodt M, Hakim Meibodi K, Kizner L, Börgermann J, Gummert J. Temporary right ventricular mechanical circulatory support for the management of right ventricular failure in critically ill patients. J Thorac Cardiovasc Surg. 2013 ;146:186–91.

[27] Beckmann A1, Benk C, Beyersdorf F, Haimerl G, Merkle F, Mestres C, Pepper J, Wahba A; ECLS Working Group. Position article for the use of extracorporeal life support in adult patients. Eur J Cardiothorac Surg. 2011;40:676–80.

[28] Affronti A, di Bella I, Carino D, Ragni T. Levosimendan may improve weaning outcomes in venoarterial ECMO patients. ASAIO J. 2013;59:554–7.

[29] Files MD, Kajimoto M, O'Kelly Priddy CM, Ledee DR, Xu C, Des Rosiers C, Isern N, Portman MA. Triiodothyronine facilitates weaning from extracorporeal membrane oxygenation by improved mitochondrial substrate utilization. J Am Heart Assoc. 2014; 3:e000680.

[30] Kajimoto M1, Ledee DR, Xu C, Kajimoto H, Isern NG, Portman MA. Triiodothyronine activates lactate oxidation without impairing fatty acid oxidation and improves weaning from extracorporeal membrane oxygenation. Circ J. 2014;28. [Epub ahead of print].

[31] Petroni T, Harrois A, Amour J, Lebreton G, Brechot N, Tanaka S, Luyt CE, Trouillet JL, Chastre J, Leprince P, Duranteau J, Combes A. Intra-aortic balloon pump effects on macrocirculation and microcirculation in cardiogenic shock patients supported by venoarterial extracorporeal membrane oxygenation. Crit Care Med. 2014; 42:2075–82.

[32] Aissaoui N, El-Banayosy A, Combes A. How to wean a patient from veno-arterial extracorporeal membrane oxygenation. Intensive Care Med. 2015 ;41:902–5.

Permissions

All chapters in this book were first published in EMO, by InTech Open; hereby published with permission under the Creative Commons Attribution License or equivalent. Every chapter published in this book has been scrutinized by our experts. Their significance has been extensively debated. The topics covered herein carry significant findings which will fuel the growth of the discipline. They may even be implemented as practical applications or may be referred to as a beginning point for another development.

The contributors of this book come from diverse backgrounds, making this book a truly international effort. This book will bring forth new frontiers with its revolutionizing research information and detailed analysis of the nascent developments around the world.

We would like to thank all the contributing authors for lending their expertise to make the book truly unique. They have played a crucial role in the development of this book. Without their invaluable contributions this book wouldn't have been possible. They have made vital efforts to compile up to date information on the varied aspects of this subject to make this book a valuable addition to the collection of many professionals and students.

This book was conceptualized with the vision of imparting up-to-date information and advanced data in this field. To ensure the same, a matchless editorial board was set up. Every individual on the board went through rigorous rounds of assessment to prove their worth. After which they invested a large part of their time researching and compiling the most relevant data for our readers.

The editorial board has been involved in producing this book since its inception. They have spent rigorous hours researching and exploring the diverse topics which have resulted in the successful publishing of this book. They have passed on their knowledge of decades through this book. To expedite this challenging task, the publisher supported the team at every step. A small team of assistant editors was also appointed to further simplify the editing procedure and attain best results for the readers.

Apart from the editorial board, the designing team has also invested a significant amount of their time in understanding the subject and creating the most relevant covers. They scrutinized every image to scout for the most suitable representation of the subject and create an appropriate cover for the book.

The publishing team has been an ardent support to the editorial, designing and production team. Their endless efforts to recruit the best for this project, has resulted in the accomplishment of this book. They are a veteran in the field of academics and their pool of knowledge is as vast as their experience in printing. Their expertise and guidance has proved useful at every step. Their uncompromising quality standards have made this book an exceptional effort. Their encouragement from time to time has been an inspiration for everyone.

The publisher and the editorial board hope that this book will prove to be a valuable piece of knowledge for researchers, students, practitioners and scholars across the globe.

List of Contributors

Marie-Eve Brunner
Geneva University Hospitals, Intensive Care, Department of Anesthesiology, Pharmacology and Intensive Care, Genève, Switzerland

Carlo Banfi
University Hospitals, Division of Cardiovascular Surgery, Department of Surgery, Geneva, Switzerland

Raphaël Giraud
Geneva University Hospitals, Intensive Care, Department of Anesthesiology, Pharmacology and Intensive Care, Genève, Switzerland

Antonio Loforte, Giacomo Murana, Mariano Cefarelli, Jacopo Alfonsi, Giuliano Jafrancesco and Giuseppe Marinelli
Department of Cardiovascular Surgery and Transplantation, S. Orsola-Malpighi Hospital, Bologna University, Bologna, Italy

Francesco Grigioni
Department of Cardiology and Transplantation, S. Orsola-Malpighi Hospital, Bologna University, Bologna, Italy

Lucio Careddu, Emanuela Angeli and Gaetano Gargiulo
Department of Pediatric Cardiac Surgery and Transplantation, S. Orsola-Malpighi Hospital, Bologna University, Bologna, Italy

Christopher Duke
Department of Paediatric Cardiology, King Faisal Cardiac Centre, National Guard Health Affairs, Jeddah, Saudi Arabia and East Midlands Congenital Heart Disease Centre, Glenfield Hospital, Leicester, UK

Chris J. Harvey
Department of Cardiothoracic Surgery, Glenfield Hospital, Leicester, UK

Vikram Kudumula and Suhair O. Shebani
East Midlands Congenital Heart Disease Centre, Glenfield Hospital, Leicester, UK

Elved B. Roberts
Department of Cardiology, Glenfield Hospital, Leicester, UK

Ronson Hughes, James Cipolla, Peter G. Thomas and Stanislaw P. Stawicki
Regional Level I Trauma Center and Department of Surgery, Section of Cardiovascular Surgery, St. Luke's University Health Network, Bethlehem, Pennsylvania, USA

Susana M. Bowling and Joao Gomes
Department of Neurology, Division of Internal Medicine, Summa Health Care System – Akron City Hospital, Akron, OH, USA

Michael S. Firstenberg
Department of Surgery – Cardiothoracic, Summa Health Care System – Akron City Hospital, Akron, OH, USA

SV Satyapriya, ML Lyaker, AJ Rozycki and Papadimos
Department of Anesthesiology, Ohio State University Wexner Medical Center, Columbus, OH, United States of America

Young-Jae Cho
Division of Pulmonary and Critical Care Medicine, Department of Internal Medicine, Seoul National University Bundang Hospital, Seongnam-Si, South Korea

David Stahl MD and Victor Davila MD
Department of Anesthesiology, The Ohio State University, Columbus, OH, USA

Vladimir I. Ganyukov
Laboratory of Interventional Cardiology, State Research Institute for Complex Issue of Cardiovascular Diseases, Kemerovo, Russia

Roman S. Tarasov
Laboratory of Reconstructive Surgery, State Research Institute for Complex Issue of Cardiovascular Diseases, Kemerovo, Russia

Dmitry L. Shukevich
Laboratory of Critical Conditions, State Research Institute for Complex Issue of Cardiovascular Diseases, Kemerovo, Russia

Nodar Khodeli, Zurab Chkhaidze, Jumber Partsakhashvili and Dimitri Kordzaia
Tbilisi State University, Tbilisi, Georgia

Otar Pilishvili
Israel Georgian Medical Research Clinic Helsicor, Tbilisi, Georgia

Nadia Aissaoui
Service de Réanimation Médicale, Hôpital Européen Georges Pompidou Assistance Publique–Hôpitaux de Paris and Université Paris Descartes, Paris, France

Christoph Brehm
Department of Medicine, Division of Cardiology, Penn State College of Medicine, Heart and Vascular Institute, Penn State Milton S. Hershey Medical Center, Hershey, Pennsylvania, USA

Aly El-Banayosy
INTEGRIS Baptist Medical Center, Oklahoma City, USA

Alain Combes
Service de Réanimation Médicale, Institut de Cardiologie, Groupe Hospitalier Pitié-Salpêtrière and Université Paris 6, Paris, France

Index